Andrographolide and its Analogs: Botanical Sources, Phytochemistry, Pharmacology, and Biotechnology

Edited by

S. Karuppusamy
Department of Botany, The Madura College
Madurai-625011
Tamil Nadu, India

Vinod K. Nelson
Centre for Global Health Research
Saveetha Medical College and Hospital
Saveetha Institute of Medical and Technical Sciences
Chennai 602105, Tamil Nadu, India

&

T. Pullaiah
Department of Botany
Sri Krishnadevaraya University, Anantapur - 515003
Andhra Pradesh, India

Andrographolide and its Analogs: Botanical Sources, Phytochemistry, Pharmacology, and Biotechnology

Editors: S. Karuppusamy, Vinod K. Nelson & T. Pullaiah

ISBN (Online): 978-981-5256-56-7

ISBN (Print): 978-981-5256-57-4

ISBN (Paperback): 978-981-5256-58-1

Published by Bentham Science Publishers Pte. Ltd. Singapore. All Rights Reserved.

First published in 2024.

need for a court order if at any point you breach any terms of this License Agreement. In no event will any delay or failure by Bentham Science Publishers in enforcing your compliance with this License Agreement constitute a waiver of any of its rights.

3. You acknowledge that you have read this License Agreement, and agree to be bound by its terms and conditions. To the extent that any other terms and conditions presented on any website of Bentham Science Publishers conflict with, or are inconsistent with, the terms and conditions set out in this License Agreement, you acknowledge that the terms and conditions set out in this License Agreement shall prevail.

Bentham Science Publishers Ltd.
Executive Suite Y - 2
PO Box 7917, Saif Zone
Sharjah, U.A.E.
Email: subscriptions@benthamscience.net

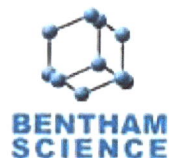

CONTENTS

Vinod K. Nelson, Juturu Mastanaiah, Nazemoon Reddy, Manohar Reddy, P.
Divya Bargavi, Sheik Nasar Ismail, Ravishankar Ram Mani, Vinyas Mayasa, Hari
Hara sudan, Nem Kumar Jain, Alagusundaram Muthumanickam and Kranthi Kumar
Kotha

*Sunkara Surya Lakshmi, Geetha Birudala, Beda Durga Prasad, Praveen Kumar
Kusuma, Moturi Anvesh Raj, Kranthi Kumar Kotha, Shaik Shakir Basha, Vinyas
Mayasa, Sandeep Kanna* and *Vinod K. Nelson*
*Chitikela P. Pullaiah, Vinod K. Nelson, T.S. Mohamed Saleem, Sasikala Chinnappan,
Ravishankar Ram Mani, Srilakshmi Bada Venkatappa Gari, S.P. Preethi Priyadharshni,
K. Balaram Kumar* and *Jamal Basha Dudekula*

PREFACE

In ancient days, human beings mainly depended on plants and plant-derived compounds for various kinds of treatments. In the intricate tapestry of nature's pharmacy, certain compounds emerge as hidden gems, offering a wealth of potential for human health and well-being. One such compound is andrographolide. This compound is well studied and has shown multiple pharmacological effects, such as anticancer, antidiabetic, antifungal, neuroprotective, cardioprotective, and hepatoprotective effects. Hence, we aimed to give a comprehensive review of andrographolide and its analogs in different aspects like chemistry, pharmacology, and biotechnology. The book "Andrographolide and its Analogs: Botanical Sources, Phytochemistry, Pharmacology, and Biotechnology" specifically provides updated information on medicinally important andrographolide and its analogs, sources from various species of *Andrographis* and its botanical identifications, traditional and ethnobotanical uses of *Andrographis* across the world by different cultures, phytochemical extraction and isolation methods, accounts on the pharmacological benefits of andrographolides, and experimental pharmacology of andrographolides against liver diseases and cancer. The book also focuses on biosynthesis, biotechnological production, bioavailability, and pharmacological actions of the andrographolide drug. The book concentrates explicitly on the current experimental research on molecular mechanisms of drug action and target-based drug delivery through phytonanomedicine. The book is a valuable reference source for cancer researchers, pharmacologists, phytochemists, biotechnologists, and those interested in the biomedical field who will benefit from this ready reference for working on andrographolide drugs. We thank all the contributors for their cooperation and erudition.

S. Karuppusamy
Department of Botany, The Madura College
Madurai-625011
Tamil Nadu, India

Vinod K. Nelson
Centre for Global Health Research
Saveetha Medical College and Hospital
Saveetha Institute of Medical and Technical Sciences
Chennai 602105, Tamil Nadu, India

&

T. Pullaiah
Department of Botany
Sri Krishnadevaraya University, Anantapur - 515003
Andhra Pradesh, India

List of Contributors

Amit Upadhyay	Amity Institute of Pharmacy, Amity University Gwalior, Madhya Pradesh 474005, India
Alagusundaram Muthumanickam	Department of Pharmaceutics, School of Pharmacy, ITM University, Gwalior, Madhya Pradesh, India
Arijit Chaudhuri	Department of Pharmaceutics, School of Pharmacy, ITM University, Gwalior, Madhya Pradesh, India
Alugubelli Gopi Reddy	Department of Pharmaceutical Chemistry, Sana College of Pharmacy, Kodad, Suryapet Dist, Telangana, India
Angala Parameswari Sundaramoorthy	Department of Pharmaceutical Analysis, Ratnam Institute of Pharmacy, Pidathapolur, Nellore, Andhra Pradesh, India
Arghya Kusum Dhar	School of Pharmacy, The Neotia University, Sarisha, West Bengal-743368, India
Beere Vishnusai	Department of Pharmacology and Toxicology, National Institute of Pharmaceutical Education and Research, Hajipur, Bihar, India
Beda Durga Prasad	Department of Pharmaceutical Chemistry, GITAM School of Pharmacy, Hyderabad, Telangana, India
B. Shivananthini	Centre for Plant Biotechnology, Department of Botany, St. Xavier's College (Autonomous), Palayamkottai – 627002, Tamil Nadu, India
Boyina Hemanthkumar	University Institute of Pharma Sciences, Chandigarh University, Gharuan Mohali 140413, Punjab, India
Chandrasekaran	Department of Pharmaceutical Chemistry, Krishna Teja Pharmacy College, Tirupati, Andhra Pradesh, India
Chitikela P. Pullaiah	Department of Pharmacology, Siddha Central Research Institute, Central Council for Research in Siddha, Ministry of AYUSH, Chennai, 600106, India
Divya Kallingil Gopi	Department of Pharmacognosy, Siddha Central Research Institute (Central Council for Research in Siddha, Ministry of AYUSH, Government of India) Chennai 600106, Tamil Nadu, India
Goli Venkateswarlu	Department of Pharmaceutics, School of Pharmacy, ITM University, Gwalior, Madhya Pradesh, India
Gopinath Papichettypalle	Department of Pharmaceutical Chemistry, GITAM School of Pharmacy, GITAM University Hyderabad Campus, Rudraram, Sangareddy, Telangana State, India
Geetha Birudala	Faculty of Pharmacy, Dr. M.G.R. Educational and Research Institute, Velappanchavadi, Chennai, India
Hari Hara sudan	Centre for Global Health Research, Saveetha Medical College and Hospital, Saveetha Institute of Medical and Technical Sciences, Chennai 602105, Tamil Nadu, India
I. Silvia Juliet	Centre for Plant Biotechnology, Department of Botany, St. Xavier's College (Autonomous), Palayamkottai – 627002, Tamil Nadu, India

Jamal Basha Dudekula	Amity Institute of Pharmacy, Amity University Gwalior, Madhya Pradesh 474005, India
Juturu Mastanaiah	Department of Pharmacology, Balaji College of Pharmacy, Anantapur, Andhra Pradesh, India
Jayaraman Rajangam	AMITY Institute of Pharmacy, AMITY University, Lucknow Campus, Uttar Pradesh-226010, India
Kona Karunya	Department of Pharmacology, Bojjam Narasimhulu College of Pharmacy, Saidabad, Hyderabad, India
Kola Venu	Seva Shikshan Prasarak Mandal's Dr. N.J. Paulbudhe College of Pharmacy, Vasant Tekadi, Savedi, Ahmed Nagar, Maharashtra, India
Kranthi Kumar Kotha	Departement of Pharmaceutics, College of Pharmaceutical Sciences, Dayananda Sagar University, Bengaluru, Karnataka 560078, India
K. Balaram Kumar	Department of Pharmaceutical Analysis, School of Pharmacy, College of Health and Medical Science (CHMS), Haramaya University, Harar, Ethiopia
L. Baskaran	Department of Botany, Government Arts College (Autonomous), Salem, Tamil Nadu 636007, India
Lakshman Kumar Dogiparthi	Department of Pharmacognosy, MB School of Pharmaceutical Sciences, Mohan Babu University, Tirupati, Andhra Pradesh, India
Mopuri Deepa	Departement of Pharmaceutical Chemistry, Annamacharya College of Pharmacy, Razampet, Andhra Pradesh, India
Mohana Vamsi Nuli	Centre for Global Health Research, Saveetha Medical College and Hospital, Saveetha Institute of Medical and Technical Sciences, Chennai 602105, Tamil Nadu, India
Manohar Reddy	Department of Pharmacology, P. Rami Reddy Memorial College of Pharmacy, Kadapa, Andhra Pradesh, India
Moturi Anvesh Raj	JSS Academy of Higher Education & Research, Rocklands, Ooty, Nilgiris, Tamil Nadu-643001, India
M. Johnson	Centre for Plant Biotechnology, Department of Botany, St. Xavier's College (Autonomous), Palayamkottai – 627002, Tamil Nadu, India
Medagam Tejaswini Reddy	Department of Biotechnology, Chaitanya Bharathi Institute of Technology, Hyderabad, Telangana, India
N. Janakiraman	Department of Botany, The Madura College, Madurai-625011, Tamil Nadu, India
Nilesh Yadav Jadhav	Seva Shikshan Prasarak Mandal's Dr. N.J. Paulbudhe College of Pharmacy, Vasant Tekadi, Savedi, Ahmed Nagar, Maharashtra, India
Narayanan Kannan	Department of Pharmacognosy, Siddha Central Research Institute (Central Council for Research in Siddha, Ministry of AYUSH, Government of India) Chennai 600106, Tamil Nadu, India
Nemallapalli Yamini	Department of Pharmacology, JNTUA-OTRI, Jawaharlal Nehru Technological University, Antnatapur-515001, Andhra Pradesh, India

Naveen Sharma	Amity Institute of Pharmacy, Amity University Gwalior, Madhya Pradesh 474005, India
Namrata Mishra	Department of Pharmaceutics, School of Pharmacy, ITM University, Gwalior, Madhya Pradesh, India
Narahari N. Palei	AMITY Institute of Pharmacy, AMITY University Lucknow Campus, Uttar Pradesh-226010, India
Nazemoon Reddy	Bharat Institute of Technology, Magalpalli, Ibrahimpatnam, Hyderabad, Telangana 501510, India
Nem Kumar Jain	Department of Pharmaceutics, School of Pharmacy, ITM University, Gwalior, Madhya Pradesh, India
N. Karmegam	Department of Botany, Government Arts College (Autonomous), Salem, Tamil Nadu 636007, India
P. Bharath Simha Yadav	Department of Botany, The Madura College, Madurai-625011, Tamil Nadu, India
Phani Deepika Polampalli	Department of Biotechnology, MNR College of Pharmacy, Sangareddy 502294, Telangana State, India
Panga Shyam	Seva Shikshan Prasarak Mandal's Dr. N.J. Paulbudhe College of Pharmacy, Vasant Tekadi, Savedi, Ahmed Nagar, Maharashtra, India
Priyanka Keshri	Department of Pharmaceutics, School of Pharmacy, ITM University, Gwalior, Madhya Pradesh, India
P. Divya Bargavi	Department of Pharmacognosy, JSS College of Pharmacy, JSS Academy of Higher Education and Research, Ooty, Nilgiris, Tamil Nadu, India
Praveen Kumar Kusuma	Department of Pharmaceutical Chemistry, School of Pharmaceutical Sciences, Govt. of NCT of Delhi, Delhi Pharmaceutical Sciences and Research University (DPSRU), Mehrauli-Badarpur Road, India
Radha Rai	Department of Pharmaceutical Chemistry, Krishna Teja Pharmacy College, Tirupati, Andhra Pradesh, India
Ravishankar Ram Mani	Faculty of Pharmaceutical Sciences, UCSI University, Cheras, Kuala Lumpur 56000, Malaysia
Ravilla Jyothsna Naidu	Department of Pharmacology, Raghavendra Institute of Pharmaceutical Education and Research (RIPER) - Autonomous, Anantapur, Andhra Pradesh, India
S. Karuppusamy	Department of Botany, The Madura College, Madurai-625011, Tamil Nadu, India
Sunil Kumar Koppala Narayana	Department of Pharmacognosy, Siddha Central Research Institute (Central Council for Research in Siddha, Ministry of AYUSH, Government of India) Chennai 600106, Tamil Nadu, India
Suryavanshu Roshini	Seva Shikshan Prasarak Mandal's Dr. N.J. Paulbudhe College of Pharmacy, Vasant Tekadi, Savedi, Ahmed Nagar, Maharashtra, India
Sasikala Chinnappan	Faculty of Pharmaceutical Sciences, UCSI University, Cheras, Kuala Lumpur 56000, Malaysia

Siddhartha Lolla	Department of Pharmacology, GITAM School of Pharmacy, Gandhi Institute of Technology and Management Deemed to be University, Hyderabad, Telangana, India
Saijyothi Ausali	MNR College of Pharmacy, MNR Higher Education and Research Academy Campus, MNR Nagar, Sangareddy-502294, India
Sheik Nasar Ismail	Department of Pharmacology, East Point College of Pharmacy, East Point Group of Institutions, Jnana Prabha Campus, Bengaluru, India
Sunkara Surya Lakshmi	Srinivasarao College of Pharmacy, Visakhapatnam, Andhra Pradesh-530041, India
Shaik Shakir Basha	Centre for Global Health Research, Saveetha Medical College and Hospital, Saveetha Institute of Medical and Technical Sciences, Chennai 602105, Tamil Nadu, India
Sandeep Kanna	Department of Pharmacology, GITAM School of Pharmacy, Gandhi Institute of Technology and Management Deemed to be University, Hyderabad, Telangana, India
Srilakshmi Bada Venkatappa Gari	Faculty of Pharmaceutical Sciences, Jawaharlal Nehru Technological University Anantapur (JNTUA), Anantapur, Andhra Pradesh, India
S.P. Preethi Priyadharshni	Department of Pharmaceutical Analysis, School of Pharmacy, College of Health and Medical Science (CHMS), Haramaya University, Harar, Ethiopia
S. Preethi	Centre for Plant Biotechnology, Department of Botany, St. Xavier's College (Autonomous), Palayamkottai – 627002, Tamil Nadu, India
T. Pullaiah	Department of Botany, Sri Krishnadevaraya University, Anantapur 515003, Andhra Pradesh, India
T.S. Mohamed Saleem	College of Pharmacy, Riyadh ELM University, Riyadh, Kingdom of Saudi Arabia
Vinod K. Nelson	Centre for Global Health Research, Saveetha Medical College and Hospital, Saveetha Institute of Medical and Technical Sciences, Chennai 602105, Tamil Nadu, India
Vinyas Mayasa	Department of Pharmacology, GITAM School of Pharmacy, Gandhi Institute of Technology and Management Deemed to be University, Hyderabad, Telangana, India
Vijetha Pendyala	Department of Pharmacognosy and Phytochemistry, Chebrolu Hanumaiah Institute of Pharmaceutical Sciences, Guntur, Pradesh, India
Vijeta Bhattacharya	Department of Pharmaceutics, School of Pharmacy, ITM University, Gwalior, Madhya Pradesh, India
V. Soundarya	Department of Botany, Government Arts College (Autonomous), Salem, Tamil Nadu 636007, India
Vidyarani George	Centre for Plant Biotechnology, Department of Botany, St. Xavier's College (Autonomous), Palayamkottai – 627002, Tamil Nadu, India
Varimadugu Aruna	Department of Biotechnology, Chaitanya Bharathi Institute of Technology, Hyderabad, Telangana, India

Vadakavila Geethikalal   Department of Biotechnology, Chaitanya Bharathi Institute of Technology, Hyderabad, Telangana, India

CHAPTER 1

Andrographolides – An Overview

S. Karuppusamy[1,*], **T. Pullaiah**[2] and **Vinod K. Nelson**[3]

[1] *Department of Botany, The Madura College, Madurai-625011, Tamil Nadu, India*

[2] *Department of Botany, Sri Krishnadevaraya University, Anantapur 515003, Andhra Pradesh, India*

[3] *Centre for Global Health Research, Saveetha Medical College and Hospital, Saveetha Institute of Medical and Technical Sciences, Chennai 602105, Tamil Nadu, India*

Abstract: The genus *Andrographis* is usually bitter and is the source of several diterpenoids, of which water-soluble labdane diterpenoid is andrographolide. Among the various diterpene lactones reported from most of the species of *Andrographis*, andrographolide is considered one of the major bioactive secondary metabolites. The genus *Andrographis* possesses diverse phytochemical constituents with significantly interesting biological potentials. Diterpenes, flavonoids, xanthoflavones, iridoids, and other groups of miscellaneous compounds have been characterized from the various species of *Andrographis*. Andrographolide has been isolated as a notable major phytochemical compound among the andrographolides, which is a common diterpene flavonoid with phytochemical constituents and therapeutic activities.

Keywords: Andrographolide, *Andrographis*, Anticancer, Ethnobotany, Pharmacology, Propagation.

INTRODUCTION

Plant-derived phytochemicals hold a significant role in cancer drug discovery and chemotherapy, addressing numerous challenging human health problems. Remarkably, phytomolecules like vincristine, vinblastine, paclitaxel, camptothecin derivatives, and epipodophyllotxins have been instrumental in modern medicine. The quest for novel potential therapeutic natural compounds from higher plant sources for cancer treatment is ongoing, with numerous plant species continuously screened for discovering effective therapeutic molecules [1].

Andrographis paniculata (Burm.f.) Wall. ex Nees (Acanthaceae) is one such medicinal plant with a prominent position in the traditional healthcare system and

---

* **Corresponding author S. Karuppusamy:** Department of Botany, The Madura College, Madurai-625011, Tamil Nadu, India; E-mail: ksamytaxonomy@gmail.com

modern drug development. It has been effectively used against cancer, diabetes, high blood pressure, ulcers, leprosy, bronchitis, skin diseases, flatulence, colic, influenza, dysentery, dyspepsia, and malaria across the globe [2]. *Andrographis* is a native of the tropical Asian genus and represents 26 taxa in India, of which 20 species are endemic to India; among these, 16 species are endemic to the Western Ghats. Most of the *Andrographis* species are native to Bangladesh, India, Myanmar, Nepal, Sri Lanka, and West Himalaya, mainly distributed in southern India and Sri Lanka, with the majority of the species confined to India except *A. panicualata* [3]. All the *Andrographis* species possess a common medicinal compound known as andrographolide.

Ethnobotany of *Andrographis*

Andrographis species, particularly *A. paniculata*, play a significant role in local traditional systems across several countries, including India, China, Bangladesh, Hong Kong, Pakistan, Philippines, Malaysia, Indonesia, and Thailand. These species are renowned for their therapeutic potential and are utilized for treating a variety of ailments, such as the common cold, diarrhoea, fever, jaundice, tumour, and cancer [4]. In India, *A. paniculata* is a crucial component of traditional medicinal systems like Unani and Ayurvedic medicine [5]. It is employed for managing conditions like snake bites, bug bites, diabetes, dysentery, fever, and malaria. The extensive use of this plant in traditional practices underscores its importance in primary healthcare, which is closely linked to its local abundance and the prevalence of seasonal diseases. Despite its widespread traditional use and the existence of commercial preparations from its extracts, there is a pressing need for standardizing these crude preparations [6]. Establishing phytochemical and pharmacological standards would significantly enhance the efficacy and reliability of these herbal medicines. Moreover, scientific standardization in terms of dosage, mode of administration, and accurate disease diagnosis is essential to validate traditional knowledge, particularly in developing countries. This would ensure the safe and effective use of *A. paniculata* and related species in contemporary medicine.

PHYTOCHEMISTRY OF ANDROGRAPHOLIDES

The genus *Andrographis* contains various phytochemical constituents with significant biological properties, including diterpenes, flavonoids, xanthones, iridoids, and other compounds. Among these, *A. paniculata* is particularly notable for its andrographolides, which are largely responsible for its therapeutic properties [7]. Other significant diterpenoids isolated from the aerial part of *Andrographis* include deoxyandrographolide, neoandrographolide, 20 different diterpenoids, and over 10 flavonoids [8, 9]. These diterpenoids and their glycoside derivatives often share a similar carbon skeleton, which is reported from different *Andrographis* species. The key bitter compounds among them are andrographolide, neoandrographolide, isoandrographanolide, 14-deoxy 11, 12-didehydroandrographolide, and andrograpanin [10]. Some other major diterpenoids have been reported, such as deoxyandrographolide, neoandrographolide, 14-deoxy-11,12-didehydroandrographide, and isoandrographolide. Four different xanthones *viz* ., 1,8-di-hydroxy-3,7-dimethoxy-xanthone, 4,8-dihydrox--2,7-dimethoxy-xanthone,1,2-dihydroxy -6,8-dimethoxy-xanthone, and 3,7,8-trimethoxy-1-hydroxy xanthone are isolated from the roots of *A. paniculata* [11]. Recent combinatorial chemistry libraries of major andrographolide analogs have been synthesised by tailoring the a,b-unsaturated c-butyrolactone moiety, the two double bonds D8 (17) and D12, (13), and the three hydroxyls at C-3 (secondary), C-14 (allylic) and C-19 (primary) positions [12]. In recent days, andrographolides and their derivatives have been effectively quantified by using HPLC coupled with a DAD detector.

PHARMACOGNOSY

The study on botanical pharmacognosy, especially focusing on the various parts of medicinal plants such as the stem, root, leaves, and other useful parts, is crucial for establishing quality control parameters for crude drugs. The utilization of macro and microscopic analysis, powder characteristics, quantitative measurements, and fluorescence standards of plant extracts help in identifying and authenticating plant drugs [13]. *A. paniculata* exhibits notable morphological and anatomical features. The leaves show eucamptodromous pinnate venation, which is characterized by veins curving towards the margin and not forming a continuous marginal vein. The upper epidermis lacks stomata, while the abaxial surface has diacytic stomata, where a small palisade ratio and less stomatal index are also noted. The presence of large cystoliths in both the upper and lower epidermis is a distinctive feature [14]. The stem of *A. paniculata* is quadrangular, with dense collenchyma strands located at the angles, providing structural support. Medullary rays are uniseriate, containing significant amounts of lignified fibres. There is an abundant deposition of calcium oxalate crystals in the epidermal tissues of the lamina, as well as in the ground tissues of the petiole and stem. Secondary xylem vessels of the root also show significant deposition of calcium oxalate, contributing to the diagnostic characteristic of the species [15]. The anatomical features are specific to *A. paniculata* and serve as diagnostic markers. However, similar detailed characterization for other species within the same genus or related taxa is often lacking. Establishing such standards for a wider range of species would enhance the identification and quality control of medicinal plants and their extracts, ensuring their authenticity and therapeutic efficacy.

PHARMACOLOGY

Andrographolide, a major bioactive constituent of *A. paniculata*, has been recognized for its diverse therapeutic potential. These include immunomodulatory, antibacterial, anti-inflammatory, laxative, depurative, prophylactic, hepatoprotective, and cardiovascular effects. Research has confirmed andrographolides' broad pharmacological properties such as anti-inflammatory, antibacterial, antiviral, antitumor, antidiabetic, antimalarial, and hepatoprotective. Due to its impressive range of biological properties, significant efforts have been made to enhance its efficacy through structural modifications, leading to the development of numerous andrographolide derivatives [16]. In recent decades, a plethora of these derivatives have been synthesized, and their pharmacological properties have been systematically screened. However, comprehensive studies focusing solely on *A. paniculata* and its active compounds remain limited [17]. Continuous investigation into the biological properties of *A. paniculata* involves analysing both the crude extracts and andrographolide fractions, revealing enhanced efficacy in developing herbal-based medicines [18, 19].

Specific biological activities, including antioxidant, anticancer, antihypertensive, and anti-inflammatory effects, have been evaluated to understand their correlation with the quantification of andrographolide fractions. Among the various extracts, the 50% methanolic fraction of *A. paniculata* exhibited the highest cytotoxic activities against CACO-2 cells, as well as the most potent anti-inflammatory and antihypertensive effects. This fraction also contained the highest level of andrographolide and its derivatives, such as 14-deoxy-11,12-didehydroandro-ra-pholide, neoandrographolide, and andrograpanin [12]. Experimental models have demonstrated the anti-inflammatory effects of andrographolides in conditions like asthma, stroke, and arthritis and in patients with upper respiratory tract infections. These effects are likely mediated through the inhibition of the NF-$_\kappa$B signaling pathway, resulting in reduced production of cytokines, chemokines, adhesion molecules, nitric oxide, and lipid mediators [20].

Moreover, synthetic analogs of andrographolides have been shown to have superior anticancer activity compared to the natural compound. Andrographolide has been proven to inhibit cell cycles [21], induce apoptosis [22, 23], and possess immunomodulating [24] and antineoplastic [25, 26] properties. Notably, 14-aryloxy analogs (ZAD-1 to ZAD-3) have demonstrated significant antiviral activity against Zika virus (ZIKV) and Dengue virus (DENV), with ZAD-1 showing greater efficacy than natural andrographolide [27, 28]. The extensive pharmacological potential of andrographolides and their derivatives continues to drive research aimed at enhancing their therapeutic efficacy, particularly in the development of new herbal-based medicines.

PHARMACODYNAMICS

Andrographolide, a bioactive diterpenoid lactone derived from the plant parts of *A. paniculata*, has demonstrated significant anticancer properties through various molecular mechanisms. Some of the key research findings regarding the anticancer activity of andrographolides are as follows:

1. Inhibition of key signalling pathways: Andrographolide derivatives can inhibit several crucial signalling pathways implicated in cancer progression, including the Janus Tyrosine Kinases-Signal Transducers and Activators of Transcription (JAK-STAT) pathway, Phosphatidylinositol 3-Kinae (PI3K) pathway, and Nuclear Factor Kappa-light-chain-enhancer of activated B cells (NK-$_κ$B) signalling pathway.

2. Targeting of cellular proteins and enzymes: These derivatives also suppress the activity of heat shock protein 90 (HSP90), Cyclins and cyclin-dependent kinase (CDKs), Matrix metalloproteinases (MMPs) and various growth factors.

3. Induction of tumour suppressor proteins: Andrographolide promotes the induction of tumour suppressor proteins such as p53 and p21, which are vital for regulating cell cycle arrest and apoptosis, thereby inhibiting cancer cell proliferation, survival, metastasis, and angiogenesis [29].

4. Mechanism of action of NF-$_κ$B: Andrographolide interacts with the nucleophilic cysteine residue (Cys62) of NF-$_κ$B p50 through a Michael addition at the $Δ12(13)$ exocyclic double bond, forming a covalent bond. Further research using computer docking, site-directed mutagenesis, and mass spectrometry revealed that noncovalent interactions with additional binding site residues are also crucial for this covalent incorporation.

5. Other therapeutic potentials: Andrographolide has shown promising antiasthmatic properties in various studies [30]. Oral administration of andrographolide in rats indicated pharmacokinetic interactions that correlate with its anti-arthritic effects [31].

There is a need for extensive studies to explore the pharmacodynamic properties of andrographolide across different ailments treated by these derivatives to better understand its therapeutic potential and optimize its clinical applications.

PRODUCTION METHODS OF ANDROGRAPHOLIDES

The natural variability in andrographolide content and the low rate of seed setting in the plant present challenges for meeting commercial demand in the pharmaceutical market. To address these challenges, researchers have developed *in vitro* protocols for increasing andrographolide accumulation in seedling culture [32]. Additionally, techniques such as microfluidization have been employed to enhance the production efficiency of andrographolides. The optimization of isolation factors, such as pressure and homogenization cycles, has also been explored to maximize production yields [33]. The adventitious root culture of *A. paniculata* has shown promise for higher production and accumulation of andrographolide compared with wild plants [34]. This method, along with other *in vitro* techniques, offers the potential for mass production of active compounds from medicinal plants like *A. paniculata*. These advancements in production techniques are essential for meeting the growing demand for andrographolide and other plant-derived pharmaceuticals.

CONCLUSION

The genus *Andrographis*, a highly valued medicinal plant group, contains a variety of bioactive compounds, with andrographolide being the most significant due to its abundance and wide range of biological properties. The key compounds of andrographolides and their analogs are 14-deoxy-11,12-didehydroan-ro-grapholide, neoandrographolide, and 14-deoxyandrographolide, which have immunostimulatory, anti-infective, anti-atherosclerotic, anti-inflammatory, anti-infective, anti-hepatotoxic and antiatherosclerotic activities. Less abundant compounds in *A. paniculata* are andrograpanin, 14-deoxy-14,15-dehydroan-ro-grapholide, isoandro-grapholid, and 3,19-isopropylideneandro-grapholide. These compounds also have proven activities such as anti-inflammatory, anti-infective, and tumor-suppressive properties. Various bioactivities of andrographolides and their analogs suggest a strong potential for developing new anti-inflammatory and anticancer drugs. The diversity in bioactive properties, ranging from anti-inflammatory to antitherosclerotic effects, highlights the medicinal values of the genus *Andrographis* and supports further research and drug development initiatives centred on andrographolide and its derivatives.

REFERENCES

[1]   Varma A, Padh H, Shrivastva N. Andrographolide: a new plant-derived antineoplastic entity on horizon. Evidence-based Complementary and Alternative Medicine. 2011; ID 815390.
       [http://dx.doi.org/10.1093/ecam/nep135]

[2]   Okhuarobo A, Ehizogie Falodun J, Erharuyi O, Imieje V, Falodun A, Langer P. Harnessing the medicinal properties of *Andrographis paniculata* for diseases and beyond: a review of its phytochemistry and pharmacology. Asian Pac J Trop Dis 2014; 4(3): 213-22.

[http://dx.doi.org/10.1016/S2222-1808(14)60509-0]

[3]   Gnanasekaran G, Murthy GVS. Taxonomy, lectotypification and distribution of *Andrographis stenophylla* (Acanthaceae), a little known endemic species from southern India. Phytotaxa 2014; 156(3): 175-81.
[http://dx.doi.org/10.11646/phytotaxa.156.3.8]

[4]   Hossain MdS, Urbi Z, Sule A, Rahman KMH. *Andrographis paniculata* (Burm.f.) Wall. ex Nees: A review of ethnobotany, phytochemistry and pharmacology. Hindawi Pub.Co. The Scientific World Js 2014; 274905.
[http://dx.doi.org/10.1155/2014/274905]

[5]   Burkill IH, Birtwistle W, Foxworthy F, Scrivenor J, Watson J. A Dictionary of the Economic Products of the Malay Peninsula. Kuala Lumpur, Malaysia: Ministry of Agriculture and Co-operatives 1966.

[6]   Kumar S, Singh B, Bajpai V. *Andrographis paniculata* (Burm.f.) Nees: Traditional uses, phytochemistry, pharmacological properties and quality control/quality assurance. J Ethnopharmacol 2021; 275: 114054.
[http://dx.doi.org/10.1016/j.jep.2021.114054] [PMID: 33831465]

[7]   Gorter MK. The bitter constituent of *Andrographis paniculata* Nees. Rec Trav Chim 1911; 30: 151-60.

[8]   Hari Kishore P, Vijaya Bhaskar Reddy M, Kesava Reddy M, Gunasekar D, Caux C, Bodo B. Flavonoids from *Andrographis lineata.* Phytochemistry 2003; 63(4): 457-61.
[http://dx.doi.org/10.1016/S0031-9422(02)00702-1] [PMID: 12770598]

[9]   Li J, Huang W, Zhang H, Wang X, Zhou H. Synthesis of andrographolide derivatives and their TNF-α and IL-6 expression inhibitory activities. Bioorg Med Chem Lett 2007; 17(24): 6891-4.
[http://dx.doi.org/10.1016/j.bmcl.2007.10.009] [PMID: 17962017]

[10] Cheung HY, Cheung CS, Kong CK. Determination of bioactive diterpenoids from *Andrographis paniculata* by micellar electrokinetic chromatography. J Chromatogr A 2001; 930(1-2): 171-6.
[http://dx.doi.org/10.1016/S0021-9673(01)01160-8] [PMID: 11681575]

[11] Dua VK, Ojha VP, Roy R, *et al.* Anti-malarial activity of some xanthones isolated from the roots of *Andrographis paniculata.* J Ethnopharmacol 2004; 95(2-3): 247-51.
[http://dx.doi.org/10.1016/j.jep.2004.07.008] [PMID: 15507344]

[12] Lim JCW, Chan TK, Ng DSW, Sagineedu SR, Stanslas J, Wong WSF. Andrographolide and its analogs: versatile bioactive molecules for combating inflammation and cancer. Clin Exp Pharmacol Physiol 2012; 39(3): 300-10.
[http://dx.doi.org/10.1111/j.1440-1681.2011.05633.x] [PMID: 22017767]

[13] Xia YF, Ye BQ, Li YD, *et al.* Andrographolide attenuates inflammation by inhibition of NF-κ B activation through covalent modification of reduced cysteine 62 of p50. J Immunol 2004; 173(6): 4207-17.
[http://dx.doi.org/10.4049/jimmunol.173.6.4207] [PMID: 15356172]

[14] Trivedi NP, Rawal UM. Hepatoprotective and antioxidant property of *Andrographis paniculata* (Nees) in BHC induced liver damage in mice. Indian J Exp Biol 2001; 39(1): 41-6.
[PMID: 11349524]

[15] Sudhakaran MV. Botanical pharmacogonosy of *Andrographis paniculata* (Burm. f.) Wall. ex Nees. Pharmacogn J 2012; 4(32): 1-10.
[http://dx.doi.org/10.5530/pj.2012.32.1]

[16] Xu J, Li Z, Cao M, *et al.* Synergetic effect of *Andrographis paniculata* polysaccharide on diabetic nephropathy with andrographolide. Int J Biol Macromol 2012; 51(5): 738-42.
[http://dx.doi.org/10.1016/j.ijbiomac.2012.06.035] [PMID: 22766034]

[17] Oktay M, Gülçin İ, Küfrevioğlu Öİ. Determination of *in vitro* antioxidant activity of fennel (*Foeniculum vulgare*) seed extracts. Lebensm Wiss Technol 2003; 36(2): 263-71.
[http://dx.doi.org/10.1016/S0023-6438(02)00226-8]

[18]   Shen YC, Chen CF, Chiou WF. Suppression of rat neutrophil reactive oxygen species production and adhesion by the diterpenoid lactone andrographolide. Planta Med 2000; 66(4): 314-7.
[http://dx.doi.org/10.1055/s-2000-8537] [PMID: 10865445]

[19]   Batkhuu J, Hattori K, Takano F, Fushiya S, Oshiman K, Fujimiya Y. Suppression of NO production in activated macrophages *in vitro* and *ex vivo* by neoandrographolide isolated from *Andrographis paniculata*. Biol Pharm Bull 2002; 25(9): 1169-74.
[http://dx.doi.org/10.1248/bpb.25.1169] [PMID: 12230111]

[20]   See D, Mason S, Roshan R. increased tumor necrosis factor alpha (TNF- α) and natural killer cell (NK) function using an integrative approach in late stage cancers. Immunol Invest 2002; 31(2): 137-53.
[http://dx.doi.org/10.1081/IMM-120004804] [PMID: 12148949]

[21]   Shi MD, Lin HH, Lee YC, Chao JK, Lin RA, Chen JH. Inhibition of cell-cycle progression in human colorectal carcinoma Lovo cells by andrographolide. Chem Biol Interact 2008; 174(3): 201-10.
[http://dx.doi.org/10.1016/j.cbi.2008.06.006] [PMID: 18619950]

[22]   Zhou J, Zhang S, Choon-Nam O, Shen HM. Critical role of pro-apoptotic Bcl-2 family members in andrographolide-induced apoptosis in human cancer cells. Biochem Pharmacol 2006; 72(2): 132-44.
[http://dx.doi.org/10.1016/j.bcp.2006.04.019] [PMID: 16740251]

[23]   Sukardiman H, Widyawaruyanti A, Sismindari N, Zaini NC. Apoptosis inducing effect of andrographolide on TD-47 human breast cancer cell line. Afr J Tradit Complement Altern Med 2007; 4(3): 345-51.
[PMID: 20161898]

[24]   Sheeja K, Kuttan G. Activation of cytotoxic T lymphocyte responses and attenuation of tumor growth *in vivo* by *Andrographis paniculata* extract and andrographolide. Immunopharmacol Immunotoxicol 2007; 29(1): 81-93.
[http://dx.doi.org/10.1080/08923970701282726] [PMID: 17464769]

[25]   Chen JH, Hsiao G, Lee AR, Wu CC, Yen MH. Andrographolide suppresses endothelial cell apoptosis *via* activation of phosphatidyl inositol-3-kinase/Akt pathway. Biochem Pharmacol 2004; 67(7): 1337-45.
[http://dx.doi.org/10.1016/j.bcp.2003.12.015] [PMID: 15013849]

[26]   Jiang CG, Li JB, Liu FR, Wu T, Yu M, Xu HM. Andrographolide inhibits the adhesion of gastric cancer cells to endothelial cells by blocking E-selectin expression. Anticancer Res 2007; 27(4B): 2439-47.
[PMID: 17695536]

[27]   Lee KC, Chang HH, Chung YH, Lee TY. Andrographolide acts as an anti-inflammatory agent in LPS-stimulated RAW264.7 macrophages by inhibiting STAT3-mediated suppression of the NF-κB pathway. J Ethnopharmacol 2011; 135(3): 678-84.
[http://dx.doi.org/10.1016/j.jep.2011.03.068] [PMID: 21497192]

[28]   Li X, Yuan W, Wu J, Zhen J, Sun Q, Yu M. Andrographolide, a natural anti-inflammatory agent: An Update. Front Pharmacol 2022; 13: 920435.
[http://dx.doi.org/10.3389/fphar.2022.920435] [PMID: 36238575]

[29]   Sato H, Hiraki M, Namba T, *et al.* Andrographolide induces degradation of mutant p53 *via* activation of Hsp70. Int J Oncol 2018; 53(2): 761-70.
[http://dx.doi.org/10.3892/ijo.2018.4416] [PMID: 29845212]

[30]   Nguyen Dinh Cat A, Montezano AC, Burger D, Touyz RM. Angiotensin II, NADPH oxidase, and redox signaling in the vasculature. Antioxid Redox Signal 2013; 19(10): 1110-20.
[http://dx.doi.org/10.1089/ars.2012.4641] [PMID: 22530599]

[31]   Balap A, Atre B, Lohidasan S, Sinnathambi A, Mahadik K. Pharmacokinetic and pharmacodynamic herb–drug interaction of *Andrographis paniculata* (Nees) extract and andrographolide with etoricoxib

after oral administration in rats. J Ethnopharmacol 2016; 183(183): 9-17.
[http://dx.doi.org/10.1016/j.jep.2015.11.011]

[32]   Das D, Bandyopadhyay M. Novel approaches towards over-production of andrographolide in *in vitro* seedling cultures of *Andrographis paniculata*. S Afr J Bot 2020; 128: 77-86.
[http://dx.doi.org/10.1016/j.sajb.2019.10.015]

[33]   Asasutjarit R, Sooksai N, Fristiohady A, Lairungruang K, Ng SF, Fuongfuchat A. Optimization of production parameters for andrographolide-loaded neoemulsion preparation by microfluidization and evaluations of its bioactivities in skin cancer cells and UVB radiation exposed skin. Pharmaceutics 2021; 13(8): 1290.
[http://dx.doi.org/10.3390/pharmaceutics13081290] [PMID: 34452250]

[34]   Praveen N, Handhar SH, Naik PM, Nayeem A, Jeeng JN, Murthy HN. Production of andrographolide form adventitious root culture of *Andrographis paniculata*. Curr Sci 2009; 96(5): 694-5.

CHAPTER 2

Botany of *Andrographis* Wall. ex Nees (Andrographinae: Acanthaceae)

P. Bharath Simha Yadav[1] and **S. Karuppusamy**[1,*]

[1] *Department of Botany, The Madura College, Madurai-625011, Tamil Nadu, India*

Abstract: The genus *Andrographis* Wall. ex Nees is recognized for its potential medicinal properties, playing a vital role in traditional and indigenous medicinal systems, particularly in India. It is used for treating various common ailments such as cold, fever, diarrhea, jaundice, cancer, and tumor. In addition, *Andrographis* is valued as a health tonic for fever and cardiovascular health as an antioxidant. Its applications extend to improving sexual dysfunctions and acting as a contraceptive. The therapeutic properties of *Andrographis* are primarily attributed to the major phytochemical andrographolide, although the composition of phytoconstituents can vary significantly among different species. These phytochemical variations are significantly influenced by geographical location, soil types, seasonal changes, and the specific time of harvest. The diversity in chemical composition highlights the importance of understanding the specific context and conditions under which *Andrographis* species are grown and harvested to optimize their medicinal efficacy. This chapter deals with the botany of andrographolide-yielding *Andrographis* species and their taxonomy, identification key, citation, description, and distribution for their availability and conservation.

Keywords: *Andrographis*, Distribution, India, Medicinal importance, Taxonomy.

INTRODUCTION

Andrographis Wall. ex Nees (Andrographinae: Acanthaceae) is a tropical herbaceous genus [1] native to Bangladesh, India, Myanmar, Nepal, Sri Lanka, and West Himalayas, mainly distributed in India and Sri Lanka. In India, it is represented by 26 taxa [2], of which 20 species are endemic [3]; among these, 16 species are confined to the Western Ghats [4, 5]. The current research and review provide a thorough examination of *Andrographis*, relying on a comprehensive field survey reported across their distributional range in India. The descriptions of the majority of species are derived from live collections. The short description, color photographs, distribution, and flowering and fruiting season details are provided here for easy identification and further study.

---

[*] **Corresponding author S. Karuppusamy:** Department of Botany, The Madura College, Madurai-625011, Tamil Nadu, India; E-mail: ksamytaxonomy@gmail.com

S. Karuppusamy, Vinod K. Nelson & T. Pullaiah (Eds.)

Species of the genus *Andrographis* are vastly utilized, effective medicinal plants in the world, especially *A. paniculata*. Plants of this genus are used traditionally to treat a number of ailments like cold, cough, fever, jaundice, diarrhea, and cardiovascular and hepatic diseases in both codified and noncodified medicinal systems. They are also used against jaundice, liver complaints, stomach infections, and external tumors and as antioxidants. Species of this genus have a major medicinal chemical compound, andrographolide, which is responsible for their medicinal potential [6]. Recent studies showed that *A. paniculata* extracts have been proven experimentally against inflammatory and infectious diseases with significant results [7]. Andrographolide is a well-known compound from the genus *Andrographis* with promising therapeutic applications. Many aspects of its bioactivity and mechanisms of action remain to be fully understood. Andrographolide is a major and bioactive diterpene lactone isolated from most species of *Andrographis*, particularly from *A. paniculata*. The compound has garnered significant attention due to its pharmacological potential [8]. Therefore, it has attracted considerable attention in several drug discovery laboratories as a lead molecule that is potentially useful for identifying structurally and functionally novel drugs. This chapter summarizes the taxonomy, distribution, and availability of *Andrographis* species for andrographolide extraction and conservation.

TAXONOMIC TREATMENT

Andrographis Wall. ex Nees in Wall., Pl. Asiat. Rar. 3: 77, 116. 1832. *Neesiella* Sreem. in Phytologia 15: 270. 1967 non Schiffn., 1893. *Indoneesiella* Sreem., Phytologia 16:466.1968; *Andrographis* subgen. *Indoneesiella* (Sreem.) L.H. Cramer, Kew Bull. 51:555. 1996; Gamble, Fl. Madras 2: 1050. 1924; Mathew: Fl. Tam. Car. 1150.1993; Flw. Pl. Ind. 1: 1. 2009; Pullaiah *et al.*, Fl. East. Ghats 4:385. 2011.

Herbs or rarely under shrubs; root stock woody; stem and branches terete or angular, glabrous or hairy. Leaves round, lanceolate, ovate, elliptic; apex acute, acuminate, round; margins entire, ciliate, glandular-hairy or revolute; base round, acute, cuneate, base obtuse, subcordate or rarely cuneate. Inflorescence elongate racemes, sometimes subpaniculate, racemes, paniculate, terminal panicles. Calyx lobes 5, glandular-hairy or glabrous, lanceolate or linear, glandular-hairy, pubescent, glabrous. Corolla glabrous, white, with a purple or pink tinge. Anthers bearded or not bearded, glabrous or villous, glandular-hairy. Capsules elliptic or ellipsoid, linear to oblong, glabrous or glandular-hairy, obtuse to attenuate at base, acute at the tip. Seeds ovoid, orbicular, narrowly elliptic to obovoid, rugose, base oblique or rounded, prominently pitted or not pitted, hairy or glabrous.

KEY TO THE SPECIES OF THE GENUS *ANDROGRAPHIS* IN INDIA

1a.. Capsules linear-oblong 2

1b. Capsules elliptic or ellipsoid 24

2a. Procumbent herbs or straggling herbs 3

2b. Erect herbs or undershrubs 8

3a. Racemes longer than 10 cm, many-flowered, unbranched 4

3b. Racemes shorter than 5 cm, few-flowered, little branched 5

4a. Racemes, both axillary and terminal, up to 11 cm long ....*A. rothii*

4b. Racemes always axillary, up to 14 cm .... *A. stenophylla*

5a. Inflorescence both axillary and terminal 6

5b. Inflorescence always terminal 7

6a. Racemes up to 3.8 cm long; leaves glabrous; capsules 1.5 cm long, 8-seeded ....*A. beddomei*

6b. Racemes scarcely 2.5 cm long; leaves villous; capsules 1.3 cm long, 4-seeded ....*A. glandulosa*

7a. Anthers conspicuously white-bearded; corolla pale, distinctly ventricose; anthers woolly at base .... *A. lobelioides*

7b. Anthers not at all bearded; corolla dark, not distinctly ventricose; anthers glaucous at base.. *A. lowsoni*

8a. Flowers in elongate racemes, sometimes subpaniculate but the flowers distant 9

8b. Flowers in short racemes, paniculate, terminal, and slender axillary racemes 14

9a. Anthers bearded at the base, filaments more are less hirsute 10

9b. Anthers not bearded at the base, the filaments nearly glabrous 13

10a. Plant erect; leaves lanceolate, glabrescent above .... *A. paniculata*

10b. Plants trailing or procumbent; leaves ovate or rotundate, hairy above 18

12a. Inflorescence axillary and terminal; leaves ovate-lanceolate .... *A. atropurpurea*

12b. Inflorescence always axillary; leaves narrowly elliptic-lanceolate ....*A. macrobotrys*

13a. Pedicels very short or 0; calyx-lobes glandular-pubescent or nearly glabrous ....*A. elongata*

13b. Pedicels 0.1-0.6 cm. long; calyx-lobes long, glandular-hispid ....*A. alata*

14a. Racemes short, forming terminal subcapitate panicles or in short terminal panicles 15

14b. Racemes long, forming rather large compound terminal 20

15a. Corolla pale pinkish or brownish purple; lower lip prominently tinged 16

15b. Corolla white or purplish white, lower lip tinged or not.............................. 17

16a. Leaves elliptic, acute at both ends, glabrous except for scattered jointed hairs.. *A. neesiana*

16b. Leaves elliptic-lanceolate, narrowed at both ends, strigose above, softly fulvous-tomentose beneath.. *A. stellulata*

17a. Stem and leaves hairy; corolla purplish white, lower lip prominently purple-tinged...*A. megamalayana*

17b. Stems and leaves glabrous; corolla white, lower lip yellowish hairy or not prominently tinged ....*A. theniensis*

18a. Leaves strigose or puberulous... 19

18b. Leaves ovate or rarely lanceolate, glabrous; calyx-lobes 0.3 cm. long; corolla very little ventricose ....*A. viscosula*

19a. Leaves ovate, wedge-shaped or blunt at base, acute or acuminate apex; strigose and black above and grey beneath when dry; calyx lobes glandular hairy...*A. gracilis*

19b. Leaves rounded or suborbicular, minutely puberulous on both surfaces; calyx glandular hispid. ....*A. rotundifolia*

20a. Leaves thick, subsessile, glabrous, raphides minute or absent 21

20b. Leaves submembranous, petioled, lanceolate, acuminate at both ends, up to 11 cm long, 4 cm broad, lineolate... 22

21a. Racemes up to 15 cm long; corolla prominently ventricose; anthers woolly at base...*A. lineata*

21b. Racemes less than 6 cm long; corolla slightly ventricose; anthers pilose at the base ....*A. affinis*

22a. Corolla prominently ventricose 23

22b. Corolla not ventricose ....*A. chendurunii*

23a. Calyx-lobes 0.4 cm. long, prominently glandular; leaves glabrous above...*A. producta*

23b. Calyx-lobes 0.8 cm. long, scarcely glandular; leaves usually strigose above...*A. explicata*

24a. Capsules hairy, 4-seeded 25

24b. Capsules glabrous, 8-seeded ....*A. serpyllifolia*

25a. Inflorescence shorter or equal to the leaves, peduncle less than 1.5 cm long; seeds deeply pitted .... *A. echioides*

25b. Inflorescence longer than the leaves, peduncle up to 4 cm long; seeds deeply pitted .... *A. longipedunclata*

SYSTEMATIC ENUMERATION

Andrographis affinis Nees in Wall. Pl. Rar. 3: 116. 1832; Gamble, Fl. Madras 2:1050.1924; Matthew, Fl. Tam. Car. 1150.1983 & Flow. Pl. Ind. 1: 1. 2009; Pullaiah *et al.*, Fl. East. Ghats 4:386. 2011. *Andrographis neesiana* Wight var. *affinis* (Nees) C.B. Clarke in Hook. f., Fl. Brit. India 4: 504. 1884.

Subshrub up to 2.5 m tall; rootstock woody. Leaves elliptic-lanceolate, to 4.5 × 2 cm, entire, apex acute; petiole to 0.5 cm long. Racemes paniculate, terminal, and axillary, 20 cm long. Flowers many, compact; bracts lanceolate. Calyx lobes 5, glandular–hispid, 5 mm long. Corolla pale with purple veins, 1.5 cm wide, glandular-hairy, tube 9 mm long, 2-lipped. Stamens 2. Ovary puberulous, 2-celled, ovules 4–6 per cell. Capsule 1.5 cm long, hairy; seeds ovoid.

Distribution: India (Karnataka, Kerala, and Tamil Nadu).

Flowering and Fruiting: November-February.

Note: Endemic Western Ghats, India.

Andrographis alata (Vahl) Nees in DC. Prodr. 11:516.1847; C.B. Clarke in Hook. f., Fl. Brit. India 4: 502. 1884; Gamble, Fl. Madras 2: 1049. 1924; Pullaiah *et al.*, Fl. East. Ghats 4:386. 2011. *Justicia alata* Vahl, Enum. Pl. 1: 139. 1084.

A branched subshrub; branches divaricate. Leaves elliptic or obovate, 6.5 × 3 cm, puberulous, base acute, margin entire, acute at apex; petiole 0.6 cm long. Panicles axillary and terminal, 12 cm long; bracts lanceolate, bracteoles 2. Calyx 5–lobed, glandular hairy. Corolla with white and purple lines. Stamens 2, anther 2.5 mm. Ovary oblong, 1.5 mm, style 1cm, hairy. Capsules oblong, 1.5 × 0.3 cm, acute, glandular-hairy; seeds ovoid.

Distribution: India (Andhra Pradesh, Karnataka, Kerala, and Tamil Nadu) and Sri Lanka.

Flowering and Fruiting: Throughout the year.

Andrographis atropurpurea (Dennst.) Alston, Taxon 26: 539. 1977; Mohanan, Fl. Quilon Dist. 299. 1984; Antony, Syst. Stud. Fl. Kottayam Dist. 297. 1989; Subram., Fl. Thenmala Div. 267. 1995; Sivar. & Mathew, Fl. Nilambur 489. 1997; Sasidh., Fl. Periyar Tiger Reserve 291. 1998; *Justicia atropurpurea* Dennst., Schluss. Hort. Malab. 35. 1818. *Andrographis wightiana* Anders. ex Nees in DC., Prodr. 11: 517. 1847; C.B.Clarke in Hook. f., Fl. Brit. India 4: 503. 1884; Gamble, Fl. Madras 1048. 1924; M. Mohanan & Henry, Fl. Thiruvanthapuram 343. 1994.

Suberect under shrubs; stems hairy. Leaves 10 × 4 cm, ovate, acuminate at apex, base broad, glabrous; nerves 4 to 5 pairs, sub-prominent; petiole 0–4 mm long. Inflorescence panicle with long, lax racemes, scabrid; bracts and bracteoles subulate. Flowers distant. Calyx 4 mm long, subulate, hairy. Corolla 15–18 mm long, glabrous, upper lip orbicular, retuse, dark brown, lower lip shallowly lobed, light pink with brown spots; lower anther bases bearded. Capsule 20 × 3 mm, oblong, glandular-hairy; seeds 8, orbicular, glabrous.

Distribution: India (Karnataka, Kerala and Tamil Nadu).

Flowering and Fruiting: July-September.

Andrographis beddomei C.B. Clarke in Hook. f., Fl. Brit. India 4: 506. 1884; Gamble, Fl. Madras: 1050.1924; M.P. Nayar *et al.*, Indian J. Forest. 7: 37. 1984; Ahmedullah & M.P. Nayar, Endemic Pl. Ind. Reg.:146. 1986; R.R.V. Raju & R.V. Reddy, J. Indian Bot. Soc. 70: 437. 1991; Moulali in Pullaiah & Moulali, Fl. Andhra Pradesh 2: 692. 1997; Karthik. *et al.*, Fl. Pl. India – Dicotyl. 1: 2. 2009; Pullaiah *et al.*, Fl. East. Ghats 4: 386. 2011. *Andrographis nallamalayana* J.L. Ellis, Bull. Bot. Surv. India 8: 362. 1967; M.P. Nayar *et al.*, Indian J. Forest. 7: 37. 1984; Ahmedullah & M.P. Nayar, Endemic Pl. Ind. Reg.: 146. 1986;

Herb, branched; branches terete to angular. Leaves elliptic or obovate, 2.5–7.5×2.2–3.7 cm, glabrous, base acute–cuneate, margins entire, apex acute or obtuse, lateral nerves 2 pairs; petioles sessile or subsessile. Racemes axillary, few-flowered, 0.5 cm long; pedicel and calyx stalked glandular (blackish brown) pubescent; pedicel to 5 mm long. Calyx 5–lobed, 5 mm long, lobes linear-lanceolate. Corolla white with purple spots on the lower lip. Stamens 2, filaments 1.5 mm long, anthers 2.25 mm long, bearded, with villous hairs, tip acute. Ovary 0.5 mm, style 1.5 mm long. Capsules 1.5 cm long, seeds 8 (Fig. **1A**).

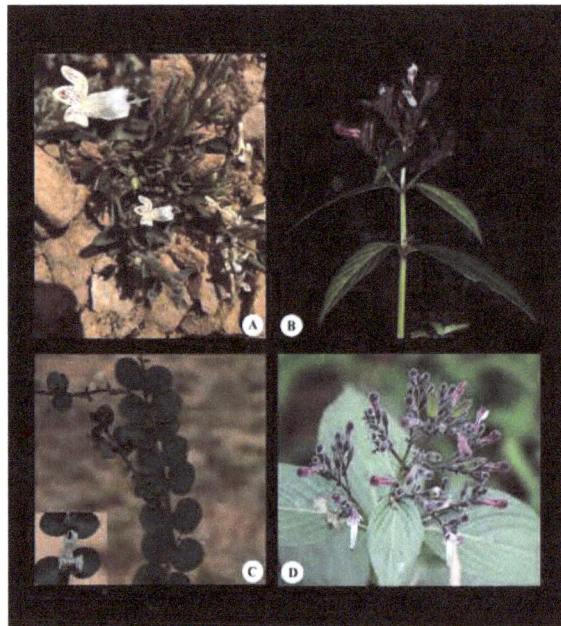

Fig. (1). A. *Andrographis beddomei*; B. *Andrographis megamalayana*; C. *Andrographis serpyllifolia*; D. *Andrographis neesiana.*

Distribution: India (Andhra Pradesh, Telangana).

Flowering and Fruiting: August-April.

Andrographis chendurunii E.S.S.Kumar *et al.*, Nordic J. Bot. 22: 683. 2002; Karthikeyan *et al.*, Fl. Pl. India – Dicotyl. 1: 2. 2009.

Perennial herbs or sub-shrubs; stems creeping and rooting at lower nodes, quadrangular. Leaves 6–12 × 2–5 cm, broadly ovate–obovate or elliptic–oblanceolate, base acute and apex acute to acuminate, glabrous above, minutely pubescent along the nerves beneath; lateral nerves 5–7 pairs; petiole 2 cm long. Flowers in branched terminal panicles, 20–45 cm long; bracts and bracteoles ovate–subulate. Calyx 5-lobed to the base; lobes 2–3.1 mm long, glandular-hairy without and glabrous within. Corolla bilabiate, greenish-white; tube to 6.5–7 mm long, slightly curved; lower lip of limb to 6.5 × 4.5 mm long; upper lip of limb 7 × 8 mm long; lobes ovate-oblong, to 5 × 3.5 mm, obtuse or rounded at apex, middle lobe larger than others, all spotted reddish-brown at base. Stamens 2, exserted; filaments to 6.5 mm long, not dilated at base, minutely puberulous at base; anthers 2-celled, glabrous. Capsule linear–obovate, to 1.5 × 0.3 cm; seeds 4-6, brown, to 1.8 × 1 mm, sub-quadrate, rugose, glabrous.

Distribution: Endemic to India (Kerala).

Flowering and Fruiting: December-February.

Andrographis echioides (L.) Nees in Wall., Pl. Asiat. Rar. 3: 117. 1832; Hook. f., Fl. Brit. India 4: 505. 1884; Gamble, Fl. Madras 1051. 1924; Vajr., Fl. Palghat Dist. 341. 1990. *Justicia echioides* L., Sp. Pl. 16. 1753. *Neesiella echioides* (L.) Sreem., Phyt. 15: 271. 1967. *Indoneesiella echioides* (L.) Sreem., Phytologia 16: 466. 1968; Manilal & Sivar., Fl. Calicut 215. 1982; Pullaiah *et al.*, Fl. East. Ghats 4: 435. 2011.

Erect herbs, 10–60 cm tall, villous. Leaves opposite decussate, 2.5–5.5 × 0.5–2 cm, elliptic oblong, apex obtuse to round, base attenuate. Inflorescence axillary, short unilateral racemes, simple or 1–2-branched, as long as or shorter than leaves. Calyx deeply 5–lobed; lobes 0.6–1.1 cm long, linear. Corolla tube 0.7–1 cm long, white, 2–lipped; lip with violet blotches; upper lip 2–lobed, 0.5–0.8 cm long, lower 0.5–0.8 cm long, 3–lobed. Stamens 2; filaments broad, hairy at base; anthers 2–celled. Style slender; stigma 2–fid. Capsules 0.6–1.4 cm long, 0.2–0.3 cm wide, compressed, broadened towards the tip, attenuated at the base, sparsely hairy towards the tip. Seeds 0.1–0.2 cm across, black, pitted without spiny retinacula.

Distribution: India (Andhra Pradesh, Telangana, Karnataka, Kerala, Tamil Nadu and Maharashtra) and Sri Lanka.

Flowering and Fruiting: April-July.

Andrographis elongata (Vahl) T. And., J. Linn. Soc. Bot. 9: 503. 1867; C.B.Clarke in Hook.f., Fl. Brit. India 4: 502. 1884; Gamble, Fl. Madras 2: 1048. 1924; Karthik. *et al.*, Fl. Pl. India – Dicotyl. 1: 2. 2009; Pullaiah *et al.*, Fl. East. Ghats 4: 388. 2011. *Justicia elongata* Vahl, Enum. Pl. 1: 130. 1804.

Erect herb, 65 cm tall, annual, branched; branches divaricate, acutely quadrangular. Leaves chartaceous, ovate-lanceolate, pubescent, 5×2.5 cm, base decurrent, margin entire, apex obtuse or acute; petiole 2.5–5 mm. Racemes irregular, 30 cm long, bracts in a pair. Calyx 5–lobed. Corolla white with purple dots and pink lines. Stamens 2, occasionally 4, anther exerted. Capsule linear-lanceolate; seeds rugose.

Distribution: India (Andhra Pradesh, Odisha, Kerala and Tamil Nadu).

Flowering and Fruiting: March-May.

Andrographis explicata (Clarke) Gamble, Fl. Madras 1049. 1924; Sasidh., Fl. Periyar Tiger Reserve 292. 1998; Karthik. *et al.*, Fl. Pl. India – Dicotyl. 1: 2. 2009; *Andrographis viscosula* Nees var. *explicata* C.B. Clarke in Hook. f., Fl. Brit. India 4: 504. 1884.

Erect woody undershrubs, about 1 m tall; stems glabrous. Leaves to 16 × 5 cm, elliptic, acuminate at both ends, strigose; nerves 7–10 pairs; petiole 2–2.5 cm long. Panicle 15–30 × 18 cm, pyramidal; branches glandular–strigose; bracts and bracteoles minute. Flowers many. Calyx lobes 5 mm long, lanceolate, subulate, glandular hairy. Corolla 15–20 mm long, tube gradually broadening above, not or slightly bellied; upper lip 2–lobed, dark–purple; lobes of lower lip equal, obtuse, hairy. Anthers acute at base, glabrous, filaments attached near the base of the corolla, glabrous. Style puberulous. Capsule 20–25 × 2–4 mm, linear–oblong, hairy, retinacula acute; seeds 12.

Distribution: Endemic to India (Tamil Nadu).

Flowering & Fruiting: June – December.

Andrographis glandulosa Nees in Wall. Pl. Asiat. Rar. 3: 115. 1832; C.B. Clarke in Hook.f., Fl. Brit. India 4: 505. 1884; Gamble, Fl. Madras 2: 1051. 1924; Karthik. *et al.*, Fl. Pl. India – Dicotyl. 1: 2. 2009; Pullaiah *et al.*, Fl. East. Ghats 4: 388. 2011.

A straggling herb; branches gray–pubescent, stem 4–tetragonous. Leaves elliptic or ovate, 2–2.5×0.8 cm, subsessile, villous, entire, often minutely lineolate. Flowers pedicellate, axillary, few-flowered racemes. Calyx lobes glandular. Corolla pale purple. Stamens 2, anthers strongly bearded. Capsule linear-oblong, 1.3 cm long; seeds 4–8.

Distribution: India (Andhra Pradesh).

Flowering & Fruiting: July – November.

Andrographis gracilis Nees in A.P. de Candolle. 11: 516. 1847; Gnansekaran, J. Jpn. Bot. 91: 351. 2016.

Herb, up to 70 cm high, stems slender, 4–angled, glabrous. Leaves ovate 3–8 × 0.5–2 cm, strigulose and black above and grey beneath when dry. Inflorescence racemose, 3–10 cm long, flowers borne in leaf axils, axis hairless, 4–6-flowered, distantly arranged one-sided. Flowers 2-lipped, about 1.3 cm across, white with pink shade; tube prominently ventricose, glandular-hairy, upper lip spoon-shaped, oblong, about 7×2.7 mm, glandular-hairy outside, 5–veined; lower lip 3–lobed, 6–7×5.5 mm, glandular hairy outside, dark purple–striped; middle lobe narrowly ovate, 2.5–3 × 2.5 cm, lateral lobes oblong, 1.4–1.6 mm across. Capsules are inverted, 18–20 x 3–3.5 mm, pointed at the tip.

Distribution: Endemic to India (Karnataka, Kerala, and Tamil Nadu).

Flowering and Fruiting: August -January.

Andrographis lineata Wall. ex Nees in Wall. Pl. Asiat. Rar. 3: 116. 1832; C.B.Clarke in Hook.f., Fl. Brit. India 4: 504. 1834; Gamble, Fl. Madras 2: 1049. 1924; Karthik. *et al.*, Fl. Pl. India – Dicotyl. 1: 3. 2009. *Andrographis lineata* var *lawii* C.B. Clarke in Hook. f. Fl. Brit. India 4: 505. 1884.

Erect branched herb, 1 m tall. Leaves elliptic-oblong, 3–5 × 2–2.5 cm, subsessile, base obtuse, margin entire, apex acute; petiole to 0.5 cm long. Panicles terminal or subterminal, bracts lanceolate. Calyx lobes 5, glandular, hispid. Corolla purple, tube 7 mm long, bifid at apex, lower lip 7 mm. Stamens 2, stalk 8 mm long, anther 2 mm, bearded. Capsule linear, glandular hairy (Fig. **2G**).

Distribution: India (Andhra Pradesh, Karnataka, Kerala, and Tamil Nadu).

Flowering and Fruiting: August-May.

Andrographis lawsonii Gamble, Bull. Misc. Inform. Kew 1923: 375. 1923 & Fl. Madras 1050(736). 1924; Sasidh. & Anto in Manoharan *et al.*, Silent

Valley–Whispers Reason 136. 1999; Biju in Manoharan *et al.*, Silent Valley–Whispers Reason 162. 1999; Karthik. *et al.*, Fl. Pl. India – Dicotyl. 1: 2. 2009.

Undershrubs, branches erect. Leaves opposite, 1.6 × 1 cm, ovate or elliptic, apex acute, base rounded or cuneate, margins recurved, villous along. Flowers in long paniculate racemes. Calyx lobes 5, lanceolate, 5–7 mm long, glandular hispid. Corolla slightly ventricose, dark brownish–purple. Anthers not bearded. Capsule linear-oblong, 1.8 × 3 mm, densely glandular-hispid (Fig. **2E**).

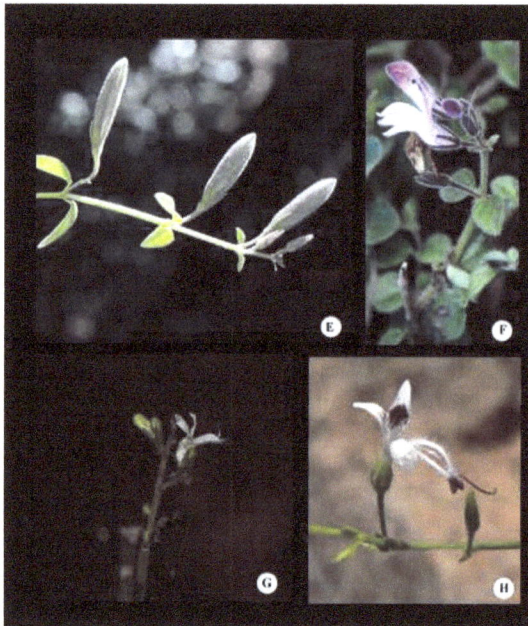

Fig. (2). E. *Andrographis lawsonii*; F. *Androgaphis lobelioides*; G. *Andrographis lineata*; H. *Andrographis longipedunculata.*

Distribution: India (Karnataka, Kerala and Tamil Nadu).

Flowering & Fruiting: September to December.

Andrographis lobelioides Wight, Ill. Ind. Bot. t. 164b, f. 11.1850 & Icon. Pl. Ind. Orient. t. 1557. 1850; C.B. Clarke in Hook. f., Fl. Brit. India 4; 505. 1884; Karthik. *et al.*, Fl. Pl. India – Dicotyl. 1: 3. 2009;

Herb, rusty pubescent or nearly glabrous at maturity; rootstock woody; stems numerous, procumbent. Leaves 0.8–2 cm, broadly ovate, cordate at base, petiole short, 0.2 mm long, silky pubescent on both surfaces. Inflorescence axillary panicles 2.5–10.5 cm. Flowers large, ventricose, purplish pink to dark purple, silky pubescent outside. Sepals 0.8 cm. Anthers exserted, conspicuously white–barbate. Capsules 1.6x0.3 cm (Fig. **2F**).

Distribution: Endemic to India (Tamil Nadu - Nilgiris).

Flowering and Fruiting: September to December.

Andrographis longipedunculata (Sreem.) L.H. Cramer, Kew Bull. 51: 555. 1996; Karthik. *et al.*, Fl. Pl. India 1: 3. 2009. *Neesiella longipedunculata* Sreem., Phytologia 15: 271. 1967, nom. Illeg. *Indoneesiella longipedunculata* Sreem., Phytologia 16: 466. 1968; Matthew, Fl. Tamilnadu Carnatic 3: 1182. 1983; Kumari in A.N. Henry *et al.*, Fl. Tamil Nadu 2: 150. 1987; Moulali in Pullaiah & Moulali, Fl. Andhra Pradesh 2: 715. 1997; Matthew, Fl. Palni Hills: 940. 1999; Pullaiah *et al.*, Fl. East. Ghats 4: 436. 2011.

Herb, about 80 cm tall; stems 4–angled, densely glandular–villous. Leaves sessile ovate-lanceolate, 2–7 × 0.5–2.5 cm, margins entire, base obtuse acute or slightly cordate, apex acute or obtuse; lateral veins 5–7 pairs, long glandular hairy on both sides. Flowers in racemes, axillary, 5–11 cm long; flowers distantly arranged, bracts 2, bracteoles 2. Calyx 5–lobed; lobes linear, subequal, 4.5–7.5 × 3 0.2–0.5.5 mm, margins hairy, apex acute to subacuminate, glandular-hairy outside. Corolla 2-lipped, 0.8–1.3 cm across, white; tube prominently ventricose, 6.5–7.2 × 1–1.8 mm, glandular–hirsute above; upper lip spathulate, minutely 2–lobed; lower lip 3–lobed, dark purple–striped with yellow shade at the center; middle lobe narrowly ovate; lateral lobes oblong, 3–veined. Stamens 2, exserted; filaments 5–7 mm long. Capsules ellipsoid, 7–11 × 3–4.1 mm, Capsules ellipsoid, 8–10 x 3–4 mm, compressed at right angles to septum; 4-seeded; seeds narrowly elliptic–obovoid (Fig. **2H**).

Distribution: India (Andhra Pradesh, Bihar, Diu and Daman, Goa, Gujarat, Haryana, Jammu and Kashmir, Jharkhand, Karnataka, Kerala, Madhya Pradesh, Maharashtra, Odisha, Punjab, Rajasthan, Tamil Nadu, Telangana, Uttar Pradesh and West Bengal), Myanmar.

Flowering and Fruiting: July-March

Andrographis macrobotrys Nees in DC., Prodr. 11: 516. 1847; C.B. Clarke in Hook. f., Fl. Brit. India 4: 503. 1884; Gamble, Fl. Pres. Madras 1048. 1924;

Herbs, erect; stem stout, glabrous. Leaves 8–12.5 × 3–4.5 cm, elliptic-lanceolate, coriaceous, glabrous, nerves up to 10 pairs; petiole 6 mm long. Flowers in axillary racemes, 19 cm long. Calyx lobes 3 mm long, glandular-hairy. Corolla 2 cm long, tube ventricose; upper lip entire, middle lobe of the lower lip broader than lateral lips, hairy; filaments bulged at the base. Capsule 2.5 cm long, linear-oblong, glandular-hairy, retinacula acute; seeds–8, glabrous.

Distribution: India (Karnataka, Kerala and Tamil Nadu), Myanmar.

Flowering and Fruiting: July-February.

Andrographis megamalayana Gnanasek. *et al.*, Phytotaxa 244: 89. 2016.

Herb, up to 60 cm high. Stems 4–angled, glandular-pubescent throughout, rarely glabrous. Leaves sessile or shortly petiolate; leaf blades variable in shape, lower ones narrowly elliptic or ovate, upper ones lanceolate or oblong, 2.5–7 × 0.5–3cm, base obtuse, subcordate or rarely cuneate, margins entire or rarely revolute, apex acute or abruptly acuminate, strigose towards margins above when young. Inflorescences racemose, axillary and terminal, branched, up to 5.5 cm long. Bracts narrowly ovate to oblong, 2–3.2 × 0.6–0.8 mm. Bracteoles 2, linear, 1.8–2 × 0.3–0.4 mm, hairy on the margin. Calyx 5–lobed; lobes subequal, linear, 5–6.5 × 0.4– 0.7 mm, hairy on the margin, acuminate at apex, glandular–hirsute outside. Corolla 2–lipped, 1.5–1.7 × 1.2–1.4 cm, white, purple-tinged; tube prominently ventricose, 6–7.7 × 1.7–3 mm, glandular-hirsute above, glabrous below; upper lip spathulate-oblong, minutely 2–lobed at apex, 8–9 × 2–3.2 mm, 6–veined; lower lip 3–lobed, 7–7.5 × 5.5–6.2 mm, purple–striped; middle lobe ovate, 2.4–2.8 × 2.6–3 mm, 3–veined; lateral lobes oblong, 2.2–3 × 1.3–1.6 mm, 3–veined. Stamens 2, exserted, adnate to base; filaments 9–10 mm long, distinctly dilated at base; anthers oblong, 1.8–2.3 × 0.6–0.8 mm, pilose at base, deep purple. Capsules linear-oblong, 18–22 × 3–4.5 mm; Seeds 10–12, subglobose to obovoid, 1.7–2.2 × 1.2–1.6 mm (Fig. **1B**).

Distribution: Endemic to India (Kerala and Tamil Nadu).

Flowering and Fruiting: June to December.

Andrographis neesiana Wight, Icon. Pl. Ind. Orient. 4: t. 1561. 1850; Karthik. *et al.*, Fl. Pl. India – Dicotyl. 1: 3. 2009.

Herbs; branches strigose. Leaves simple, opposite, 2–4 × 2 cm, ovate-elliptic, base and apex acute, glabrous, margin ciliate, nearly sessile; veins 5 pairs. Inflorescence panicle 2–5 × 4 cm, congested, terminal, strigose; flowers densely arranged. Calyx lobes 6.5 mm long, linear, acuminate, glandular hairy. Corolla 10–14 mm long, brownish–purple, tube not ventricose, upper lip emarginate; lobes of lower lip obtuse, hairy. Stamens 2, filaments broadened below; anthers attenuate at base; style hairy. Capsule 13–16 × 2.5– 3 mm, oblong, acute, hairy; seeds–6, glabrous (Fig. **1D**).

Distribution: Endemic to India (Kerala and Tamil Nadu).

Flowering and Fruiting: September to February.

Andrographis paniculata (Burm.f.) Wall. ex Nees in Wall. Pl. Asiat. Rar. 3: 116. 1832; C.B. Clarke in Hook. f., Fl. Brit. India 4: 501. 1884; Gamble, Fl. Madras 2: 1048. 1924. *Justicia paniculata* Burm. f., Fl. Indica 9. 1768. *Andrographis subspathulata* C.B. Clarke in Hook.f. Fl. Brit. India 4: 502. 1884; Karthik. *et al.*, Fl. Pl. India – Dicotyl. 1: 3. 2009; Pullaiah *et al.*, Fl. East. Ghats 4: 391. 2011.

Erect branched herb, 30 to 90 cm tall; branches quadrangular, grooved, slightly winged. Leaves linear–obovate, 5–8×1–2 cm, glabrous or minutely puberulous beneath, margin entire, base cuneate, apex acuminate; petiole to 1.5 cm long. Panicle branches zigzag, to 15 cm; flowers unilateral, distant bracts lanceolate, acute, bracteoles 2. Calyx lobes 5, sparsely glandular–hairy, acute. Corolla white, with pink tinge, 5×3 mm. Stamens 2, adnate to the throat of corolla, filaments hairy, bearded, anthers obovoid, 2 mm long. Capsule oblong, 1.5×0.3 cm, compressed, minutely hairy; seeds subquadrate, rugose, 1x0.6 mm.

Distribution: India, Bangladesh, Nepal, Sri Lanka.

Flowering & Fruiting: July – March.

Andrographis producta (C. B. Clarke) Gamble, Fl. Madras: 1049. 1924; Karthik. *et al.*, Fl. Pl. India – Dicotyl. 1: 3. 2009. *A. neesiana* Wight var. *producta* C.B.Clarke in Hook. f. Fl. Brit. India 4: 504. 1884.

Subshrubs, erect 1.2–1.5 m high. Leaves opposite, 4.5–14.5 × 2–5.5 cm, elliptic, lanceolate, base attenuate, apex acute, glabrous; lateral nerves 4–10 pairs; petioles 2.5–6 mm long. Flowers in paniculate axillary or terminal racemes; peduncle trichotomously branched, peduncle with glandular and pubescent hairs; bracts lanceolate, elliptic, acute, 0.5–1.5 × 0.1–0.4 cm, tomentose along margins, caduceus. Calyx 5–lobed, lanceolate filaments, 2.5–5 mm long, with glandular hairs on the outer surface. Corolla–tube 6–8 × 1.5–2 mm; white with pink lines, blipped; upper lip 4.5–7 × 2.2 mm, lower lip 3–lobed, 4.5–8.2 mm long, ca 3 mm wide, dark purple spots on the lower lip, outer surface pubescent and glandular-hairy. Stamens 2; filaments 1–1.2 cm long, membranous, white, with pink lines, hirsute; anthers 1.2–3 mm long, bearded at the base, closely arranged. Ovary 2.2–5.5 mm long, dark red; style 1–2 cm long, pubescent; stigma simple. Capsules 1.5–2.5 cm long, 1.5–4 mm thick, surface with glandular hairs, tip pointed; seeds 5–11, ovoid, glabrous.

Distribution: Endemic to India (Karnataka, Kerala, and Tamil Nadu).

Flowering and Fruiting: September-February.

Andrographis rothii C.B. Clarke in Hook.f., Fl. Brit. India 4: 506. 1884; Gamble, Fl. Madras 1050. 1924; Ahmedullah & M.P. Nayar, Endemic Pl. Ind. Reg.: 146. 1986; Kumari in A.N. Henry *et al.*, Fl. Tamil Nadu 2: 140. 1987; Vajr. *et al.*, J. Econ. Taxon. Bot. 10: 284. 1987; Karthik. *et al.*, Fl. Pl. India – Dicotyl. 1: 3. 2009; T.S. Nayar *et al.*, Fl. Pl. Western Ghats 1: 14. 2014. *Andrographis lobelioides* (Wall. ex Nees) Wight var. *composita* C.B. Clarke in Hook. f., Fl. Brit. India 4: 505. 1884; Kumari in A.N. Henry *et al.*, Fl. Tamil Nadu 2: 139. 1987; Karthik. *et al.*, Fl. Pl. India – Dicotyl. 1: 3. 2009; T.S. Nayar *et al.*, Fl. Pl. Western Ghats 1: 13. 2014,

Decumbent herbs, up to 80 cm high; stem 4–angled, densely glandular–pubescent throughout. Leaves ovate to elliptic or orbicular, 0.5–3.5 × 0.4–1.5 cm, base attenuate or obtuse, margins undulate and glandular-hairy, apex acute or obtuse; lateral veins 3–5 pairs glandular-pubescent on both sides; petioles absent, or to 3 mm long. Inflorescence a raceme, axillary, at times branched, 5.5–14 cm long; flowers distantly arranged. Bracts 2, ovate, elliptic or rotund, 1–5 × 0.5–2.5 mm. Bracteoles 2, subulate, 0.5–0.8 × 0.1–0.3 mm. Calyx 5–lobed; lobes subequal, linear, 4.5–5 × 0.3–0.6 mm, glandular-pubescent above, antrorsely strigulose beneath. Corolla 2–lipped, 1.2–1.5 cm across, white with yellow shade; upper lip spathulate–oblong, entire at margins, minutely 2–lobed at apex, 6–veined; lower lip 3–lobed, entire at margins, obtuse at apex, dark purple–striped with yellow eye spots; middle lobe narrowly ovate 3–veined; lateral lobes oblong 3–veined. Stamens 2, exserted; filaments 5– 7 mm long, anthers linear, 3–4 × 0.4–0.8 mm, woolly at the base, deep purple. Capsules linear-oblong, 10–15 × 2.5–4 mm, mucronate to apiculate, densely glandular-hairy; seeds narrowly ellipsoid–obovoid, 2–3 × 1.5 mm, oblique at base.

Distribution: Endemic to India (Tamil Nadu, Tirunelveli).

Flowering and Fruiting: October-April.

Andrographis rotundifolia (Sreem.) Sreem. Phytologia 37: 416. 1977; Karthik. *et al.*, Fl. Pl.India – Dicotyl. 1: 2. 2009. *Andrographis neesiana* var. *rotundifolia* Sreem., Bull. Bot. Surv. India 8: 91. 1966.

Erect herbs, up to 50 cm tall; 4-angled often rooting at lower nodes. Leaves 1.3–3.5 × 1–3.3 cm, opposite, rounded or suborbicular, chartaceous, minutely puberulous on both surfaces, obtuse at apex, rounded or subcordate at base, margins entire with scattered bulbous-based, hook-like, hairs; nerves 4–5 pairs.

Flowers many, in terminal condensed subcapitate panicles. Bract 2 mm, ovate-lanceolate, acute, densely glandular–hispid. Bracteoles two, each 1.5 × 0.5 mm, linear-oblong or oblong-lanceolate, acute, glandular–hispid. Calyx–lobes five, each 5 × 1 mm, cleft almost to the base, linear-oblong, acute, glandular–hispid. Corolla 1.2– 1.4 cm long, pale creamy–yellow with purple streaks and spots within, upper lip slightly bifid, lower prominently three-lobed, densely glandular-pubescent without, less densely so within. Stamens two; filaments densely hispid at the base, sparsely towards the tip; anthers of the two stamens adhering together in the bud, dithecous, thecae subequal, bearded. Capsules 1.8– 2 × 0.5 cm, linear-oblong to oblong, densely glandular–hispid. Seeds 2 mm in diameter, ellipsoid, pitted, several in each capsule.

Distribution: Stenoendemic to India (Tamil Nadu - Boluvampatti hills in Coimbatore District).

Flowering and Fruiting: September.

Note: Possibly extinct; after type collection, there is no recollection; description adopted from the original protologue.

Andrographis serpyllifolia (Rottl. ex. Vahl) Wight, Ic. t. 517. 1842; C.B. Clarke in Hook. f., Fl. Brit. India 4: 506. 1884; Gamble, Fl. Madras 2: 1051. 1924; Karthik. *et al.*, Fl. Pl. India – Dicotyl. 1: 2. 2009. *Justicia serpyllifolia* Rottl. ex Vahl, Enum. Pl. 1: 169. 1804.

Prostrate herb, branches raising from a woody rootstock; branchlets densely hairy. Leaves round–orbicular, sub-reniform 3×2.5 cm, villous when young, glabrous when mature except at margins, base obtuse or subcordate, margin entire, apex obtuse, lateral nerves 3–4 pairs; petiole 1 mm. Flowers axillary, solitary of few-flowered, 2.8–3 cm long racemes; bracts orbicular, 3 × 2 mm; calyx glandular-pubescent, sepal 5, linear, corolla whitish–pink, tube 8 mm, upper lip 5.5 mm, minutely bifid, lower lip purple, 7 mm; stamens 2, 6 mm, anthers unequal, bearded. Capsule 1.5 cm, elliptic–obovoid, glabrous, with short, blunt acuminate tips; seeds 8, pale, rugose, retinacula spathulate.

Distribution: Endemic to India (Andhra Pradesh, Telangana, Karnataka, Kerala, and Tamil Nadu).

Flowering and Fruiting: March-October.

Andrographis stellulata C.B. Clarke in Hook. f., Fl. Brit. India 4: 504. 1884; Karthik. *et al.*, Fl. Pl. India – Dicotyl. 1: 4. 2009.

Herbs; branches elongate, obscurely quadrangular, closely villous. Leaves 6.5 × 2.5 cm, fulvous, multicellular hairy above, villous beneath; petiole 0–0.8 cm. Inflorescence heads 2.5–5 cm. Corolla pale pink with purple spots on the lower lip. Filaments somewhat flattened, hairy upwards. Capsule 2 × 0.4 cm, hairy, compressed. Seeds osseous, rugose, glabrous, not compressed.

Distribution: Endemic to India (Nilgiris hill of Tamil Nadu).

Flowering & Fruiting: February – October.

Note: Much similar to the *A. neesiana* and *A. megamalayana* but distinguished by the long substellate sepal.

Andrographis stenophylla C.B. Clarke in Hook. f., Fl. Brit. India 4: 503. 1884; Karthik. *et al.*, Fl. Pl. India – Dicotyl. 1:4. 2009.

Herb, rootstock woody; annual stems numerous, erect and diffuse, quadrangular. Leaves 2.5–4 × 0.2–0.4 cm; raphides 0 or obscure. Inflorescence racemes 5–13 cm, axillary and terminal, not distinctly panicled; pedicles mostly nearly as long as the calyx. Calyx 0.4 cm linear to lanceolate, glabrous to or very nearly so. Corolla with a pink tinge, 4 × 2 mm. Capsules 1.6 × 0.4 cm, compressed.

Distribution: Endemic to India (Tamil Nadu).

Flowering and Fruiting: June-February.

Note: Description taken from the original protologue

***Andrographis* theniensis** Karupp. & P. Bharath, Nord. J. Bot. e04218: 3. 2024.

Herbs to 60 cm high; stems 4–angled, nodes swollen, a few rows of elongated hairs at nodes, internodes glabrous. Leaves sessile or sub-sessile, narrowly elliptic to elliptic-lanceolate, 1.5–5.5 × 0.8–2.1 cm, base obtuse, margin entire, revolute, apex acute or acuminate, midrib conspicuous beneath, lateral veins 3–5 pairs; petiole 0-1 mm long, glabrous. Inflorescence terminal subcapitate panicle. Flowers closely arranged; pedicel slender, 0.3-0.4 mm long, glandular-hairy; bracts 2 × 0.5 mm, lanceolate, green in color. Calyx 5-lobed, lobes almost equal, 8–10 × 1 mm, linear-lanceolate, glandular-hairy throughout, margin entire, acuminate at apex. Corolla tube to 7 mm long, 2–lipped, white, ventricose at lower lip; upper lip 2–lobed, lobes 1 mm long, glabrous inside, margin entire, outside glandular-hairy; lower lip glabrous inner side except slightly pale yellowish hairy at middle lobe, purple tinge is absent, pale pink tinge rarely present, margin entire, outside glabrous, 9-veined; stamens 2, adnate to ventricose tube at base, exerted; filament 1 cm long, flattened, twisted at base, tapering towards apex, short white hairs at margins, base dilated and white villous; anthers oblong 2.2 × 1 mm, long pilose hairy at base, anther lobes pale yellow. Ovary 1.2 × 0.8 mm, rounded to elliptic, glandular-hairy, green, ovules 5-6 in each cell; style 1.3 cm long, slender, partially hairy, whitish green; stigma linear, green, glabrous. Capsule 2 cm, linear lanceolate, glandular hairy, seeds 10–12. Seeds oblongoid-obovate, subquadrate, grooved irregularly, minutely puberulate, yellowish brown.

Distribution: Theni district of Tamil Nadu, Western Ghats.

Flowering & Fruiting: July - August.

Note: *Andrographis theniensis* Karupp. & P. Bharath is a more recently described species and it is closely allied to *A. megamalayana* Gnanasek., Karupp. & G.V.S. Murthy, but it can be easily recognized from glabrous leaves and stems, calyx green, lower lips with 9-veined, anthers pale yellow, style white, pale yellowish hairy on the middle lobe of the lower lip, and scattered pale pink tinge.

Andrographis viscosula Nees in Wall., Pl. Asiat. Rar. 3:116. 1832; C.B. Clarke in Hook. f., Fl. Brit. India 4: 504. 1884; Karthik. *et al*., Fl. Pl. India – Dicotyl. 1:4. 2009.

Erect branched herb, 40 to 100 cm tall; branches quadrangular, slightly winged. Leaves linear–obovate, 3–7 × 1–2.5 cm, hairy viscous beneath, margin entire, base rounded, apex acuminate; petiole to 1.2 cm long. Panicle branches linear, to 10 cm; flowers unilateral, distant bracts lanceolate, acute, bracteoles 2; calyx lobes 5, conspicuously viscous glandular-hairy, acute; corolla white, with light pink tinge at the throat, 5 × 3 mm; stamens 2, adnate to the throat of corolla, filaments hairy, bearded, anthers obovoid, 2 mm, long. Capsule oblong, 1.8 × 0.4 cm, compressed, glandular-hairy; seeds subquadrate, rugose.

Distribution: India, Bangladesh, Myanmar, Nepal, and Sri Lanka. Common in South Western Ghats.

Flowering and Fruiting: November-January.

TAXONOMIC UPDATE

Flowering Plants of India- Dicotyledons enumerated about 28 species of *Andrographis*, where *A.ceylonica, A. lobelioides* var. *composita,* and *A. lineata* var. *lawii* were reduced as synonyms to *A. macrobotrys, A. rothii* and *A. lineata,* respectively [9]. Very recently, a new species *Andrographis megamalayana* was found from the Megamalai Wildlife Sanctuary, Tamil Nadu [10]. *Andrographis nallamalayana* J.L. Ellis has been reduced as a synonym *A. beddomei* C.B. Clarke, a little-known endemic species [5]. *Andrographis ovata* and *Andrographis laxiflora* are nested into the genus *Haplanthus,* and a new combination is proposed as *Haplanthus ovatus* and *Haplanthus laxiflora* [11]. *Andrographis rotundifolia* was not recollected after type collection, and it was presumed that the species was possibly extinct [12]. More recently, one new species, *A. theniensis,*was described in the Theni district of Tamil Nadu by the authors [13]. All the above information synthesizes the availability of andrographolide-yielding species in Southeast Asia, particularly India, which is helpful in locating the species for further extraction, characterization, and structural elucidation of pharmacologically important active compounds from *Andrographis* species.

CONCLUSION

Andrographolide is a major and bioactive diterpene lactone isolated from most of the species of *Andrographis.* The compound has garnered significant attention due to its pharmacological potential. Alternate sources of this therapeutically important compound should be the prime research topics. Research should also be carried out on genetics, molecular biology, and breeding of *Andrographis* species for enhanced production of andrographolide and its analogs.

REFERENCES

[1]   Mabberley DJ. Mabberley's Plant-Book: A Portable Dictionary of Plants, Their Classifications, and Uses. Cambridge: Cambridge University Press 2008.

[2]   *Plants of the World Online.* Facilitated by the Royal Botanic Gardens, Kew. Published on the Internet; 2023; http://www.plantsoftheworldonline.org/(Continuously updated).

[3]   Gnanasekaran G, Murthy GVS. Taxonomy, lectotypification and distribution of *Andrographis stenophylla* (Acanthaceae), a little known endemic species from southern India. Phytotaxa 2014; 156(3): 175-81.
[http://dx.doi.org/10.11646/phytotaxa.156.3.8]

[4]   Nayar TS, Beegam RA, Sibi A. Flowering Plants of the Western Ghats, India. 2 Vols. Jawaharlal Nehru Tropical Botanic Garden. 2014.

[5]   Gnanasekaran G, Rajakullayiswamy K, Murthy GVS. *Andrographis nallamalayana*, a heterotypic synonym of a little-known endemic species *A. beddomei* (Acanthaceae). Rheedea 2015; 25(1): 47-53.

[6]   Okhuarobo A, Ehizogie Falodun J, Erharuyi O, Imieje V, Falodun A, Langer P. Harnessing the medicinal properties of *Andrographis paniculata* for diseases and beyond: a review of its phytochemistry and pharmacology. Asian Pac J Trop Dis 2014; 4(3): 213-22.
[http://dx.doi.org/10.1016/S2222-1808(14)60509-0]

[7]   Intharuksa A, Arunotayanun W, Yooin W, Sirisa-ard P. A comprehensive review of *Andrographis paniculata* (Burm. f.) Nees and its constituents as potential lead compounds for COVID-19 drug discovery. Molecules 2022; 27(14): 4479.
[http://dx.doi.org/10.3390/molecules27144479] [PMID: 35889352]

[8]   Li, x., Yuan, W., Wu, J., Zhen, J., Sun, Q., Yu, M. Andrographolide, a natural anti-inflammatory agent: an update. Frontiers in Pharmacology 2022; 13.
[http://dx.doi.org/10.3389/fphar.2022.920435]

[9]   Karthikeyan S, Sanjappa M, Moorthy GVS. Flowering Plants of India–Dicotyledons, Volume 1 (Acanthaceae – Avicenniaceae). Botanical Survey of India, Kolkata, 2009.

[10]   Gnanasekaran G, Karuppusamy S, Murthy GVS. *Andrographis megamalayana* (Andrographinae: Acanthaceae), a new species from the southern Western Ghats, India. Phytotaxa 2016; 244(1): 089-95.

[11]   Gnanasekaran G, Murthy GVS, Deng YF. Resurrection of the genus *Haplanthus* (Acanthaceae: Andrographinae). Blumea 2016; 61(3): 165-9.
[http://dx.doi.org/10.3767/000651916X693185]

[12]   Gnanasekaran G, Murthy GVS. Is *Andrographis rotundifolia* (Acanthaceae) possibly extinct? Nelumbo 2015; 57(0): 46-9.
[http://dx.doi.org/10.20324/nelumbo/v57/2015/87086]

[13]   Karuppusamy S, Yadav PBS. *Andrographis theniensis* (Acanthaceae), a new species from the southern Western Ghats of India. Nord J Bot 2024; 3: e04218.
[http://dx.doi.org/10.1111/njb.04218]

CHAPTER 3

Ethnobotany of the Genus *Andrographis* Wall. ex Nees (Acanthaceae)

S. Karuppusamy[1,*]

[1] *Department of Botany, The Madura College, Madurai-625011, Tamil Nadu, India*

Abstract: Various species of the Genus *Andrographis* are used in multiple tribal and community medicinal systems in India and adjoining countries for more than 20 different local ailments. *A. paniculata* is predominantly used for treating jaundice, liver diseases, fever, cardiovascular diseases, cancer, stomach problems, and common cold and as a blood purifier. This chapter gives an overview of the ethnobotanical uses of various species of *Andrographis* by several tribal communities and local inhabitants in almost all the states of India and other countries.

Keywords: *Andrographis*, Ethnomedicine, Fever, Jaundice, Liver diseases, Snake bites, Traditional medicine.

INTRODUCTION

Species of *Andrographis* Wall. ex Nees (Acanthaceae) are widely used worldwide to treat various human ailments. The plants of different species of *Andrographis* are used as a traditional herbal medicine in Bangladesh, China, Hong Kong, India, Pakistan, Philippines, Malaysia, Indonesia, and Thailand [1]. They are ethnobotanically used to treat snake bites, bug bites, diabetes, dysentery, fever, and malaria [2]. In the Unani and Ayurvedic medicines, *A. paniculata* is a mainly used medicinal plant [3]. Commercial preparations of this plant's extracts have recently been used in certain countries. However, the preparations need to be standardized for the better efficacy of pharmacological standards. The aerial part of *A. paniculata* is most commonly used for various ailments. Whole plant leaves and roots are also used as a folklore remedy for diseases in Asia and Europe [4]. The tribal communities primarily depend on the forest for their livelihood and primary healthcare needs [5]. Indigenous traditional knowledge is integral to local communities' folk culture and history. Ethnic people have rich indigenous conventional wisdom of using local vegetation to remedy and treat several local

* **Corresponding author S. Karuppusamy:** Department of Botany, The Madura College, Madurai-625011, Tamil Nadu, India; E-mail: ksamytaxonomy@gmail.com

ailments. This knowledge includes the uses, beliefs, management systems, classification systems, and language that modern and traditional cultures attribute to their local ecosystem [6]. Amongst the genus *Andrographis*, *A. paniculata* is widely used for medicinal purposes and is also a pre-clinically and clinically well-studied species. It is a well-known Ayurvedic herb that is medicinally used in various traditional, folklore, unani and homeopathic medicinal systems in India, China, and Thailand [7]. In traditional Chinese medicine, *A. paniculata* treats "heat", especially in the lungs, throat, and urinary tract, and skin-related ailments, such as sores and carbuncles [8]. In China, the herbal formulation derived from the leaves or aerial parts of *A. paniculata* is Chuanxinlian, Yijianxi, or Lanhelian. It treats the common cold and is considered antipyretic, detoxicant, anti-inflammatory, and detumescent. *A. paniculata* is used for the treatment of pharyngolaryngitis, diarrhea, dysentery, cough with thick sputum, carbuncle, sores, and snake bites by the locals of China [9].

Andrographis paniculata extract has been used pharmacologically and experimentally, providing its traditional usage for rheumatoid arthritis, inflammation, cold, fever, and diarrhea [10 - 14]. The World Health Organization (WHO) published the monograph on *A. paniculata* in 2003 that mentioned the uses for prophylaxis and symptomatic treatments of respiratory infection, bronchitis, pharyngotonsillitis, urinary tract infections, and acute diarrhea. This plant species also has other traditionally known medicinal uses mentioned in pharmacopeia [15]. *A. panicaluata* is a multipurpose medicinal plant used widely in Southeast Asia for curing primary ailments, predominantly in remote village areas [16].

ANDROGRAPHIS IN THE INDIAN MEDICINAL SYSTEM

Ayurvedic system of medicine has long been widely practiced in India. In this system, *A. paniculata* is often used in combination with other herbs to treat diverse spectrums of organ pathologies and mental health problems. It is estimated that *A. paniculata* is used in more than 50 different herbal formulations commercialized in India for hepatoprotective treatments [17]. This herb is classified as Rasayana, which helps maintain the digestive system and regulate energy metabolism and immune functions [18, 19]. Rasayana herbs are now pharmacologically classified as herbal adaptogens or adaptogenic and anti-stress activity agents, which has also been proven in *A. paniculata* extracts. The leaves and roots have been used in Ayurvedic medicine as an adjunct treatment for cholera, diabetes, dysentery, enteritis, gastritis, malaria, pneumonia, pyelonephritis, and rabies. The leaf juice has been utilized as a tonic to relieve pain and stomach distress, expel parasites, promote bile flow, and reduce fever, as well as as an antiseptic, antispasmodic, and laxative. As a traditional household remedy, the leaf juice is used for diarrhea, dysentery, dyspepsia, general debility, and loss of appetite. Two ayurvedic drugs, namely Kalmeghnamayas and Kalmeghashiva, are prepared from *A. paniculata*. Churnas such as Katu churna and Swetradiphala churna, which contain *A. paniculata* as a significant ingredient [20].

Andrographis is Mentioned in Pharmacopeias.

A. paniculata has been used in various medicinal systems, and this herb is mentioned in multiple pharmacopeias for treating several human ailments. These include pharmacopeias like *Indian Pharmacopoeia* (7th edition) [21], *Malaysian Herbal Monograph* (Volume 1) [22], *Medicinal Plants of Myanmar* (Volume 1) [23], *Pharmacopoeia of the People's Republic of China* [24], *Thai Herbal Pharmacopoeia* (Volume 1), *WHO Monographs on Selected Medicinal Plants* [25], and the *United States Pharmacopeia* (USP 37) [26].

Ethnobotany of *Andrographis* Species

A study documented the ethnomedicinal uses of the genus *Andrographis* in the Nilgiri Biosphere Reserve. Nine species of *Andrographis* were used to treat everyday ailments like colds, fever, poisonous bites, and skin diseases by hill tribes of Kotas, Irulas, Kaatunayakkas, Kurumbas, and Todas [27]. Ethnobotany of *Andrographis* is well surveyed in the Eastern Ghats of Tamil Nadu [28]. Tribal people residing in the Eastern Ghats of India used many species of *Andrographis* for treating various ailments like snake bites, colds, coughs, diabetes, fever, malaria, scabies, warts, and skin diseases [29].

Ethnobotany of *A. affinis*

A decoction of the whole plant is administered orally for snake bites, sugar control, and jaundice by the Kota tribes of Nilgiri Hills [27].

Ethnobotany of *A. alata*

The juice of the leaf is mixed with water, which is used to cure snake bites. Fresh leaf juice is given orally twice daily for four to six days for treating fever, diabetes, and diarrhea by Malayalis [30]. Leaf decoction is orally administered for snake bites, scorpion and centipede bites, and heavy fever like malaria and typhoid by Kurumba tribes of Nilgiri hills [27]. Leaf paste is externally used for poisonous bites by the Malayali tribes of Kolli Hills [31].

Ethnobotany of *A. beddomei*

The plant's root extract is used to cure leucorrhoea by Adivasis in Gundlabrameshwaram Wildlife Sanctuary of Eastern Ghats [32, 33].

Ethnobotany of *A. echioides*

Leaves decoction of *A. echioides* is taken orally with hot water for fever and stomach ache problems, and the leaf paste is applied externally on cuts and wounds by Malayalis [34]. Leaf juice is mixed with hot water and given for snake bites and eczema; it is also used as an anthelmintic by tribals in Sirumalai hills [29]. Leaf juice is used as an antipyretic and anthelmintic by Malayali tribes in Shervarayan hills, and it can cure stomach problems [30]. Most of the tribes and remote villagers in India used these plant parts as antivenoms with several formulas for treating poisonous bites as antivenoms [35]. The tribes of Eastern Ghats used the whole plant extract for treating liver diseases [36]. Plant powder is given orally for treating fever by people in the Amaravati district in Maharashtra [37].

Ethnobotany of *A. lawsonii*

According to local older men, it is a substitute or mixed with *A. paniculata* powder for treating various ailments by Kurumbas and Badagas of Nilgiri hills [27].

Ethnobotany of *A. lineata*

The whole plant is considered antipoisonous and effective against jaundice by Paliyars of Sirumalai Hills [38]. Leaf paste is applied externally to cure scorpion stings and snake bites, and leaf powder mixed with milk is taken orally by Paliyans to cure diabetes [39]. Leaf powder is orally given to treat sugar complaints among the Irulars of the Coimbatore district [40]. The plant parts are used in the form of decoction, juice, paste, and powder among the Malayali tribes in Eastern Ghats of Tamil Nadu for treating sicknesses like diabetes, jaundice, snake bites, and skin diseases and as anti-diabetic, antipyretic, anti-inflammatory and antivenom agents [38]. The extract of the whole plant is used to cure snake bites by the Malayalis of Kolli Hills [41].

Ethnobotany of *A. lobelioides*

Leaf decoction is used orally with buffalo milk to treat viral fever, snake bites, and jaundice by Todas of Nilgiri Hills [27].

Ethnobotany of *A. neesiana*

Leaf juice is taken orally as an aphrodisiac and to treat jaundice, skin allergy, and fever by the Kurumba and Kaatunayakka tribes of Nilgiri hills [27]. Young twigs are crushed to paste, and 20-30 gms paste is taken three times daily after meal for 2-3 weeks by Paliyars of Sathuragiri Hills to treat liver infection [42].

Ethnobotany of *A. ovata*

Leaves decoction is taken orally with water as an antipyretic and to treat jaundice, snake bites, and scorpion stings by tribals in Sirumalai hills [38]. Leaf juice is externally applied to treat scabies among the Kontha tribes in Mahendragiri hills in Odisha [43].

Ethnobotany of *A. paniculata*

One teaspoon of fresh plant juice or one to two grams of shade-dried plant powder is taken twice a day for seven days by the Kanis of Tirunelveli Hills to treat snake bites and scorpion stings [44]. A handful of leaves are taken, and an extract is made, which, mixed with milk, is taken by Valayans of Alagar Hills to cure snake bites [45]. Roots are used as a potential antidote for snake bites by Paliyars of Sirumalai Hills [38]. Leaf powder is taken to treat diabetes by Paliyars of Virudhunagar district [46]. Leaf extract is used by Malayali tribes in Kolli Hills to treat blood sugar [47]. Irulas used to cure fever from the leaves [48]. Leaves are mixed with the root of *Aristolochia indica* and ground into a paste. The paste thus obtained is applied over the body to treat fever. Fresh leaves are decocted orally thrice a day for two days to treat poisonous bites by tribes in the Theni district [49]. The decoction of the leaves is taken to treat dyspepsia and stomach aches by villagers of Kolli Hills [50]. The leaf infusion is used to cure cough by Nadars of Kanyakumari district [52]. The juice of the leaves is used for diabetes by the people residing in Jawathu Hills [53]. The whole plant paste is applied externally totreat skin diseases, snake bites, and poisonous bites by tribals in Sirumalai Hills [54]. Daily, leaf decoction is taken orally with hot water for snake bites and scorpion stings. The leaf paste is applied externally to cure skin diseases and snake bites by Malayalis [51]. The plant extract is used to treat snake bites by tribes of the Sigur plateau in Nilgiris [55]. Leaf juice mixed with milk is taken orallyby Irulas of Bolampatty Valley in Nilgiris to treat snake bites. The root is helpful in diarrhea [56]. Leaf paste is taken orally by local people in the Ariyalur district for snake bites and to reduce pain [57]. Plant extract is orally administered to treat snake bites by the people of Nilgiri Biosphere Reserve [58]. Crushed leaf paste is taken twice daily as an antidote against snake bites by the hill people of Tiruvallur district [59]. Plant extract is orally given for curing fever by Paliyars and Muthuvars of Agamalai Hills [60]. The Kani tribe in Keeriparai of

Kanyakumari district uses the leaf extract to treat rheumatism and respiratory illness [61]. Paliyars of Agamalai Hills use leaf paste and common salt to treat fever [62]. Leaf powder is taken as a contraceptive by local tribes in the Suruli hills of the Theni district [63]. The decoction of the leaves is anthelmintic and also administered against dyspepsia and stomach ache. Decoction of the root is given as a tonic to cure fever by Malayali tribes in Shervarayan hills [34]. Leaf decoction is taken orally by the Kani tribes in Pechiparai to treat fever and stomach ache [64]. Leaves are mixed with the root of *Aristolochia indica* and ground into a paste. The paste obtained is applied over the body to treat chronic fever. The decoction of fresh leaves is taken orally for two days, thrice a day, to treat poisonous bites by Paliyars of Kurangani hills. Fresh leaves are ground with the seeds of *Cuminum cyminum* and seeds of *Piper nigrum*, and leaves of *Piper betel* are made into a paste, and it is applied on the tongue of goats twice a day for two days for fever [65]. Fresh tender leaves are collected, ground well, and made into a paste. The paste is applied on the forehead to treat headaches by Kanis of the Kalial range in the Kanyakumari district [66]. Leaf paste is taken orally for treating snake bite by Irulars of Walayar Valley [58] and Malayalis of Kolli Hills [54].

Ethnobotany of *A. serpyllifolia*

A paste of leaves is applied to the affected part in snake and scorpion bites. Decoction of the leaves is used by Malayalis to cure fever and cough [53]. Plant extract is used to treats snake bites by the tribes of the Sigur plateau in Nilgiris [65]. A whole plant extract is administered orally for snake bites, dog bites, fever-like malaria, and typhoid by the Kota tribes of Nilgiri Hills [27]. The whole plant is pounded, and the paste is applied externally on poisonous worms/insect bite sites to alleviate the burning sensation. The root paste is mixed with lemon juice and given orally for 7-8 days to neutralize the snake venom [67].

Ethnobotany of *A. stellulata*

Leaf extracts are orally administered with buffalo milk to treat poisonous bites, common cold fever, and jaundice by the Toda tribes of Nilgiris [27].

Ethnobotany of *A. stenophylla*

Leaf decoction is mixed with cow's milk and orally taken for treating infectious fever and snake bites by Irulas of Nilgiris [27].

Ethnobotany of *A. producta*

Leaf juice is applied externally to treat skin diseases and psoriasis by Todas of Nilgiris [27].

ETHNOMEDICINAL USES OF *ANDROGRAPHIS*

Snake Bites and Poisonous Bites

A. paniculata is a well-known medicinal plant for treating poisonous snake bites [68]. Fresh leaves of *A. paniculata* are used as an antidote for snake venom, whereas a poultice of fresh leaves is applied to the affected area [69]. Malayali tribes of Kolli Hills and Jawadhu Hills in Tamil Nadu use *A. alata* and *A. paniculata* to treat snake bites [70]. Some Malayalis in Shervaroyan Hills treat snake bites with the external application of *A. paniculata* extract [71]. Paliyars of Palni Hills used the leaf paste of *A. paniculata* and hot water taken orally to treat snake bites, and it also works on menstrual problems in women [72]. Paliyars of Western Ghats in the Madurai district used *A. paniculata* to treat unknown poisonous bites [68]. Malayali tribes in the Eastern Ghats of Salem district in Tamil Nadu used *A. echioides*, *A. paniculata*, and *A. serpyllifolia* for treating snake bites and scorpion stings [73 - 75]. *A. paniculata* treats snake bites in almost all the local communities in Tamil Nadu [76, 77]. Valayan tribes of the Madurai district in Tamil Nadu treat snake bites by chewing the fresh leaves of *A. alata* [78]. *A. serpyllifolia* plant decoction is taken orally to treat snake bites and scorpion stings in the northern part of Tamil Nadu and Karnataka [79]. The tribes of Nilgiris use the whole plant infusion of *A. paniculata* to treat snake bites [80]. Local inhabitants of Gingee Hills of Villupuram district in Tamil Nadu used the *A. echioides* leaves to treat snake bites [81]. In contrast, in the Palamalai hills of Salem district, Malayali tribes use it for treating scorpion stings [82]. Urali tribes in the Nilgiri biosphere reserve used the *A. paniculata* to treat poisonous bites [83]. Tribes in the Kallar forest division of Kerala used the whole plant extract of *A. paniculata* as an antidote for snake bites [84]. The people in the Pathanamthitta district of Kerala also use *A. paniculata* decoction to treat snake bites and other common ailments like body pain and joint pain [85]. Roots of *A. paniculata* are used to treat snake bites among the people of eastern Shimoga in Karnataka [86]. Jenu Kuruba tribes in Karnataka used the leaves and roots of *A. paniculata* as an antidote for snake bites [87]. Plant juice with buttermilk is orally given to treat snake bites by the people of the Vijayapur district in Karnataka [88]. People in the Tumkur district of Karnataka used the *A. serpyllifolia* root extract to neutralize snake venom [67]. The root paste of *A. paniculata* is mixed orally with lemon juice to alleviate snake venom by local inhabitants of the Challakere district of Karnataka [89]. Leaf decoction of *A. paniculata* is combined with *A. alata* whole plant. A decoction or extract is used by the Khamti tribe of Arunachal Pradesh, India, for snake bites. Plant paste with mustard oil is used for wounds by the Korku community in central India to treat the same [90 - 92].

Liver Diseases and Jaundice

Malayali tribes of Shervaroy Hills used leaf extracts of *A. affinis*, *A. alata*, *A. lineata*, *A. neesiana*, *A. ovata*, *A. paniculata*, and *A. serpyllifolia* for treating liver complaints in different formulations [93]. *A. paniculata* is predominantly used for treating jaundice by the tribes and local communities of Tamil Nadu. Chenchu tribe of Eastern Ghats treats liver diseases with the plant extract of *A. echioides* [36]. The hill-residing people in the Eastern Ghats of Namakkal district use four species of *Andrographis-A. affinis*, *A. lineata*, *A. ovata*, and *A. macrobotrys* - to treat liver complaints and jaundice in addition to epilepsy [94].

Meich, Rava, Santhal, Garo, and Oraon tribes of Coochbehar district in West Bengal used *A. paniculata* leaf extract given orally for treating jaundice and body pain [95]. Leaf juice of *A. paniculata* with ginger is given orally for three days to cure jaundice by traditional healers of Andhra Pradesh [96]. Yerukala, Yanadi, and Sugalis of Seshachalam hills of Andhra Pradesh have reported that *A. paniculata* leaf decoction is used to cure jaundice [97]. Leaves of *A. paniculata* and *Phyllanthus amarus* are taken in equal quantities and boiled. The ground paste is made into pills of soapnut seed size. Two pills are administered daily twice for seven days to cure jaundice by Vaidyas in East Godavari district of Andhra Pradesh [98]. *A. paniculata* leaf juice is given orally for treating jaundice in Bellary district of Karnataka [99]. Leaf juice is taken orally to treat jaundice by the Rajgond tribes in the Bidar district of Karnataka [100]. About 20 ml of *A. paniculata* leaf juice is given daily on an empty stomach for 41 days to cure jaundice by people in the Davanagere district in Karnataka [101]. The people residing in the Uttarakhand region of Eastern Himalaya used *A. paniculata* leaf decoction against liver diseases and jaundice [102].

Blood Purifier

Sholaga tribes in the Kathiri hills of the Erode district used *A. paniculata* as a blood purifier against stomach problems [103]. Fresh leaf juice is given to prevent excessive bleeding during periods by local people in the Kaprada forest division in Gujarat [104].

Diabetes

Leaf powder of *A. paniculata* is used by Malayali tribes to treat blood sugar in the Kolli hills of Tamil Nadu [103]. Fresh leaves of *A. paniculata* are taken orally on an empty stomach for treating diabetes by the Malayali tribes of the Pachamalai hills of Eastern Ghats [105]. Leaf powder of *A. lineata* is taken internally to treat diabetes by Hoorali tribes in the Kadambur hills of the Nilgiri biosphere reserve [106]. Various tribal communities, such as Bagata, Gadaba, Kammara, Konda Doras, Khondus, Kotia, Kulia, Malis, Manne Dora, Mukha Dora, Porja, and Reddi Doras, of Andhra Pradesh to treat diabetes with *A. paniculata* plant extract in different formulations [107]. Local vaidyas in the Ahobilam forest of Andhra Pradesh used the *A. paniculata* leaves to treat fever, cough, bronchitis, and diabetes [108]. Koya tribes of Warangal district in Andhra Pradesh prepared the formulation with *A. paniculata* leaf powder for treating diabetes [109]. The Sugali tribe in Yerramalais of Andhra Pradesh treats diabetes with leaf decoction of *A. paniculata* [110]. Leaf decoction of *A. paniculata* is used to control diabetes by the Bodo tribes of Assam [111]. Dried leaf powder and seeds of *A. paniculata* are soaked in hot water overnight, and filtrate is orally administered for seven days to cure malaria by the Bodo tribes in Manas Biosphere Reserve in Assam [112]. Leaf paste with *Piper nigrum*, made as an herbal drink, treats skin diseases, and 50 ml leaves decoction is given with *Piper nigrum* to treat diabetes [113]. People inhabiting Gandamardhan Hills of Odisha utilize the leaf juice of *A. paniculata* to reduce their diabetic condition [114]. The tribal communities of Khyber province in Pakistan use the *A. paniculata* extract for treating diabetes [115].

Fever

A. paniculata leaves boiled with water and filtered decoction are taken orally for treating dengue fever [73, 74, 116]. The plant extract is used to cure viral fever, vermifuge, and eczema by the local inhabitants of the Kanyakumari district in Tamil Nadu [117]. Sholaga tribes of Western Ghats in Tamil Nadu used the *A. paniculata* leaf extract for treating fever and skin diseases [118]. Tribes of Jharkhand used to treat malarial fever with *A. paniculata* extract [119]. During COVID-19, local people of Thiruvannamalai district, Tamil Nadu, used the *A. paniculata* leaf extract to reduce fever [120]. Konda Dora, Satapu, and Savara tribes in Kotia hills of Andhra Pradesh used the *A. paniculata* leaf and root extract for treating malarial fever [121]. In the Adilabad district of Telangana, the leaves of *A. paniculata* with sugar candy are given orally to treat infant fever [122]. Yanadhi tribes in Nellore district of Andhra Pradesh treated malarial fever and worm infection with whole plant extract of *A. paniculata* [123]. The leaves of *A. paniculata* are used for treating fever by Yanadhi tribes in Kavali of Andhra Pradesh [124]. Local vaidyas in the Ahobilam forests of Andhra Pradesh treat fever, cough, and bronchitis with leaves of *A. paniculata* [125]. The whole plant extract of *A. paniculata* is administered orally to treat malaria, typhoid, and viral fevers by Gonds of Adilabad district in Telangana [126]. Kani tribals in the Agasthiyamalai range of Kerala used the *A. paniculata* plant extract to treat cough and cold [127]. *A. serpyllifolia* plant paste is taken internally to treat rheumatic fever by Narikiravar communities of the Erode district in Tamil Nadu [128]. Decoction of *A. paniculata* leaves with cumin or ginger is a good remedy for fever, cough, and fatty liver. The decoction of leaves with *Tinospora* stem is also used as a remedy for fever and reducing blood glucose by local practitioners in Kerala [129]. Leaf decoction of *A. paniculata* is administered against dyspepsia, anthelmintics, and stomach aches. Root decoction is given as a tonic to cure fever by the Malayali tribes in the Shervarayan hills of the Eastern Ghats [34]. Juice prepared from the leaves of *A. paniculata* is used to treat fever by local inhabitants of the Belgaum district in Karnataka [130]. Leaves of *A. paniculata*are grind with seeds of *Piper nigrum* and bulbs of *Allium sativum* and consumed as a paste with hot water by the residents of the Tumkur district in Karnataka to manage malarial fever [131]. Whole plant decoction of *A. paniculata* is used to treat fever and weakness by the people residing in Bagalkot in Karnataka [132]. Chiru tribes in Assam treat liver diseases and fever by drinking *A. paniculata* plant decoction for seven days [133]. Manipuri communities in Assam prescribed *A. paniculata* leaf juice and honey for treating fever [134]. Leaf decoction of *A. paniculata* is given to treat diarrhea, about 10 ml once daily until cure and 10 ml twice daily for three days for fever and cough. Root decoction is given in malaria by Deori communities in Assam [135]. Whole plant powder in decoction is taken to cure fever and edema by Maharashtra's vaidyas of the Bhadravati region [136]. The roots of *A. paniculata* are boiled in water, and the water is taken to reduce fever; whole plant powder dissolved in water is taken to control fever by the people of Wardha district in Maharashtra [137]. The people residing in the Nashik district of Maharashtra used whole plants to treat bronchitis, influenza, dysentery, fever, and liver diseases [138]. Gond tribes in the Bhandara district of Maharashtra used the whole plant decoction of *A. paniculata* to cure malarial fever and common fever [139]. Banjara, Gawali, and Gond tribes of the Yavatmal district in Maharashtra used to cure dyspepsia and fever with whole plant decoction [140]. Villagers of Jaipur district in Odisha used the *A. paniculata* leaf juice against diabetes, malaria, and fever [141]. Two to 3 spoonfuls of leaf decoction *A. paniculata* is taken twice a day for four days against malaria by the tribes of Odisha [142]. Tribes in coastal Odisha used to cure malaria with the leaves of *A. paniculata* and Neem leaf extract, which were administered orally for three days [143].

Cancer

A. paniculata is used to treat cancer by the local communities residing in Nainamalai of Erode district in Tamil Nadu [144]. *A. macrobotrys* leaf paste is consumed with hot water by hill tribes of the Namakkal district in the Eastern Ghats to treat mouth and intestinal cancer [84]. Local inhabitants in Tekkali,

Srikakulam district in Andhra Pradesh, used to treat cancer with *A. paniculata* whole plant extract [145]. Whole plant extract of *A. paniculata* is used to treat cancer by the six tribal communities in the Malappuram district in Kerala [146].

Nervous Problems

Traditional healers of Dharmapuri district in Tamil Nadu used *A. affinis* for treating nervous problems [147]. The tribals in the Pachamalai hills of Eastern Ghats used *A. affinis* leaf extract for treating nervous-related ailments [148]. The leaf juice of *A. panicuata* is used to treat skeleton-muscular disorders by local residing people of Karnataka [149].

Stomach Problems

Decoction of *A. paniculata* leaves is taken orally to cure stomach problems by tribals of Sathyamangalam reserve forests in the Karnataka range [150]. Villagers of Kolli Hills in Eastern Ghats used *A. paniculata* to treat stomach aches and dyspepsia [51]. Konda Reddis of Andhra Pradesh prepared the pills with garlic and *Hemidesmus* root paste and took them orally for three days to treat jaundice [151]. *A. paniculata* leaves are eaten raw for indigestion and other stomach problems among the local inhabitants of West Bengal [152]. Stem and leaves of *A. paniculata* are useful in treating dysentery by different tribes (Jaintia, Riang, Chorai, Mizo, Vaiphei, Kari, Naga, and Kuki) of Cachar district in Assam, and leaf juice is given orally for all kinds of stomach problems [153]. Plant decoction of *A. paniculata* is used for treating gastrointestinal problems among Bodo communities in Chakrashila Wildlife Sanctuary of Assam [154]. Dimasa Kachari and Dima Hasa communities of Assam used *A. paniculata* plant decoction against dysentery and diarrhea [155]. Whole plant extract of *A. paniculata* is used for treating dysentery, bronchitis, influenza, fever, and liver diseases by the people of the Nashik district in Maharashtra [156]. The tribes in Jharkhand used the *A. paniculata* plant juice to treat stomach problems [157].

Miscellaneous Medicinal Uses

Leaf juice of *A. paniculata* is used to cure excess bleeding during menstruation by Paliyar tribes in the Madurai district of Tamil Nadu [39]. Leaf paste of *A. paniculata* is used to heal cut wounds by local inhabitants of Virudhunagar district in Tamil Nadu [158]. Tribal communities in Andhra Pradesh, such as Chenchu, Kondas, Sugalis, Lambadis, and Dhoras, used the whole plant extract of *A. paniculata* for treating body pain, urinary infection, and common cold [159]. The people in the Rayalaseema area of Andhra Pradesh used *A. echioides*, *A. paniculata*, and *A. serpyllifolia* for treating the common cough and cold, fever, blisters, and cut wounds [160]. *A. paniculata* is used to cure foot and mouth diseases of cattle by tribals in the Visakhapatnam and Vizianagaram districts of Andhra Pradesh [161]. Gadabas, Jatapus, Savaras, Konda doras, Manne doras, Yerukulas, Goudus, and Mukha doras of Vizianagaram district in Andhra Pradesh used the stem powder of *A. paniculata* along with leaves of *Gymnema sylvestre* and *Justicia adhatoda* for treating asthma [162]. Leaf juice of *A. elongata* with 2 to 4 drops of infant urine is dropped into the ear to control earache by tribals of Rapur-Chitvel Ghat of Eastern Ghats [163]. The tribal people of Attapadai and Vakkodan hill range in Kerala used the *A. paniculata* plant extract externally to cure the burning sensation [164]. The extract of *A. paniculata* is taken orally for postnatal care by the people of Kozhikode in Kerala [165]. The leaves of *A. paniculata* are ground well with the leaves of *Psidium guajava*, *Clerodendrum*, *Olea*, *Breynia*, and *Ludwigia*. The juice is taken to cure stomach acidity by the tribes of the Wayanad district of Kerala [166]. *A. echioides* leaf paste is applied externally for treating hair fall, ringworm, and muscular fitness by the Malayali tribe in the Kalvarayan hills of Eastern Ghats [167].

A. paniculata is used for curing fever, dysentery, and dyspepsia and to deworm by using hot water extract orally. It is also used for treating liver disorders, and the plant is powdered in mustard oil and used externally to stop itching [168]. The leaves of *A. paniculata*, *Tinospora cordifolia*, and *Solanum surattense* are taken for five days for curing fever, and water extract of dried leaf of *A. paniculata* is used orally as febrifuge, tonic, and anthelmintic. The review of ethnomedicine of Thailand mentioned the use of *A. paniculata* leaf decoction for treating high blood pressure [169]. *A. paniculata* leaf paste is used to treat cut wounds by the tribes of the Uttara Kannada district of Karnataka [170]. Leaf juice of *A. paniculata* is orally given to treat itching among the tribes of Shimoga district in Karnataka [171]. In Assam, local tribal people used to expel the intestinal worms with the intake of plant juice of *A. paniculata* [172]. Whole plant extract of *A. paniculata* is used to treat skin problems among the tribes of Odisha [173]. Leaf infusion of *A. paniculata* is used for wound healing and treating skin infections by the Juang tribes of Keonjhar district in Odisha [174]. The people of Jammu & Kashmir rarely used *A. paniculata* for treating kidney disorders [175].

CONCLUSION

The endemic species of the genus *Andrographis* in India need further studies to confirm the hypothesis that traditional medicine plants are still important in remote villages and hilly areas. It also supported the usefulness of primary health care in the community culture and is directly related to the local abundance, life forms, and seasonal diseases. Scientific standardization about disease diagnosis dosage, administration, and accuracy is needed to validate traditional knowledge in developing countries. Furthermore, there is a need for legal regulations about the conservation and protection of medicinally potential species of *Andrographis* because many species have restricted distribution in southern Peninsular India. Therefore, indigenous knowledge of potential medicinal herb usage must be recorded before it is lost.

REFERENCES

[1]   Hossain MS, Urbi Z, Sule A, Rahman KMH. *Andrographis paniculata* (Burm. f.) Wall. ex Nees: a review of ethnobotany, phytochemistry, and pharmacology. ScientificWorldJournal 2014; 2014: 1-28.
        [http://dx.doi.org/10.1155/2014/274905] [PMID: 25950015]

[2]   Burkill IH, Birtwistle W, Foxworthy F, Scrivenor J, Watson J. A Dictionary of the Economic Products of the Malay Peninsula. Kuala Lumpur, Malaysia: Ministry of Agriculture and Co-operatives 1966.

[3]   Akbar S. *Andrographis paniculata*: a review of pharmacological activities and clinical effects. Altern Med Rev 2011; 16(1): 66-77.
        [PMID: 21438648]

[4]   Jarukamjorn K, Nemoto N. Pharmacological aspects of *Andrographis paniculata* on health and its major diterpenoid constituent andrographolide. J Health Sci 2008; 54(4): 370-81.
        [http://dx.doi.org/10.1248/jhs.54.370]

[5]   Suresh K, Kottaimuthu R, Norman TSJ, Kumuthakalavalli R, Simon SM. Ethnobotanical study of medicinal plants used by Malayali tribals in Kolli Hills of Tamil Nadu, India. Int J Res Ayurveda Pharm 2011; 2(2): 502-8.

[6]   Gritto MJ, Nadanagopalan V, Doss A. Ethnobotanical survey of medicinal plants used by traditional healers in Shobanapuram village of Pachamalai hills, Tamil Nadu. Adv Appl Sci Res 2015; 6(3): 153-64.

[7]   Aminuddin, Girach RD, Wasiuddin. Medicinal potential of *Andrographis paniculata* (Bhuneem) - A less known medicinal plant in Unani medicine . Hamdard 1992; 40(2): 55-58.

[8]   Bensky D, Gamble A. Chinese Herbal Medicine Materia Medica. 1st ed. Washington, Eastland Press, USA. 1986; 136.

[9]   Rajasekaran A, Arivukkarasu R, Mathew L. A systematic comprehensive review on therapeutic potential of *Andrographis paniculata* (Burm. f.) Wall. ex Nees. J Pharmacogn Phytochm 2016; 5(5): 189-99.

[10]   Kumar S, Singh B, Bajpai V. *Andrographis paniculata* (Burm.f.) Nees: Traditional uses, phytochemistry, pharmacological properties and quality control/quality assurance. J Ethnopharmacol 2021; 275: 114054.
        [http://dx.doi.org/10.1016/j.jep.2021.114054] [PMID: 33831465]

[11]   Burgos RA, Hancke JL, Bertoglio JC, *et al.* Efficacy of an *Andrographis paniculata* composition for the relief of rheumatoid arthritis symptoms: a prospective randomized placebo-controlled trial. Clin Rheumatol 2009; 28(8): 931-46.
        [http://dx.doi.org/10.1007/s10067-009-1180-5] [PMID: 19408036]

[12]   Chandrasekaran CV, Gupta A, Agarwal A. Effect of an extract of *Andrographis paniculata* leaves on inflammatory and allergic mediators *in vitro*. J Ethnopharmacol 2010; 129(2): 203-7.
        [http://dx.doi.org/10.1016/j.jep.2010.03.007] [PMID: 20307638]

[13]   Chandrasekaran CV, Thiyagarajan P, Deepak HB, Agarwal A. *In vitro* modulation of LPS/calcimycin induced inflammatory and allergic mediators by pure compounds of *Andrographis paniculata* (King of bitters) extract. Int Immunopharmacol 2011; 11(1): 79-84.
        [http://dx.doi.org/10.1016/j.intimp.2010.10.009] [PMID: 21034865]

[14]   Shen T, Yang WS, Yi YS, *et al.* AP-1/IRF-3 targeted antiinflammatory activity of andrographolide isolated from *Andrographis paniculata*. Evid Based Complement Alternat Med 2013; 2013: 1-16.

[http://dx.doi.org/10.1155/2013/210736] [PMID: 23840248]

[15]   WHO Herba andrographidis.WHO Monographs on Selected Medicinal Plants, WHO. Geneva, Switzerland: World Health Organization 2013; pp. 12-25.

[16]   Rai PK, Lalramnghinglova H. Ethnomedicinal Plants of India with Special Reference to an Indo-Burma Hotspot Region: An overview. Ethnobot Res Appl 2011; 9: 379-420.
       [http://dx.doi.org/10.17348/era.9.0.379-420]

[17]   Govindarajan R, Vijayakumar M, Pushpangadan P. Antioxidant approach to disease management and the role of 'Rasayana' herbs of Ayurveda. J Ethnopharmacol 2005; 99(2): 165-78.
       [http://dx.doi.org/10.1016/j.jep.2005.02.035] [PMID: 15894123]

[18]   Thakur AK, Chatterjee SS, Kumar V. Andrographolides and traditionally used *Andrographis paniculata* as potential adaptogens: Implications for therapeutic innovation. TANG [HUMANITAS MEDICINE] 2014; 4(3): 15.1-15.14.
       [http://dx.doi.org/10.5667/tang.2014.0002]

[19]   Williamson EM. Major Herbs of Ayurveda. London, England: Churchill Livingstone 2002; p. 361.

[20]   Vijay D, Seetharam YN. *Andrographis paniculata* Nees A well known hepatoprotective drug: a review. Intern J Pharmaceut Clin Res 2018; 1(1): 12-6.

[21]   India Pharmacopoeia Commission Indian Pharmacopoeia. 7th ed., Ghaziabad, India: India Pharmacopoeia Commission 2014.

[22]   Ismail Z, Ismail N, Lassa J. Malaysian Herbal Monograph. Kuala Lumpur, Malaysia: Malaysian Monograph Committee 1999; Vol. 1.

[23]   Department of Traditional Medicine Medicinal Plants of Myanmar. Yangon, Myanmar: Ministry of Health 2008; Vol. 1.

[24]   Chinese Pharmacopoeia. Vol. I. Chemical Industry Press. China 2015.

[25]   World Health Organization, WHO Consultation on Selected Medicinal Plants, WHO Consultation on Selected Medicinal Plants (2nd, Ravello-Salerno, Italy) 1999. 1999.

[26]   United States Pharmacopeia Convention United States Pharmacopeia, 37th Revision. Rockville, MD: United States Pharmacopeia Convention 2014.

[27]   Samydurai P, Rajendran A, Sarvalingam A, Rajasekar C. Ethnobotanical knowledge of threatened plant species *Andrographis* in Nilgiri Biosphere Reserve, Tamil Nadu, India. Int J Herb Med 2017; 5(6): 103-7.

[28]   Alageesaboopathi C. Ethnobotany of *Andrographis lineata* Wallich ex Nees – an endemic medicinal plant of India. Int J Recent Sci Res 2012; 3(2): 71-4.

[29]   Karuppusamy S, Pullaiah T. Ethnomedicinal plants of Eastern Ghats and adjacent deccan region.Ethnobotany of India. USA: CRC press 2017; pp. 214-84.

[30]   Alagesaboopathi C. Ethnomedicinal plants and their utilization by villagers in Kumaragiri Hills of Salem district of Tamilnadu, India. Afr J Tradit Complement Altern Med 2009; 6(3): 222-7.
       [PMID: 20448846]

[31]   Sri DS, Manivasakan S, Hemalatha P, Fernandaz CC. Ethnobotanical study of medicinal plants in Kolli hills. Pharma Innov 2022; 11(7): 381-6.
       [http://dx.doi.org/10.22271/tpi.2022.v11.i7e.13665]

[32]   Venkataratnam K, Raju RRV. Folk medicines from Gundlabrameshwaram Wild Life Sanctuary, Andhra Pradesh, India. Ethnobotany 2004; 16: 33-9.

[33]   Venkataratnam K, Raju RRV. Folk medicine used for common women ailments by Adivasis in the Eastern Ghats of Andhra Pradesh. Indian J Tradit Knowl 2005; 4(3): 267-70.

[34]   Soniya S, Raju K. Traditional herbal remedies the herbs of Malayali in Shervarayan hills (Yercaud),

Salem district, Tamil Nadu. Int J Eng Res Appl 2017; 7(11): 86-91.

[35] Upasani SV, Beldar VG, Tatiya AU, Upasani MS, Surana SJ, Patil DS. Ethnomedicinal plants used for snakebite in India: a brief overview. Integr Med Res 2017; 6(2): 114-30.
[http://dx.doi.org/10.1016/j.imr.2017.03.001] [PMID: 28664135]

[36] Sabjan G, Sundaram G, Dharaneeshwara R, Muralidhara Rao D. Ethnobotanical crude drugs used in treatment of liver diseases by Chenchu tribes in Nallamalais, Andhra Pradesh, India. American J Ethnomed 2014; 1(3): 115-21.

[37] Dhole PA, Bhogaonkar PY, Chavhan VN, Kashirsagar PP. Some ethnomedicinal plants in Amaravati district (M.S), India. Indian J Adv Res Biol Sci 2021; 8(1): 61-75.
[http://dx.doi.org/10.22192/ijarbs.2021.08.01.009]

[38] Karuppusamy S, Muthuraja G, Rajasekaran KM. Lesser known ethnomedicinal plants of Alagar Hills, Madurai district of Tamil Nadu, India. Ethnobotanical Leaflets 2009; 13: 1426-33.

[39] Ignacimuthu S, Ayyanar M, Sivaraman K S. Ethnobotanical investigations among tribes in Madurai District of Tamil Nadu (India). J Ethnobiol Ethnomed 2006; 2(1): 25.
[http://dx.doi.org/10.1186/1746-4269-2-25] [PMID: 16689985]

[40] Jeganathan GK, Hoa THT, Bao-Lin L. Ethnobotanical survey of Irulars tribes in Pillur valley, Coimbatore (Tamil Nadu), India. Int J Herb Med 2016; 4(1): 1-11.

[41] Xavier TF, Fred Rose A, Dhivyaa M. Ethnomedicinal survey of Malayali tribes in Kolli hills of Eastern Ghats of Tamil Nadu. Indian J Tradit Knowl 2011; 10(3): 559-62.

[42] Adhan K, Anand SP. Wild ethnopharmacognosy plants utilize for the treatment of jaundice by Paliyars tribe in Sathuragiri hills, a part of Western Ghats, Tamil Nadu, India. Int J Pharma Health Res Sci 2019; 6(1): 2109-18.

[43] Giarch RD. Ethnobotanical notes on some plants of Mahendragiri hills, Orissa. Ethnobotany 2001; 13: 80-3.

[44] Mohan VR, Rajesh A, Athiperumalsami T, Sudha S. Ethnomedicinal plants of the Tirunelveli district, Tamil Nadu, India. Ethnobotanical Leaflets 2008; 12: 79-95.

[45] Ganesan S, Ramar Pandi N, Banumathy N. Ethnomedicinal survey of Alagarkoil hills (reserved forest), Tamil Nadu, India. J Indian Medicine 2008; 1: 1-18.

[46] Ignacimuthu S, Ayyanar M, Sankarasivaraman K. Ethnobotanical study of medicinal plants used by Paliyar tribals in Theni district of Tamil Nadu, India. Fitoterapia 2008; 79(7-8): 562-8.
[http://dx.doi.org/10.1016/j.fitote.2008.06.003] [PMID: 18678232]

[47] Kadirvelmurugan V, Raju K, Ravikumar S. Ethnobotany of medi-flora of Kolli hills, Tamil Nadu. Arch Appl Sci Res 2014; 6(1): 159-64.

[48] Umapriya T, Rajendran A, Aravindhan V. Binu Thomas, Maharajan. Ethnobotany of Irula tribes of Palani Hills, Coimbatore, Tamil Nadu. Ind J Nat Prod Res 2011; 2(2): 250-5.

[49] Lalitha Rani S, Kalpana Devi V, Tresina Soris P, Maruthupandian A, Mohan VR. Ethnomedicinal plants used by Kanikkars of Agasthiyamalai Biosphere Reserve, Western Ghats. J Ecobiotechnol 2011; 3(7): 16-25.

[50] Jeyaprakash K, Ayyanar M, Geetha KN, Sekar T. Traditional uses of medicinal plants among the tribal people in Theni District (Western Ghats), Southern India. Asian Pac J Trop Biomed 2011; 1(1): S20-5.
[http://dx.doi.org/10.1016/S2221-1691(11)60115-9]

[51] Murugesan P, Raja G, Suresh Kumar M, Selvam BP. Ethnobotanical study of medicinal plants used by villagers of Kolli hills of Namakkal district of Tamil Nadu, India. Int J Pharm Sci Rev Res 2011; 10(1): 170-6.

[52] Jeeva S, Femila V. Ethnobotanical investigation of Nadars in Atoor village, Kanyakumari district, Tamilnadu, India. Asian Pac J Trop Biomed 2012; 2(2): S593-600.

[http://dx.doi.org/10.1016/S2221-1691(12)60280-9]

[53]   Thirumalai T, Beverly CD, Sathiyaraj K, Senthilkumar B, David E. Ethnobotanical Study of Anti-diabetic medicinal plants used by the local people in Javadhu hills Tamilnadu, India. Asian Pac J Trop Biomed 2012; 2(2): S910-3.
       [http://dx.doi.org/10.1016/S2221-1691(12)60335-9]

[54]   Alagesaboopathi C. Ethnobotanical studies on useful plants of Sirumalai hills of Eastern Ghats, Dindigul district of Tamil Nadu, southern India. Int J Biosci 2012; 2(2): 77-84.

[55]   Pradheeps M, Poyyamoli G. Ethnobotany and utilization of plant resources in Irula villages (Sigur plateau, Nilgiri Biosphere Reserve, India). J Med Plants Res 2012; 7(6): 267-76.

[56]   Kalaiselvan M, Gopalan R. Ethnobotanical studies on selected wild medicinal plants used by Irula tribes of Bolampatty valley, Nilgiri Biosphere Resereve (NBR), southern Western Ghats, India. Asian J Pharm Clin Res 2014; 7(1): 21-6.

[57]   Sathishpandian S, Prathap S, Vivek P, *et al.* Ethnobotanical study of medicinal plants used by local people in Ariyalur district, Tamil Nadu, India. Intern J ChemTech Res 2014; 6(9): 4276-84.

[58]   Venkatachalapathi A, Sangeeth T, Ali MA, Tamilselvi SS, Paulsamy S, Al-Hemaidc FMA. Ethnomedicinal assessment of Irula tribes of Walayar valley of southern Western Ghats, India. Saudi J Biol Sci 2018; 25(4): 760-75.
       [http://dx.doi.org/10.1016/j.sjbs.2016.10.011] [PMID: 29740242]

[59]   Tamilvannan MV, Kadirvelmurugan V, Ravikumar S. Ethnobotanical survey of Gudiyum forests, Tiruvallur district, Tamil Nadu, India. Int J Ethnobiol & Ethnomed 2016; 2(1): 1-9.

[60]   M J, S K. Preliminary phytochemical investigation on *Tylophora subramanii* Henry (Apocynaceae) – an endemic medicinal plant species of southern India. Kongunadu Research Journal 2015; 2(2): 84-7.
       [http://dx.doi.org/10.26524/krj99]

[61]   Ida JC, Arul AA. Ethnobotanical study of Kani tribes in Keeriparai of Kanyakumari district, south India. Int Educ Res J 2016; 2(3): 49-52.

[62]   Maheshwaran S, Sivarathinavel RA, Pounraj P, Suresh K. Ethnobotanical studies on Agamalai hills, southern Western Ghats. J Emerg Technol Innov Res 2019; 6(3): 13-7.

[63]   Nehrurajan M, Hari Prakash M, Suresh K. Study of medicinal plants used by local tribes in Suruli hills of Theni district, Tamil Nadu. J Emerg Technol Innov Res 2019; 6(3): 18-23.

[64]   Sukumaran S, Sujin RM, Geetha VS, Jeeva S. Ethnobotanical study of medicinal plants used by the Kani tribes of Pechiparai hills, Western Ghats, India. Acta Ecol Sin 2021; 41(5): 365-76.
       [http://dx.doi.org/10.1016/j.chnaes.2020.04.005]

[65]   B A, P R. Documentation of ethnomedicinal and ethnoveterinary plants used by Paliyar Tribes, Kurangani Hills, Western Ghats, Theni District, Tnadu, India. Kongunadu Research Journal 2021; 8(1): 51-64.
       [http://dx.doi.org/10.26524/krj.2021.8]

[66]   Siva Pradeesh D, Sukumaran S, Jeeva S. Jenisha R Ethnobotanical studies of Kanies in Mothiramalai, Kilamalai reserve forest, Kalial range, Kanyakumari forest division. Tamil Nadu: High Technology Letter 2021.

[67]   Lakshmana, Sreenath KP. Phytoantidotes of Tumkur district, Karnataka, India. Global J Biol Agric Health Sci 2014; 3(4): 122-30.

[68]   Perumal Samy R, Thwin MM, Ponnambalam G, Ignacimuthu S. Ethnobotanical survey of folk plants for the treatment of snake bites in southern part of Tamil Nadu, India. J Ethnopharmacol 2007; 17(115(2)): 302-12.
       [http://dx.doi.org/10.1016/j.jep.2007.10.006]

[69]   Ahmed M, Talukder SA. Studies on the hypoglycemic activity of Kalmegh (*Andrographis paniculata* Nees) on the blood sugar level of rats. Bangladesh Pharm J 1977; 62: 21-3.

[70] Magendiran M, Vijayakumar KK. Ethnobotanical survey of medicinal plants used by Malayali tribes in Jawadhu hills of Eastern Ghats, Tamilnadu, India. Journal of Medicinal Herbs and Ethnomedicine 2022; 8: 7-11.
[http://dx.doi.org/10.25081/jmhe.2022.v8.7711]

[71] Udayan PS, George S, Tushar KV, Balachandran I. Medicinal plants used by the Malayali tribe of Servarayan hills, Yercad, Salem district, Tamil Nadu, India. Zoos' Print J 2006; 21(4): 2223-4.
[http://dx.doi.org/10.11609/JoTT.ZPJ.1426a.2223-4]

[72] Ganesan S, Suresh N, Kesavan L. Ethnomedicinal survey of lower Palni hills of Tamil Nadu. Indian J Tradit Knowl 2004; 3(3): 299-304.

[73] Alagesaboopathi C. Medicinal plants used for the treatment of liver diseases by Malayali tribes in Shevaroy hills, Salem district, Tamil Nadu, India. World J Pharm Res 2015; 4(1): 816-28.

[74] Alageesaboopathi C, Prabakaran G, Subramanian G, Vijayakumar RP. Ethnomedicinal studies of plants growing in the Salem district of Tamil Nadu, India. Int J Pharm Biol Sci 2018; 8(3): 503-11.

[75] Thirunarayanan T. Ethnobotanical survey on Folk Medicine in the management of animal bite poisons in the forest tract of Salem region of Tamil Nadu, India. Int J Pharmacol Clin Sci 2013; 2: 41-6.

[76] Alagesaboopathi C, Diwakaran P, Ramachandran VS. *Andrographis paniculata* Nees in tribal medicine of Tamil Nadu. Anc Sci Life 1999; 19(1-2): 28-30.
[PMID: 22556914]

[77] Saranraj P, Bhavani L, Suganthi K. Ethnobotanical survey of medicinal plants from Vellore district, Tamil nadu, India. International Journal of Advanced Research in Biological Sciences (IJARBS) 2016; 3(9): 238-46.
[http://dx.doi.org/10.22192/ijarbs.2016.03.09.032]

[78] Kottaimuthu R. Ethnobotany of the Valayans of Karandamalai, Dindigul district, Tamil Nadu, India. Ethnobotanical Leaflets 2008; 12: 195-203.

[79] Krishnaswamy S, Kushalappa BA. Systematic review and meta-analysis of *Andrographis serpyllifolia* (Rottler ex Vahl) Wight: An ethnopharmaco-botanical perspective. Pharmacogn J 2018; 10(6s): s14-26.
[http://dx.doi.org/10.5530/pj.2018.6s.3]

[80] Dhivya S, Kalaichelvi K. Ethnomedicinal plants used to treat skin diseases and poisonous bites by the tribals of Karamadai range, Western Ghats, Tamil Nadu, India. International Journal of Plant, Animal and Environmental Sciences 2016; 6: 3.
[http://dx.doi.org/10.21276/Ijpaes]

[81] Arulappan MT, Britto SJ, Ruckmani K, Kumar RM. An ethnobotanical study of medicinal plants used by ethnic people in Gingee hills, Villupuram district, Tamil Nadu, India. American J Ethnomed 2022; 5: 2022.

[82] Ranjani N, Kannan R, Kokila D, Bhuvaneswari V. Ethnobotanical survey of medicinal plants used by Malayali tribes in Palamalai hills Salem district, Tamil Nadu, India. Biol Forum 2023; 15(1): 222-9.

[83] Vadivalagan A, Kannan R. Ethnopharmacological studies on the medicinal plants used by Urali tribes of Kadambur hills, Sathyamangalam, Erode district, Tamil Nadu, India. J Plant Sci Res 2020; 7(1): 191-5.

[84] Sulochana A, Raveendran D, Krishnamma A, Oommen O. Ethnomedicinal plants used for snake envenomation by folk traditional practitioners from Kallar forest region of South Western Ghats, Kerala, India. J Intercult Ethnopharmacol 2015; 4(1): 47-51.
[http://dx.doi.org/10.5455/jice.20141010122750] [PMID: 26401384]

[85] Nitheesh A, Paul A, Fathima KM, Arvind R, Nair SG. A study of medicinal plants in Kozhlenchery taluk, Pathinamthitta district, Kerala. Int J Pharm Sci Rev Res 2017; 4(1): 274-99.

[86] Rajakumar N, Shivanna MB. Ethno-medicinal application of plants in the eastern region of Shimoga

district, Karnataka, India. J Ethnopharmacol 2009; 126(1): 64-73.
[http://dx.doi.org/10.1016/j.jep.2009.08.010] [PMID: 19686831]

[87]   Nanjunda DC. Ethno-medico-botanical survey of Jenu Kuruba ethnic group of Karnataka state, India. Bangladesh Journal of Medical Science 1970; 9(3): 161-9.
[http://dx.doi.org/10.3329/bjms.v9i3.6479]

[88]   Laddimath A. Ethnomedicinal plants used to treat snakebites (antidote) of Vijayapur (Bijapur) district of Karnataka, India. Global J Biol Agric Health Sci 2021; 10: 4.
[http://dx.doi.org/10.35248/2319-5584.21.10.112]

[89]   Lakshmana S, Dwraknath V. Shravana Kumar S. Folklore medicinal plants of Challakere taluk of Chitradurga district, Karnataka, India. Int J Life Sci Res 2018; 6(4): 185-93.

[90]   Das AK, Tag H. Ethnomedicinal studies of the Khamti tribe of Arunachal Pradesh. Indian J Tradit Knowl 2006; 5(3): 317-22.

[91]   Kadel C, Jain AK. Folklore claims on snakebite among some tribal communities of Central India. Indian J Tradit Knowl 2008; 7(2): 296-9.

[92]   Morvin Yabesh JE, Prabhu S, Vijayakumar S. An ethnobotanical study of medicinal plants used by traditional healers in silent valley of Kerala, India. J Ethnopharmacol 2014; 154(3): 774-89.
[http://dx.doi.org/10.1016/j.jep.2014.05.004] [PMID: 24832113]

[93]   Alageesaboopathi C. Medicinal plant used by tribal and non-tribal people of Dharmapuri district, Tamil Nadu, India. Int J Curr Res Biosci Plant Biol 2015; 1(2): 64-73.

[94]   Indumathi M, Aswini R, Murugesan S. Studies on ethnobotanical survey of medicinal plants in Palaniyappar hills, Namakkal district Eastern Ghats, Tamil Nadu, India. Intern J Pharma Res Health Sci 2018; 6(1): 2191-00.

[95]   Datta T, Patra AK, Dastidar SG. Medicinal plants used by tribal population of Coochbehar district, West Bengal, India–an ethnobotanical survey. Asian Pac J Trop Biomed 2014; 4(1) (Suppl. 1): S478-82.
[http://dx.doi.org/10.12980/APJTB.4.2014C1122] [PMID: 25183132]

[96]   Ramakrishna N, Saidulu Ch. Medicinal plants used by ethnic people of Adilabad district, Andhra Pradesh, India. Intern J Pharmaceut Res Allied Sci 2014; 3(2): 51-9.

[97]   Rajagopal Reddy S, Madhusuthana Reddy A, Philomina NS, Yasodamma N. Ethnobotanical survey of Seshachalam hill range of Kadapa district, Andhra Pradesh, India. Indian J Fundam Appl Life Sci 2011; 1(4): 324-9.

[98]   Suneetha J, Koteswara Rao J, Prabhakara Rao P, Seetharami Reddi TVV. Ethnomedicine for jaundice by tribals of East Godavari district, Andhra Pradesh. J Nat Rem 2013; 13(2): 142-7.

[99]   Murthy SMS, Vidyasagar GM. Traditional herbal remedies for Jaundice in Bellary district, Karnataka, India. Pearl : A Journal of Library and Information Science 2012; 4(4): 240-4.
[http://dx.doi.org/10.5958/j.0975-4261.4.4.029]

[100] Pooja S, Vidyasagar GM. Ethnomedicinal plants used by Rajgond tribes of Kaladhere village in Bidar district, Karnataka, India. Int J Pharm Pharm Sci 2015; 7(8): 216-20.

[101] Murthy SM. Traditional medicinal plants used to treat human ailments in Harapanahalli taluk of Davanagree district, Karnataka. J Med Plants Studies 2015; 3(5): 27-31.

[102] Sharma J, Gairola S, Gaur RD, Painuli RM. The treatment of jaundice with medicinal plants in indigenous communities of the Sub-Himalayan region of Uttarakhand, India. J Ethnopharmacol 2012; 143(1): 262-91.
[http://dx.doi.org/10.1016/j.jep.2012.06.034] [PMID: 22759701]

[103] Kadirvelmurugan V, Dhamotharan R, Ravikumar S. Ethnomedicinal study on tribal area of Kathiri hills in Erode district of Tamil Nadu, India. Central European J Exp Biol 2015; 4(1): 20-6.

[104] Patel Dharmesh C, Jat BL. An ethnobotanical survey of plants used by traditional healers of Kaprada forest (Valsad district), Gujarat, India. Int J Curr Microbiol Appl Sci 2018; 7(7): 2034-43. [http://dx.doi.org/10.20546/ijcmas.2018.707.240]

[105] Prabhu S, Vijayakumar S. Ethnobotanical study of traditionally used medicinal plants in Malayali ethnic people of Pachamalai hills, Tamil Nadu, India. J Pharmaceut Med Res 2016; 2(3): 39-42.

[106] Karuppusamy A, Parimelazhagan T. Ethnomedicinal observations among Hoorali tribes in Kadambur hills (Kalkadambur), Erode district, Tamil Nadu. Glob J Pharmacol 2011; 5(3): 117-21.

[107] Padal SB, Prayaga Murthy P, Srinivasa Rao D, Venkaiah M. Ethnomedicinal plants from Paderu division of Visakapatnam district, A.P., India. J Phytol 2010; 2(8): 79-91.

[108] Basha SK. An ethnobotanical studies of medicinal plants of Ahobilam reserve forests in Kurnool district, Andhra Pradesh, India. Intern J Scientific Dev Res 2018; 3(4): 232-325.

[109] Manjula S, Mamidala E. An ethnobotanical survey of medicinal plants used by traditional healers of Thadvai, Warangal district, Andhra Pradesh, India. Int J Med Res Health Sci 2012; 2(1): 40-6.

[110] Basha SK, Sudarsanam G, Silar Mohammad M, Niaz Parveen D. Investigation of antidiabetic medicinal plants used by Sugali tribal inhabitants of Yerramalais of Kurnool district, Andhra Pradesh, India. J Pharm Sci 2011; 4(2): 19-24.

[111] Daimari M, Roy MK, Swargiary A, Baruah S, Basumataray S. An ethnobotanical survey of antidiabetic medicinal plants used by the Bodo tribe of Kokrajhar district, Assam. Indian J Tradit Knowl 2019; 18(3): 421-9.

[112] Paul S, Devi N, Sarma GC. Ethnobotanical utilization of some medicinal plants used by Bodo people of Manas biosphere reserve in the treatment of malaria. INTERNATIONAL RESEARCH JOURNAL OF PHARMACY 2013; 4(6): 102-5. [http://dx.doi.org/10.7897/2230-8407.04622]

[113] Kumar M, Butt AT, Hussaini SA, Kumar K, Khan H, Samiulla L. Ethnomedicines in the Khordha forest division of Khordha district of Odisha, India. Int J Curr Microbiol Appl Res 2014; 3(1): 274-80.

[114] Das S, Mohaty S, Nayak S, Bhatta K. Plants of Gandhamardan in maternal care: an ethnobotanical approach. Asian J Pharm Clin Res 2021; 14(7): 70-3. [http://dx.doi.org/10.22159/ajpcr.2021.v14i7.41862]

[115] Ullah M, Mehmood S, Ali M, *et al.* An ethnopharmacological study of plants used for treatment of diabetes in the Southern and Tribal regions of Khyber Pakhtunkhwa province, Pakistan. Ethnobot Res Appl 2019; 18: 9-22. [http://dx.doi.org/10.32859/era.18.8.1-20]

[116] Selson PDS, Edison DPS, Abraham SMD. Ethnomedical survey at Puliyankudi in Tirunelveli district, Tamil Nadu, India. Res. Res J Life Sci Bioinform Pharm Chem Sci 2019; 5(1): 390. [http://dx.doi.org/10.26479/2019.0501.34]

[117] Jenisha SR, Athira PA, Sujin RM. Ethnobotanical study of the local inhabitants of Arumanai village, Kanyakumari district, Tamil Nadu, India: a quantitative approach. J Emerg Technol Innov Res 2021; 8(10): a726.

[118] Yogeshwari C, Kumudha P. Ethnobotany of Sholaga tribes of Kathri hills, Chennampatti Range, Western Ghats, India. Research Journal of Pharmacognosy and Phytochemistry 2018; 10(2): 179-82. [http://dx.doi.org/10.5958/0975-4385.2018.00028.6]

[119] Marandi RR, Britto SJ, Soreng PK. Ethnomedicinal formulations used for treatment and prophylaxis of malaria by Oraon tribals of Palamu division, Jharkhand, India. Intern J Pharmaceut Res Biosci 2015; 4(6): 145-62.

[120] Porchezhian V, Pandikuamr P, Ramya TP, Maria Packiam S. Documentation of medicinal plants used by the local people for the prevention of COVID-19 in Thiruvannamalai district, Tamil Nadu, South India. Intern J Botany Studies 2021; 6(4): 493-500.

[121] Sankara Rao B, Sarada Mani N, Sujatha B, Polumahanthi S. Ethnobotanical investigation of underground plant parts of Kotia hills of Vizianagaram district, Andhra Pradesh, India. J Med Plants Studies 2015; 3(2): 118-20.

[122] Madhu Y, Naik DSR. Ethnomedicinal uses of leaf preparations in Adilabad district, Andhra Pradesh, India. Ethnobotanical Leaflets 2006; 13: 1337-47.

[123] Sasidhar K, Brahamjirao P, Sujith Kumar A. Ethnobotanical studies on medicinal plant utilization by the Yanadhi tribe of Ananthasagaram mandal, Nellore district, Andhra Pradesh, India. Intern Adv Res J Sci Eng Technol 2016; 3(2): 75-80.

[124] B S. An ethnobotanical survey of plants used by Yanadi tribe of Kavali, Nellore district, Andhra Pradesh, India. Journal of Scientific and Innovative Research 2015; 4(1): 22-6.
[http://dx.doi.org/10.31254/jsir.2015.4106]

[125] Basha SKM, Priyadarsini I. Ethnobotanical study of Rapur-Chitvel Ghat, Eastern Ghats, Andhra Pradesh. Int J Eng Tech Res 2017; 6(3): 69-72.

[126] Murthy EN. Ethnomedicinal plants used by Gonds of Adilabad district, Andhra Pradesh, India. Int J Pharm Life Sci 2012; 3(10): 2034-43.

[127] Prakash JW, Anpin Raja RD, Aspin Anderson N, *et al.* Ethnomedicinal plants used by Kani tribes of Agasthiyamalai biosphere reserve, southern Western Ghats. Indian J Tradit Knowl 2008; 7(3): 410-3.

[128] Silambarasan R, Suresh Kumar J, Ayyanar M. Ethnomedicinal plants used by Malayali and Narikuravar communities in Erode district Tamil Nadu, India. Am J Ethnomed 2017; 4(2): 15.

[129] Pramod Kumar N, Sivan NT, Renjusha AP. Relevance of practicing ethnobotany in modern era. Devagiri J Sci 2020; 6(1): 21-8.

[130] Malabadi RB, Mulgund GS, Nataraja K. Ethnobotanical survey of medicinal plants of Belgaum district, Karnataka. Curr Res Med Aromat Plants 2007; 29: 70-7.

[131] Prakash BN, Unnikrishnan PM. Ethnomedicinal survey of herbs for the management of malaria in Karnataka, India. Ethnobot Res Appl 2013; 11: 289-98.

[132] Topalakatti DAA. Traditional uses of medicinal plants of Badami Taluk district Bagalkot. International Journal of Unani and Integrative Medicine 2021; 5(2): 82-3.
[http://dx.doi.org/10.33545/2616454X.2021.v5.i2b.174]

[133] Narayana VL, Narasimharao GM. Plant used in ethnoveterinary medicine by tribals of Visakhapatnam and Vizianagaram district, Andhra Pradesh, India. Int J Pure App Biosci 2015; 3(2): 432-9.

[134] Choudhury MD, Bawai M, Singha S. Some anti-pyretic ethnomedicinal plants of Manipuri community of Barak valley, Assam, India. Ethnobotanical Leaflets 2010; 14: 21-8.

[135] Borah S, Bora A. Ethnomedicinal plants used for the treatment of common diseases by the Deori community people of Lakshimpur district, Assam. Universal Journal of Plant Science 2020; 8(3): 39-46.
[http://dx.doi.org/10.13189/ujps.2020.080301]

[136] Rajurkar BM. Ethnobotanical studies of Bhadravati Tashil of Chandrapur district, Maharashtra State. Int J Creative Res Thoughts 2018; 6(2): 24-31.

[137] Shende JJ, Rajurkar BM, Mhaiskar MN, Dalal LP. Ethnobotanical studies of Samudrapur Tashil of Wardha district. J Pharma Biol Sci 2014; 9(6): 16-23.

[138] Gaikwad KN, Kandhbahale DS, Khalkar KM, Bhamare MR. Ethnomedicinal potential of Salher-Mulher forest Nashik district (Maharashtra). Intern J Botany Studies 2022; 7(3): 68-71.

[139] Gupta R, Vairale MG, Deshmuckh RR, Chaudhary PR, Wate SR. Ethnomedicinal uses of some plants used by Gond tribes of Bhandara district, Maharashtra. Indian J Tradit Knowl 2010; 9(4): 713-7.

[140] Samarth VD, Sinkar SR. Folkloric medicinal plants of Ralegaon region of Yavatmal district,

Maharashtra. Indian J Adv Res Biol Sci 2019; 6(5): 65-71.

[141] Panda D. Ethnobotanical study of medicinal plants in Jaipur district of Odisha, India. J Pharmacogn Phytochem 2018; 7(4): 1508-12.

[142] Pani M, Nahak G, Sahu RK. Review on ethnomedicinal plants of Odisha for the treatment of Malaria. Int. J Pharmcog Phytochem Res 2014; 7(1): 156-65.

[143] Singh H, Dhole PA, Krishna G, Saravanan R, Baske PK. Ethnobotanical plants used in malaria in tribal areas of Odisha, India. Indian J Nat Prod Resour 2018; 9(2): 160-7.

[144] Rajalakshmi P, Pugalenthi M, Vadivel V. Traditional knowledge on medicinal plants used by the Irula tribes of Kadambur hills, Erode district, Tamil Nadu, India. J Med Plants Studies 2016; 4(5): 14-7.

[145] Chandra Sekhar T, Jyoshna K, Thanuja G, Leelavathi S. Ethnobotany of selected medicinal plants of Tekkali Srikakulam district, Andhra Pradesh. J Emerg Technol Innov Res 2014; 9(8): e601-7.

[146] Chithra M, Prabhukumar KM, Geetha SP. A comparative study on ethnobotanical usage of plants for twenty selected diseases by six tribal communities in Malappuram district. Int J Herb Med 2016; 4(4): 108-13.

[147] Sundararajan G, Preamkumar K. Ethnobotanical survey of medicinal plants used by traditional healers in Krishnagiri district of Tamil Nadu. Int J Sci Res 2018; 7(11): 216.
[http://dx.doi.org/10.21275/ART20192542]

[148] Gritto MJ, Nanadagopalan V, Doss A. Ethnobotanical survey of medicinal plants used by traditional healers in Shobanapuram village of Pachamalai Hill, Tamilnadu. Adv Appl Sci Res 2015; 6(3): 157-64.

[149] Yogeesha A, Kumar KG. A review on traditional medicinal plants used against common neuro-musculo-skeletal disorders in Karnataka state, India. Int J Pharm Sci Res 2022; 13(2): 499-502.

[150] Poongodi A, Thilagavathi S, Aravindhan V, Rajendran A. Observations on some ethnomedicinal plants in Sathyamangalam forests of Erode district, Tamil Nadu, India. J Med Plants Res 2011; 5(19): 4709-14.

[151] Raju VS, Reddy KN. Ethnomedicine for dysentery and diarrhoea from Khammam district of Andhra Pradesh. Indian J Tradit Knowl 2005; 4(4): 443-7.

[152] Mazumder M, Sarkar AK. Ethnobotanical survey of indigenous leafy vegetables consumed in rural areas of Terai-Dooars region of West Bengal, India. J Threat Taxa 2019; 11(12): 14612-8.
[http://dx.doi.org/10.11609/jott.5039.11.12.14612-14618]

[153] Das AK, Dutta BK, Sharma GD. Medicinal plants used by different tribes of Cachar district, Assam. Indian J Tradit Knowl 2008; 7(3): 446-54.

[154] Talukdar S, Gupta A. Medicinal plants used by the Bodo community of Chakrashila wildlife sanctuary in Assam, India. Indian J Appl Res 2014; 4(2): 3.

[155] Parbo D, Kumar A. Ethnobotany: the ethnicity of the Dimasa Kachari, Dima Haso, Assam India. J Plant Sci Res 2021; 8(2): 1-14.

[156] Sanjayrao KS, Sanjay GV. Studies on ethnobotanical plants used by tribal community of Nashik district, Maharashtra, India. J Med Plants Studies 2019; 7(4): 200-2.

[157] Singh H. Ethnomedicinal plants of Jharkhand, India.Herbal cures – Traditional approach Avisshkar Publishes. Jaipur 2008; pp. 248-63.

[158] Shanmugam S, Rajagopal V, Balamurugan S, *et al.* Ethnobotanical indices on wound healing medicinal plants in the Arjuna River of Virudhunagar District in Tamil Nadu, Southern India. Asian Journal of Ethnobiology 2021; 4(1): 31-6.
[http://dx.doi.org/10.13057/asianjethnobiol/y040103]

[159] Sripriya D. Ethnobotanical uses of some plants by tribes in AP, India. Intern J Pharma Biol Sci 2017; 7(4): 67-74.

[160] Muralidhra Rao D, Bhaskara Rao UVU, Sudharsanam G. Ethno-medico-botanical studies from Rayalaseema region of southern Eastern Ghats, Andhra Pradesh, India. Ethnobotanical Leaflets 2006; 10: 198-207.

[161] Narayan SV, Ibemhal CI, Community C, Baruah MK. An ethnobotanical study of Chirus – a less known tribe of Assam. Indian J Trad knowl 2011; 10(3): 572-4.

[162] Chandra Babu N, Tarakeswara Naidu M, Venkaiah M. Ethnomedicinal plants used by tribals of Vizianagaram district, Andhra Pradesh. Ann Pharm Pharm Sci 2011; 2(1&2): 1-14.

[163] Basha SKM, Priyadharsini AI. Ethnobotany of Rapur-Chitvel Ghat, Eastern Ghats, Andhra Pradesh. Intern J Eng Res Technol 2017; 6(3): 178-83.

[164] Limcy TJ, Subhashini S. Ethnomedicinal practices of tribal inhabitants of Attapadai and Vakkodan hill ranges of Kerala. Int J Sci Res 2012; 2(3): 33-6.

[165] Anvar K, Haneef J. Ethnobotanical plants used for postnatal care by traditional practitioners from Kozhikode district, Kerala, India. Int J Res Pharm Chem 2015; 5(4): 570-81.

[166] David Prasad AG, Shyma TB, Raghavendra MP. Plants used by the tribes for treatment of digestive system disorders in Wayanad district, Kerala. J Appl Pharm Sci 2013; 3(8): 171-5.

[167] Pushparaj A, Andrew GD, Vinothkannan A, Mohan G, Kandavel D. Indigenous uses of medicinal plants among Malayali tribes in siriya Kalvarayan hills, Eastern Ghats, India. Intern J Botany Studies 2021; 6(5): 1243-60.

[168] Hemadri K, Rao SS. Jaundice : tribal medicine. Anc Sci Life 1984; 3(4): 209-12. [PMID: 22557408]

[169] Siddiqui MB, Hussain W. Traditional antidotes of Snake poison. Fitoterapia 1990; 61(1): 41-4.

[170] Bhat P, Hegde G, Hegde GR. Ethnomedicinal practices in different communities of Uttara Kannada district of Karnataka for treatment of wounds. J Ethnopharmacol 2012; 143(2): 501-14. [http://dx.doi.org/10.1016/j.jep.2012.07.003] [PMID: 22820243]

[171] Shivanna MB, Rajkumar N. Ethno-medico-botanical knowledge of rural folk in Bhadravathi taluk of Shimoga district, Karnataka. Indian J Tradit Knowl 2010; 9(1): 159-68.

[172] Swargiary A, Roy MK, Daimari M. Survey and documentation of ethnobotanicals used in the traditional medicines system of tribal communities of Chirang district of Assam against Helminthiasis. Biomed Pharmacol J 2019; 12(4): 1923-35. [http://dx.doi.org/10.13005/bpj/1824]

[173] Prusti AB, Beherra KK. Ethnomedicinal exploration of Malakangiri district of Odisha, India. Ethnobotanical Leaflets 2007; 11: 122-40.

[174] Khatoon G. Ethnomedicinal uses of plants: a study among the Juang tribes of Keonjhar district of Odisha. Int J Ayurveda Pharma Res 2020; 8(1): 22-9.

[175] Azad SH, Bhat AR. Ethnomedicinal plants recorded from Rajouri-Pooch districts of Jammu & Kashmir state. Indian J Life Sci 2013; 2(2): 15-30.

CHAPTER 4

Andrographolide and its Analogs

S. Karuppusamy[1,*] and N. Janakiraman[1]

[1] *Department of Botany, The Madura College, Madurai-625011, Tamil Nadu, India*

Abstract: Andrographolide is a pharmacologically significant labdane diterpenoid primarily isolated from *Andrographis paniculata*, and later, from many of its allied species. *A. paniculata* is used in many Indian traditional and alternative medicinal systems for treating several human ailments. The phytochemical studies on species has yielded a number of diterpenoids and flavonoids, which have been screened for their pharmacological potential by various scientific groups. The results proved that andrographolides and their analogs have the potential to treat cancer and cardiovascular, hepatic, and various other diseases. In this chapter, the phytochemistry of *Andrographis* and the structure and properties of major andrographolides and their analogs have been reviewed.

Keywords: Andrographolide, anticancer, toxicology, phytochemistry, pharmacology.

INTRODUCTION

Andrographis paniculata (Acanthaceae) is an indigenous medicinal species of India, popularly called "Kalmegh". Due to its bitterness, it is said to be a king of bitters among medicinal herbs. It is widely distributed all over the Indian states, Sri Lanka, and entire Southeast Asia [1]. *A. paniculata* is traditionally used for treating snake bites, poisonous stings, fever, diarrhea, jaundice, skin diseases, and respiratory problems by local communities in India. This plant species is a well-recognized ingredient in several Indian medicinal systems like Siddha, Ayurveda, Unani, and homeopathy and also in Chinese and Thai traditional systems for treating various human ailments [2 - 5]. The extracts obtained from various parts of *A. paniculata* have been reported to have several pharmacological properties like anticancer, analgesic, antidiabetic, anti-inflammatory, antimicrobial, antiviral, cardioprotective, hepatoprotective, and immunomodulatory [6 - 9]. While, in the extracts of herbs, a major class of phytochemicals such as diterpenoid lactones, flavonoids, phenolic compounds, and xanthones have been reported [10, 11]. The

---

* **Corresponding author S. Karuppusamy:** Department of Botany, The Madura College, Madurai-625011, Tamil Nadu, India; E-mail: ksamytaxonomy@gmail.com

S. Karuppusamy, Vinod K. Nelson & T. Pullaiah (Eds.)

relationship between the chemical structure and biological properties was proved by applying modern prediction tools such as pharmacophore modeling and 3D QSAR analysis of andrographolides and their analogs [12].

Phytochemistry of *A. paniculata*

The extracts of *A. paniculata*have been phytochemically profiled with several compounds from various parts, including leaves, stems, and roots. Several traditional medicinal systems use specific parts of the herb due to the active compounds accumulated in the respective plant parts. The major phytochemical compounds isolated from *A. paniculata* are labdane diterpenes, such as andrographolide, which is a bitter alkaloid that accumulates in all the parts of the plant in various proportions. It is only responsible for the major pharmacological properties of the herb. The other class of compounds have also been reported in plants, including flavonoids, iridoids, polyphenols, xantholactones, and some macro-elements. However, andrographolide, a diterpenoid lactone, is a predominant phytochemical principle found in all the parts of *A. paniculata* in higher quantities than other compounds [13]. Some other terpenoid compounds, including deoxyandrographolide and neoandrographolide have been isolated from the aerial parts of *A. paniculata*. Some phytochemical experiments profiled 20 different diterpenoids and 10 flavonoid fractions from the ethanolic and methanolic extracts of various parts of *A. paniculata* [14, 15]. Andrographolide diterpenoids and oxyflavonoids are chemical signatures of *Andrographis,* which is used as a chemotaxonomic marker of the genus. A number of other diterpenoids with common chemical skeletons and stereochemical principles were isolated by the later exploration, including Angrographolide-A, B, C, D, E, and F, neoandrographolide, isoandrographolide, deoxyandrographolide and andrographanin [16 - 18]. Sometimes, these common andrographolide rings are associated with the xanthone group, which is another class of phytochemicals, including 1,8-hydroxy-3,7-dimethoxy-xanthone, 4,8-dihydroxy-2,7-dimeth-xy-xanthone, 1,2-dihyroxy-6,8-dimehtoxy-xanthine, and 3,7,8-trimethoxy-1-hydroxy-xanthone, and are also characterized from the roots of *A. paniculata* [19]. There are two major flavonoids, 5,7,2,3-tetramethaoxy flavone and 5-hydroxy-7,2,3-trimethoxy flavone, reported from the whole plant of *A. paniculata* [20]. The ethylacetate extracts of aerial parts and roots of *A. paniculata* were reported to have seven major flavonoids, including 7-0-methylwogonin, 1,2-dimethyether flavone, hydroxy tetramethoxy flavone, dihydroxy tetramehtoxy flavone, dihyroxy trimethoxy flavone, dihydroxy-0-methylwogonin, and dimethyl ether [21 - 23].

Phytochemistry of other Species of *Andrographis*

A. affinis

The whole plant extract of *A. affinis* has been isolated with two diterpenoids, andrographanin and 14-deoxy-11,12-didehydroandrographolide, and also three flavonoids, namely 5,7,2,3,4-pentamethoxy flavone, 5-hydroxy-tetramethoxy flavone, and echiodinin-glucopyranoside [18].

A. alata

It is also an endemic herb of Southern India, which is reported to be a source of andrographolide derivatives, including five acetylated flavones and two oxygenated glycopyranosides from the whole plant [24].

A. lineata

The whole plant extract of *A. lineata* fractioned three major flavonoids, including 2,3,4-pentamethoxy flavone, 2-hydroxy, 2,4,6-trimethoxychalcone, and dihydroskullcapflavone. In addition to this, known andrographolide stereomers and six other flavonoid fractions were also reported from the whole plant extract [14]. The phytochemical analysis of the leaf, stems and roots of *A. lineata* extracted with different solvents such as aqueous, ethanol, butanol, methanol and chloroform showed the presence of alkaloids, flavonoids, phenols, coumarins, glycosides, phytosterols, saponins, resins, tannins, terpenoids and steroids [25].

A. wightiana

It is also an endemic herb of Southern India. Three known labdane diterpenoids and two new acetylated diterpenoids including 14-deoxy-3,19-diacetyl-1-,12-didehydroandrographolide with flavones such as echioidinin, skullcapflavone, and 12-methy-ether were isolated from the whole plant extract [26].

Andrographolide

Andrographolide, a common chemical skeleton of labdane diterpenoids as 14-deoxy-11,12-didehydroandrographolide, is a major compound isolated from *A. paniculata*. This compound exhibits varying degrees of the pharmacological spectrum, including antiviral, antibacterial, hepatoprotective, cardioprotective, anti-inflammatory, and anticancer activities in *in vivo* and *in vitro* models. The structure of andrographolide contains a,b-unsaturated, c-butyrolactone moiety (primary, secondary, and allylic) with two double bonds and three hydroxyls at the C3 position, C14, C18, and C19, interacted with the a,b, c-butyrolactones, where the D rings, D12 and D13, with double bonds, interact with hydroxyl and ester moiety. In D8, D17 bonded with epoxy moiety is responsible for a crucial role in pharmacological and cytotoxic activities of the andrographolides. Several other andrographolides were synthesized by the modification of reactive groups 3,19-isopropylindane andrographolide, Dehydroandrographolide, 11,12-didehydro-14- deoxyandrographolide, 11,12-didehydro-19-formyl-14-deox-andr-ographolide, and diacetoide [27]. In recent phytochemical explorations of *A. paniculata*, 14 different andrographolide derivatives, including neoandrogra-pholide, isoandrographolide, bisandrogra-pholide, deoxyandro-graphiside, didehydro-xyandrographiside, and andrographiside, were reported [28]. These chemical structures with their active chemical moieties are associated with a spectrum of pharmacological properties, including antibacterial [29], hepatoprotective [30], anti-HIV [31], anticancer [32 - 34], hypoglycaemic, and hypotensive properties [35 - 37]. In recent years, much attention has been paid to enhancing the biological properties of andrographolide molecules by structural modifications using modern techniques of docking and biosynthesis [38, 39]. The synthetic andrographolide analogs also exhibited considerable biological properties both in *in vitro* and *in vivo* experimental models, especially in cytotoxic properties [40 - 49] (Table **1**).

Table 1. Phytochemistry and pharmacology of clinically proven major Andrographolides and its analogs.

Name of the Compound	Isolated from	IUPAC Name	Pharmacological Properties Reported
Andrographolide	*Andrographis paniculata Andrographis alata Andrographis affinis Andrographis lineata Andrographis wightiana*	3-[2-[Decahydro-6-hydroxy-5-(hydroxymethyl)-5,8a-dimethyl-2-methylene-1-napthalenyl]ethylidene]dihydro-4-hydroxy-2(3H)-furanone	Anti-neoplastic [73]; Antiviral against SARS CoV-2 [74]; Antiasthmatic [57]; Antibacterial [75]; Neuroprotective [76]; Hypolipidemic [77; Gastroprotective [78]; Antidiabetic and antilipidemic [79]
Neoandrograholide	*Andrographis paniculata, Andrographis affinis Andrographis lineata Andrographis wightiana Tabernaemontana corymbosa, Potamogeton natans*	4-[2-[(1R,4aS,5R,8aS)-5,8a-dimethyl-2-methylidene-5-[[(2R,3R,4S,5S,6R)-3,4,5-trihydroxy-6-(hydroxymethyl)oxan-2-yl]oxymethyl]-3,4,4a,6,7,8-hexahydro-1H-naphthalen-1-yl]ethyl]-2H-furan-5-one	Antiviral against SARS CoV-2 [74]; Antiasthmatic [57]; Neuroprotection [76]; Anti-inflammatory [80]; Antibacterial [75]

(Table 1) cont.....

Name of the Compound	Isolated from	IUPAC Name	Pharmacological Properties Reported
14-deoxy 11, 12-didehydroandrographolide	*Andrographis paniculata Andrographis lineata*	4-[(E)-2-[(1R,4aS,5R,6R,8aR)-6-hydroxy-5-(hydroxymethyl)-5,8a-dimethyl-2-methylidene-3,4,4a,6,7,8-hexahydro-1H-naphthalen-1-yl]ethenyl]-2H-furan-5-one	Anti-inflammatory and antiasthmatic [64]; Anti-inflammatory [80]; Hepatoprotective [65]; Antiviral [81]; Anticancer [82]; Anticarcinoma cell lines [83]; Cardioprotective [84, 85]; Glucose uptake and transporter [86]; Antiplatelet aggregation [87]
14-Dexoyandrographolide	*Andrographis paniculata Andrographis affinis Andrographis wightiata*	3-[2-[(1R,4aS,5R,6R,8aS)-decahydro-6-hydroxy-5-(hydroxymethyl)-5,8a-dimethyl-2-methylene-1-naphthalenyl]ethyl]-2(5H)-furanone	Antimicrobial [66]; Hepatoprotective [67]; Antifungal [88]; Antifibrosis activity [68]; Antiasthmatic [57]; Antibacterial [75]
andrographiside	*Andrographis paniculata*	6-hydroxy-5-(hydroxymethyl)-5,8a-dimethyl-2-methylidene-3,4,4a,6,7,8-hexahydro-1H-naphthalen-1-yl]-1-[(4S)-4-hydroxy-2-oxooxoan-3-yl]ethanesulfonate	Zika virus protease inhibitor [69]; Antiasthmatic [57]; Neuroprotection [76].
3,19-Acetonylidene andrographolide	*Andrographis paniculata Andrographis lineata Andrographis alata*	2-acetyloxy-5-[(2E)-2-[(4S)-4-hydroxy-2-oxooxolan-3-ylidene]ethyl]-1,4a-dimethyl-6-methylidene-3,4,5,7,8,8a-hexahydro-2H-naphthalen-1-yl]methyl acetate	Anti-Zika and Anti- Dengue viral [72]

Name of the Compound	Isolated from	IUPAC Name	Pharmacological Properties Reported
7-O-methylwogonin	*Andrographis affinis Andrographis paniculata, Andrographis lineata, Ranunculus japonicus Scutellaria baicalensis*	5-Hydroxy-7,8-dimethoxy-2-phenyl-4-chromenone, 5-Hydroxy-7-8-dimethoxy-2-phenyl-4*H*-1-benzopyran-4-one, 5-Hydroxy-7-8-dimethoxyflavone, 7,8-Dimethoxynorwogonin, Moslosooflavone	Anti-inflammatory [89, 90]

Analogs of Andrographolides

In addition to the known diterpenoid labdane moity of andrographolide, several other andrographolide derivatives were isolated from *Andrographis,* like neoandrographolide, bisandrographolide, acetylandrographolide, deoxyandrographolide, deoxyandrographiside, and andrographanin, which are called andrographolide analogs [50]. In the genus *Andrographis*, the major class of andrographolide is closely associated with oxygenated flavones, which give several other chemical derivatives and are also highly potential for pharmacological properties. Usually, flavonoidal moiety is also an active group exhibited with andrographolides, namely hydroxy-dimethyl flavone, dihydroxy-tirmethyl flavone, dimethoxyflavones, and andrographnaidine-A (Table **1**).

Apart from the naturally occurring andrographolide derivatives, several other biosynthetic andrographolides have been added in recent years [51]. These synthetic andrographolides also possess considerable pharmacological potential. The natural product library showes about 360 different andrographolide analogs [52]. The naturally occurring andrographolide contains primary, secondary, and allyl rings, which are associated with double-bonded hydroxyl groups [53]. The structural modifications in the primary skeleton of andrographolide molecules by modern biosynthetic combinatorial docking methods were carried out to improve the anticancer properties of these compounds [54, 55]. Recently synthesized andrographolide analogs, including isopropylideneandrogrpaholide, acetylisopropylidene, andrographolide, and acetylandrographolide, were employed for the anticancer properties against various cell lines [55], among which 14-acetylandrographolide showed significant anticancer activity. However, the mechanism of action varies from that of the natural andrographolide. Another experiment observed significant improvement in the cytotoxic properties of synthesized andrographolide analog 2-bromobenzylideneandrographolide [43]. Whereas, another research team synthesized semisynthetic andrographolide molecule DRF3188, which possessed highly significant cytotoxicity against MCF-7 breast cancer cell lines comparable to mother andrographolide [54].

In another experiment, a new combination of glucoside molecule α-glucosidase inhibitors in the andrographolide moiety was synthesized for enhancing the hypoglycaemic properties [43]. It demonstrated improved biological properties of andrographolide compounds by structural modification and additions of respective active groups. Succinyl ester of andrographolide exhibited significant antiviral properties against HIV-1 and HIV-2 [56]. All the modern efforts emphasized synthetic andrographolide derivatives and analogs with improved pharmacological properties.

All the reported andrographolide analogs were changed in the structural groups in the parental andrographolide molecules, and these derivatives may be classified based on the types of additional chemical groups, including cyclophosphate derivatives, cinnamoyl derivatives, limonidinlactone derivatives, alkylidene derivatives, and methoxy derivatives. Modification in the structural groups in andrographolide moiety leads to improved biological activities [12, 57]. Sometimes, synthetic molecules exhibit superior activities compared to natural molecules. The superior anticancer activity against MCF-7 breast cancer and HCT116 colonic cancer cell lines was demonstrated with synthetic andrographolide analog dihydro-14-deoxy-11,12-didehydroandrographolide [58].

Neoandrographolide

It is a chemical β-glucoside of 19-hydroxy-8,13-labdadiene-16,15-olide and possesses an anti-inflammatory, antioxidant, lipid-lowering, hepatoprotective, cardioprotective molecule isolated from *A. paniculata* [59]. Eighty-four different neoandrographolide molecules have been registered in PubChem with different rates of biological properties. Among them, benzylideneoandrographolide and methoxybenzylideneneoandrographolide were reported tohave superior cytotoxic activity against SW620, PC-3, and A549 cancer cell lines [60]. Andrographanin is another natural analog of the hydrolyzed state of neoandrographolide isolated from *A. paniculata*. The overproduction of nitric oxide (NO) and proinflammatory cytokines is involved in the key enzymatic activity of the lipopolysaccharide pathway in activated macrophages [61]. This analog inhibits the lipopolysaccharide-induced NO production in *in vivo* mouse models and protects endotoxemia in mice by downregulating TLR4 and NF-kB mRNA expression [62].

14-deoxy 11, 12-didehydroxyandrographolide

Didehydroxyandrographolide analog is a major bitter compound in *A. paniculata*, which possesses hypotensive, anti-inflammatory, antiasthmatic, and anticancer properties. It also has a protective effect against pro-inflammation and is effective in treating spinal cord injury [63]. The compound has cytotoxic activity against

A549 and BEAS-2B human lung epithelial cell lines by MTS assay [64]. This compound inhibits asthma by inducing the production of total eosinophil count and serum ovalbumin protein in mouse models [64]. It has significant hepatoprotective effect by reducing fatty liver diseases at a dose of 0.05% to 0.1% supplementation of neoandrographolide in treated male mice [65]. 14-deoxy 11,12-didehydroxyandrographolide succinate was patented in South Korea [patent KR-1023616557-B1] for ameliorating, preventing, and treating Duchenne muscular dystrophy. This compound may be crystallized by the addition of exomethylene and oxymethylene proton singlets with a coupling constant of 1.5 Hz [66]. 14-deoxyandrographolide activates the adenylate cyclase and modulates the cyclic AMP-mediated expression in caveolin-1 and calmodulin cycle [67]. This compound has been registered in several libraries for antifungal, hepatoprotective, anticancer, cardioprotective, vaso-relaxation, anti-inflammatory, NoS inhibitor, cAMP inhibitor, and calcium channel inhibitor properties.In mouse experimental models, this compound exhibited better anti-fibrotic activity against NIH-323 mouse fibroblast cell lines [68].

Andrographisides

PubMed registered about 93 different andrographiside analogs. The major andrographisides are 11,7-bisandrographolide, 10,2-andrographolide, and 9,7-andrographiside. They have convenient protease binding sites that easily interact in animal proteins [69]. For the protein interaction with the best *in silico* dock score, important andrographisides are biandrographiside (-10.4), andrographiside (9-9.5), isoandrographolide (-9.4), and neoandrographolide (-9.1) [70]. Carbon tetrachloride-induced hepatic injury in mice was treated with neoandrographolide analog, which showed better healing effect [71].

3,19-Acetonylindene Andrographolide

There are three analogs of 14-aryloxy andrographolide characterized by *A. paniculata*, *viz.*, ZAD-1, ZAD-2, and ZAD-3. All these three analogs were used to treat Dengue and Zika viruses, which showed significant antiviral properties [72].

CONCLUSION

Andrographolide is a potential labdane diterpenoid isolated from *Andrographis* species with significant pharmacological properties, including analgesic, antiviral, anticancer, and anti-inflammatory activities. It is evidenced from modern scientific screening and clinical trials that the compound has potential therapeutic effects for treating liver diseases, respiratory problems, inflammatory conditions, viral infections, and immunosuppressive disorders. Several of its natural and synthetic analogs also have enhanced activity for targeted ailments. Neoandrographolides deoxy 11, 12-didehydroandrographolide analogs exhibited more protective effects than the other andrographolide derivatives. Most of the synthetic andrographolide analogs are being tested for their biological properties and many of them are in clinical trials. If their chemical principles and mechanisms of interactions with biological systems are understood, it will lead to safe and cost-effective medicine for new-generation diseases in the future.

REFERENCES

[1] Lee KC, Chang HH, Chung YH, Lee TY. Andrographolide acts as an anti-inflammatory agent in LPS-stimulated RAW264.7 macrophages by inhibiting STAT3-mediated suppression of the NF-κB pathway. J Ethnopharmacol 2011; 135(3): 678-84.
[http://dx.doi.org/10.1016/j.jep.2011.03.068] [PMID: 21497192]

[2] Sujarwo W, Keim AP, Savo V, Guarrera PM, Caneva G. Ethnobotanical study of Loloh: Traditional herbal drinks from Bali (Indonesia). J Ethnopharmacol 2015; 169: 34-48.
[http://dx.doi.org/10.1016/j.jep.2015.03.079] [PMID: 25861955]

[3] Jiao J, Yang Y, Wu Z, *et al.* Screening cyclooxygenase-2 inhibitors from *Andrographis paniculata* to treat inflammation based on bio-affinity ultrafiltration coupled with UPLC-Q-TOF-MS. Fitoterapia 2019; 137: 104259.
[http://dx.doi.org/10.1016/j.fitote.2019.104259] [PMID: 31319108]

[4] Singh B. Botanical leads for drug discovery. Springer Nature, 2020: Singapore.
[http://dx.doi.org/10.1007/978-981-15-5917-4]

[5] Nayak AG, Ahammad J, Kumar N, Shenoy S, Roche M. Can the methanolic extract of *Andrographis paniculata* be used as a supplement to anti-snake venom to normalize hemostatic parameters: A thromboelastographic study. J Ethnopharmacol 2020; 252(24): 112480.
[http://dx.doi.org/10.1016/j.jep.2019.112480] [PMID: 31857127]

[6] Kumar S, Ratha KK, Jaiswal S, Rao MM, Acharya R. Exploring the potential of *Andrographis paniculata* and its bioactive compounds in the management of liver diseases: A comprehensive food chemistry perspective. Food Chemistry Advances 2024; 4: 100674.

[7] Dai C, Deng P, Long Z. Fault detection and diagnosis of relative position sensor for high speed maglev train based kernel principal component analysis. Vol. 1138411th Int. Conference on Signal Processing Systems.
[http://dx.doi.org/10.1117/12.2559466]

[8] Kaushik S, Dar L, Kaushik S, Yadav JP. Identification and characterization of new potent inhibitors of dengue virus NS5 proteinase from *Andrographis paniculata* supercritical extracts on in animal cell culture and *in silico* approaches. J Ethnopharmacol 2020; 267: 113541.
[http://dx.doi.org/10.1016/j.jep.2020.113541] [PMID: 33152438]

[9] Kumar S, Singh B, Bajpai V. *Andrographis paniculata* (Burm.f.) Nees: Traditional uses, phytochemistry, pharmacological properties and quality control/quality assurance. J Ethnopharmacol 2021; 275: 114054.
[http://dx.doi.org/10.1016/j.jep.2021.114054] [PMID: 33831465]

[10] Chandra P, Kannujia R, Pandey R, *et al.* Rapid quantitative analysis of multi-components in *Andrographis paniculata* using UPLC-QqQ$_{LIT}$-MS/MS: Application to soil sodicity and organic farming. Ind Crops Prod 2016; 83: 423-30.
[http://dx.doi.org/10.1016/j.indcrop.2015.12.091]

[11] Kumar S, Singh A, Bajpai V, Sharma KR, Kumar B. Identification and characterization of terpenoid

lactones and flavonoids from ethanolic extract of *Andrographis paniculata* (Burm.f.) Nees using Liquid Chromatography/Tandem Mass Spectrometry. Separ Sci Plus 2018; 1(12): 762-70. [http://dx.doi.org/10.1002/sscp.201800106]

[12]   Pande JN, Gupta BK, Ghosh LK, Sen D. Andrographolide analogs: Pharmacophore modelling and 3D QSAR analysis. Intern J Res Allied Sci 2012; 4(1): 89-93.

[13]   Gorter MK. The bitter constituent of *Andrographis paniculata* Nees. Rec Trav Chim 1911; 30: 151-60.

[14]   Hari Kishore P, Vijaya Bhaskar Reddy M, Kesava Reddy M, Gunasekar D, Caux C, Bodo B. Flavonoids from *Andrographis lineata*. Phytochemistry 2003; 63(4): 457-61. [http://dx.doi.org/10.1016/S0031-9422(02)00702-1] [PMID: 12770598]

[15]   Li J, Huang W, Zhang H, Wang X, Zhou H. Synthesis of andrographolide derivatives and their TNF-α and IL-6 expression inhibitory activities. Bioorg Med Chem Lett 2007; 17(24): 6891-4. [http://dx.doi.org/10.1016/j.bmcl.2007.10.009] [PMID: 17962017]

[16]   Thakur AK, Chatterjee SS, Kumar V. Andrographolides and traditionally used *Andrographis paniculata* as potential adaptogens: Implications for therapeutic innovation. TANG [HUMANITAS MEDICINE] 2014; 4(3): 15.1-15.14. [http://dx.doi.org/10.5667/tang.2014.0002]

[17]   Cheung HY, Cheung CS, Kong CK. Determination of bioactive diterpenoids from *Andrographis paniculata* by micellar electrokinetic chromatography. J Chromatogr A 2001; 930(1-2): 171-6. [http://dx.doi.org/10.1016/S0021-9673(01)01160-8] [PMID: 11681575]

[18]   Bhaskar Reddy MV, Kishore PH, Rao CV, Gunasekar D, Caux C, Bodo B. New 2'-oxygenated flavonoids from *Andrographis affinis*. J Nat Prod 2003; 66(2): 295-7. [http://dx.doi.org/10.1021/np020331k] [PMID: 12608871]

[19]   Dua VK, Ojha VP, Roy R, *et al.* Anti-malarial activity of some xanthones isolated from the roots of *Andrographis paniculata*. J Ethnopharmacol 2004; 95(2-3): 247-51. [http://dx.doi.org/10.1016/j.jep.2004.07.008] [PMID: 15507344]

[20]   Koteswara Rao Y, Vimalamma G, Venkata Rao C, Tzeng YM. Flavonoids and andrographolides from *Andrographis paniculata*. Phytochemistry 2004; 65(16): 2317-21. [http://dx.doi.org/10.1016/j.phytochem.2004.05.008] [PMID: 15381002]

[21]   Kuroyanagi M, Sato M, Ueno A, Nishi K. Flavonoids from *Andrographis paniculata*. Chem Pharm Bull (Tokyo) 1987; 35(11): 4429-35. [http://dx.doi.org/10.1248/cpb.35.4429]

[22]   Chao WW, Kuo YH, Lin BF. Anti-inflammatory activity of new compounds from *Andrographis paniculata* by NF-kappaB transactivation inhibition. J Agric Food Chem 2010; 58(4): 2505-12. [http://dx.doi.org/10.1021/jf903629j] [PMID: 20085279]

[23]   Radhika P, Prasad YR, Lakshmi KR. Flavones from the stem of *Andrographis paniculata* Nees. Nat Prod Commun 2010; 5(1): 1934578X1000500115. [http://dx.doi.org/10.1177/1934578X1000500115] [PMID: 20184022]

[24]   Das B, Ramu R, Rao YK, *et al.* Acylated 5,7,2',6'-oxygenated flavone glycosides from *Andrographis alata*. Phytochemistry 2006; 67(10): 978-83. [http://dx.doi.org/10.1016/j.phytochem.2006.03.003] [PMID: 16624351]

[25]   Ratna Kumari BM, Raveesha BM. Phytochemical analysis and antibacterial activity of *Andrographis lineata* Nees (Acanthaceae). Current Botany 2024; 15: 1-6.

[26]   Sudhana JM, Munikishore R, Reddy MV, Gunasekar D, Blond A, Bodo B. A new diacylated labdane diterpenoid from *Andrographis wightiana*. Nat Prod Commun 2011; 6(11): 1934578X1100601102. [http://dx.doi.org/10.1177/1934578X1100601102] [PMID: 22224261]

[27]   Rahman M, Shakeel IA, Khursheed RA, Ara BT. Microwave-assisted synthesis of andrographolide analogs as potent β-glycosidase inhibitors. Georg Thieme Verlag Stuttgart · New York — SynOpen

2018; 2: 200–206.
[http://dx.doi.org/10.1055/s-0036-1591967]

[28]   Chen L-X, Qu GX, Qiu F. [Studies on diterpenoids from *Andrographis paniculata*.]. Zhongguo
        Zhongyao Zazhi 2006; 31(19): 1594-7.
        [PMID: 17165582]

[29]   Singha PK, Roy S, Dey S. Antimicrobial activity of *Andrographis paniculata*. Fitoterapia 2003; 74(7-
        8): 692-4.
        [http://dx.doi.org/10.1016/S0367-326X(03)00159-X] [PMID: 14630176]

[30]   Handa SS, Sharma A. Hepatoprotective activity of andrographolide against galactosamine &
        paracetamol intoxication in rats. Indian J Med Res 1990; 92: 284-92.
        [PMID: 2228075]

[31]   Calabrese C, Berman SH, Babish JG, *et al.* A phase I trial of andrographolide in HIV positive patients
        and normal volunteers. Phytother Res 2000; 14(5): 333-8.
        [http://dx.doi.org/10.1002/1099-1573(200008)14:5<333::AID-PTR584>3.0.CO;2-D]   [PMID:
        10925397]

[32]   Matsuda T, Kuroyanagi M, Sugiyama S, Umehara K, Ueno A, Nishi K. Cell differentiation-inducing
        diterpenes from *Andrographis paniculata* Nees. Chem Pharm Bull (Tokyo) 1994; 42(6): 1216-25.
        [http://dx.doi.org/10.1248/cpb.42.1216] [PMID: 8069972]

[33]   Niranjan Reddy VL, Malla Reddy S, Ravikanth V, *et al.* A new BIS-Andrographolide Ether from
        Andrographis paniculata Nees and evaluation of anti-HIV activity. Nat Prod Res 2005; 19(3): 223-30.
        [http://dx.doi.org/10.1080/14786410410001709197] [PMID: 15702635]

[34]   Siripong P, Kongkathip B, Preechanukool K, Picha P, Tunsuwan K, Taylor WC. Sci Asia 1992; 18(4):
        187-94.
        [http://dx.doi.org/10.2306/scienceasia1513-1874.1992.18.187]

[35]   Ajaya Kumar R, Sridevi K, Vijaya Kumar N, Nanduri S, Rajagopal S. Anticancer and
        immunostimulatory compounds from *Andrographis paniculata*. J Ethnopharmacol 2004; 92(2-3): 291-
        5.
        [http://dx.doi.org/10.1016/j.jep.2004.03.004] [PMID: 15138014]

[36]   Dai GF, Xu HW, Wang JF, Liu FW, Liu HM. Studies on the novel α-glucosidase inhibitory activity
        and structure–activity relationships for andrographolide analogs. Bioorg Med Chem Lett 2006; 16(10):
        2710-3.
        [http://dx.doi.org/10.1016/j.bmcl.2006.02.011] [PMID: 16504503]

[37]   Kameda Y, Asano N, Yoshikawa M, *et al.* Valiolamine, a new. ALPHA.-glucosidase inhibiting
        aminocyclitol produced by *Streptomyces hygroscopicus*. J Antibiot (Tokyo) 1984; 37(11): 1301-7.
        [http://dx.doi.org/10.7164/antibiotics.37.1301] [PMID: 6392268]

[38]   Wan L, Li Y, Liao W, *et al.* Synergistic inhibition effects of andrographolide and baicalin on
        coronavirus mechanisms by downregulation of ACE2 protein level. Scientific Reports 2024; 14:
        Article Number 4287

[39]   Jiang X, Yu P, Jiang J, *et al.* Synthesis and evaluation of antibacterial activities of andrographolide
        analogs. Eur J Med Chem 2009; 44(7): 2936-43.
        [http://dx.doi.org/10.1016/j.ejmech.2008.12.014] [PMID: 19152987]

[40]   Wang B, Li J, Huang WL, Zhang HB, Qian H, Zheng YT. Synthesis and biological evaluation of
        andrographolide derivatives as potent anti-HIV agents. Chin Chem Lett 2011; 22(7): 781-4.
        [http://dx.doi.org/10.1016/j.cclet.2011.01.015]

[41]   Nanduri S, Nyavanandi VK, Sanjeeva Rao Thunuguntla S, *et al.* Synthesis and structure–activity
        relationships of andrographolide analogs as novel cytotoxic agents. Bioorg Med Chem Lett 2004;
        14(18): 4711-7. a
        [http://dx.doi.org/10.1016/j.bmcl.2004.06.090] [PMID: 15324893]

[42] Nanduri S, Nyavanandi VK, Thunuguntla SSR, *et al.* Novel routes for the generation of structurally diverse labdane diterpenes from andrographolide. Tetrahedron Lett 2004; 45(25): 4883-6. b [http://dx.doi.org/10.1016/j.tetlet.2004.04.142]

[43] Jada SR, Matthews C, Saad MS, *et al.* Benzylidene derivatives of andrographolide inhibit growth of breast and colon cancer cells *in vitro* by inducing G $_1$ arrest and apoptosis. Br J Pharmacol 2008; 155(5): 641-54. [http://dx.doi.org/10.1038/bjp.2008.368] [PMID: 18806812]

[44] Messire G, Rollin P, Gillaizeau I, Berteina-Raboin S. Synthetic Modifications of Andrographolide Targeting New Potential Anticancer Drug Candidates: A Comprehensive Overview. Moleules 2024; 29(12): 2884.

[45] Das B, Chowdhury C, Kumar D, *et al.* Synthesis, cytotoxicity, and structure–activity relationship (SAR) studies of andrographolide analogs as anti-cancer agent. Bioorg Med Chem Lett 2010; 20(23): 6947-50. [http://dx.doi.org/10.1016/j.bmcl.2010.09.126] [PMID: 20974534]

[46] Xu C, Wang ZT. Synthesis and cytotoxic activity of 12-methyleneurea-14-deoxyandrographolide derivatives. Chin J Nat Med 2011; 9(1): 46-50. [http://dx.doi.org/10.1016/S1875-5364(11)60019-8]

[47] Fan QQ, Wang QJ, Zeng BB, Ji WH, Ji H, Wu YL. Apoptosis induction of ZBB-006, a novel synthetic diterpenoid, in the human hepatocellular carcinoma cell line HepG2 *in vitro* and in vivo. Cancer Biol Ther 2010; 10(3): 282-9. a [http://dx.doi.org/10.4161/cbt.10.3.12425] [PMID: 20543568]

[48] Fan QQ, Wang QJ, Zeng BB, Wu YL, Ji H. Synthesis and antitumor effect of novel andrographolide derivative. Zhongguo Yaoke Daxue Xuebao 2010; 41: 326-32. b

[49] Sirion U, Kasemsook S, Suksen K, Piyachaturawat P, Suksamrarn A, Saeeng R. New substituted C-19-andrographolide analogs with potent cytotoxic activities. Bioorg Med Chem Lett 2012; 22(1): 49-52. [http://dx.doi.org/10.1016/j.bmcl.2011.11.085] [PMID: 22154665]

[50] Gonde DP, Bhole BK, Kakad KS. Andrographolide, diterpenoid constituent of *Andrographis paniculata*: Review on botany, phytochemistry, molecular docking analysis, and pharmacology. Annales Pharmaceutiques Françaises 82(1): 15-43.

[51] Xu HW, Zhang J, Liu HM, Wang JF. Synthesis of andrographolide cyclophosphate derivatives and their antitumor activities. Synth Commun 2006; 36(4): 407-14. [http://dx.doi.org/10.1080/00397910500377594]

[52] Mang C, Jakupovic S, Schunk S, Ambrosi HD, Schwarz O, Jakupovic J. Natural products in combinatorial chemistry: an andrographolide-based library. J Comb Chem 2006; 8(2): 268-74. [http://dx.doi.org/10.1021/cc050143n] [PMID: 16529523]

[53] Xu HW, Dai GF, Liu GZ, Wang JF, Liu HM. Synthesis of andrographolide derivatives: A new family of α-glucosidase inhibitors. Bioorg Med Chem 2007; 15(12): 4247-55. [http://dx.doi.org/10.1016/j.bmc.2007.03.063] [PMID: 17428667]

[54] Satyanarayana C, Deevi DS, Rajagopalan R, Srinivas N, Rajagopal S. DRF 3188 a novel semi-synthetic analog of andrographolide: cellular response to MCF 7 breast cancer cells. BMC Cancer 2004; 4(1): 26. [http://dx.doi.org/10.1186/1471-2407-4-26] [PMID: 15207007]

[55] Jada SR, Subur GS, Matthews C, *et al.* Semisynthesis and *in vitro* anticancer activities of andrographolide analogs. Phytochemistry 2007; 68(6): 904-12. [http://dx.doi.org/10.1016/j.phytochem.2006.11.031] [PMID: 17234223]

[56] Basak A, Cooper S, Roberge AG, Banik UK, Chrétien M, Seidah NG. Inhibition of proprotein convertases-1, -7 and furin by diterpines of *Andrographis paniculata* and their succinoyl esters.

Biochem J 1999; 338(1): 107-13.
[http://dx.doi.org/10.1042/bj3380107] [PMID: 9931305]

[57]   Nguyen VS, Loh XY, Wijaya H, *et al.* Specificity and inhibitory mechanism of andrographolide and its analogs as antiasthma agents on NF-κB p50. J Nat Prod 2015; 78(2): 208-17.
[http://dx.doi.org/10.1021/np5007179] [PMID: 25615020]

[58]   Lim JCW, Chan TK, Ng DSW, Sagineedu SR, Stanslas J, Wong WSF. Andrographolide and its analogs: versatile bioactive molecules for combating inflammation and cancer. Clin Exp Pharmacol Physiol 2012; 39(3): 300-10.
[http://dx.doi.org/10.1111/j.1440-1681.2011.05633.x] [PMID: 22017767]

[59]   Chan WR, Taylor DR, Willis CR, Bodden RL, Fehlhaber HW. The structure and stereochemistry of neoandrographolide, a diterpene glucoside from *Andrographis paniculata* nees. Tetrahedron 1971; 27(21): 5081-91.
[http://dx.doi.org/10.1016/S0040-4020(01)90763-X]

[60]   Sharma V, Qayum A, Kaul S, *et al.* Carbohydrate modifications of neoandrographolide for improved reactive oxygen species-mediated apoptosis through mitochondrial pathway in colon cancer. ACS Omega 2019; 4(24): 20435-42.
[http://dx.doi.org/10.1021/acsomega.9b01249] [PMID: 31858026]

[61]   Liu J, Wang ZT, Ge BX. Andrograpanin, isolated from *Andrographis paniculata*, exhibits anti-inflammatory property in lipopolysaccharide-induced macrophage cells through down-regulating the p38 MAPKs signaling pathways. Int Immunopharmacol 2008; 8(7): 951-8.
[http://dx.doi.org/10.1016/j.intimp.2007.12.014] [PMID: 18486905]

[62]   Gong NB, Du LD, Lu Y. Neoandrographolide.Natural small molecule drugs from plants. Singapore: Springer 2018.
[http://dx.doi.org/10.1007/978-981-10-8022-7_71]

[63]   Tzeng Y-M, Lee Y-C, Cheng W-T, *et al.* Effects of andrographolide and 14-deoxy-11,-2-didehydroandrographolide on cultured primary astrocytes and PC12 cells. Life Sci. 2012; 13;90(7-8):257-66.
[http://dx.doi.org/10.1016/j.lfs.2011.11.004]

[64]   Guan SP, Kong LR, Cheng C, Lim JCW, Wong WSF. Protective role of 14-deoxy-11,-2-didehydroandrographolide, a noncytotoxic analogue of andrographolide, in allergic airway inflammation. J Nat Prod 2011; 74(6): 1484-90.
[http://dx.doi.org/10.1021/np2002572] [PMID: 21598983]

[65]   Liu YT, Chen HW, Lii CK, *et al.* A diterpenoid, 14-Deoxy-11, 12-Didehydroandrographolide, in *Andrographis paniculata* reduces steatohepatitis and liver injury in mice fed a high-fat and high-cholesterol diet. Nutrients 2020; 12(2): 523.
[http://dx.doi.org/10.3390/nu12020523] [PMID: 32085637]

[66]   Rashid PT, Ahmed M, Rahaman MM, Muhit MA. 14-Deoxyandrographolide isolated from *Andrographis paniculata* (Burm. f.) Nees growing in Bangladesh and its antimicrobial properties. Dhaka University Journal of Pharmaceutical Sciences 2018; 17(2): 265-7.
[http://dx.doi.org/10.3329/dujps.v17i2.39185]

[67]   Mandal S, Nelson VK, Mukhopadhyay S, *et al.* 14-Deoxyandrographolide targets adenylate cyclase and prevents ethanol-induced liver injury through constitutive NOS dependent reduced redox signaling in rats. Food Chem Toxicol 2013; 59: 236-48.
[http://dx.doi.org/10.1016/j.fct.2013.05.056] [PMID: 23764359]

[68]   Song Z, Huang S, He Y, Li J, Lin K, Xue X. Synthesis and anti-fibrosis activity study of 14-deoxyandrographolide-19-oic acid and 14-deoxydidehydroandrographolide-19-oic acid derivatives. European J Med Chem 2018; 157: 805-816.
[http://dx.doi.org/10.1016/j.ejmech.2018.08.046]

[69]   Thirumoorthy G, Tarachand SP, Nagella P, Lakshmaiah VV. Identification of potential ZIKV NS2B-

NS3 protease inhibitors from *Andrographis paniculata*: An in silico approach. J Biomol Struct Dyn. 2022; 40(21):11203-11215.
[http://dx.doi.org/10.1080/07391102.2021.1956592]

[70]   Al-Khayri JM, Dubey S, Thirumoorthy G, Nagella P, Shehata WF. In silico identification of 1-DTP Inhibitors of *Corynebacterium diphtheriae* using phytochemicals from *Andrographis paniculata*. Molecule 2023; 16; 28(2):909.
[http://dx.doi.org/10.3390/molecules28020909]

[71]   Kapil A, Koul IB, Banerjee SK, Gupta BD. Antihepatotoxic effects of major diterpenoid constituents of *Andrographis paniculata*. Biochem Pharmacol 1993; 6;46(1):182-5.
[http://dx.doi.org/10.1016/0006-2952(93)90364-3]

[72]   Li F, Khanom W, Sun X, *et al.* Andrographolide and its 14-aryloxy analogs inhibit zika and dengue virus infection. Molecules 2020; 25(21): 5037.
[http://dx.doi.org/10.3390/molecules25215037] [PMID: 33143016]

[73]   Varma A, Padh H, Shrivastava N. Andrographolide: A new plant-derived antineoplastic entity on horizon. Evidence-Based Complementary and Alternative Medicine 2011; 815390. 9.
[http://dx.doi.org/10.1093/ecam/nep135]

[74]   Lim XY, Chan JSW, Tan TYC, *et al. Andrographis paniculata* (Burm. F.) Wall. ex Nees, Andrographolide, and Andrographolide analogs as SARS-CoV-2 Antivirals? A Rapid Review. Nat Prod Commun 2021; 16(5): 1934578X211016610.journals.sagepub.com/home/npx
[http://dx.doi.org/10.1177/1934578X211016610]

[75]   Zhang L, Bao M, Liu B, *et al.* Effect of andrographolide and its analogs on bacterial infection: a review. Pharmacology 2020; 105(3-4): 123-34.
[http://dx.doi.org/10.1159/000503410] [PMID: 31694037]

[76]   Xu Y, Wei H, Wang J, Wang W, Gao J. Synthesis of andrographolide analogs and their neuroprotection and neurite outgrowth-promoting activities. Bioorg Med Chem 2019; 27(11): 2209-19.
[http://dx.doi.org/10.1016/j.bmc.2019.04.025] [PMID: 31014564]

[77]   Yang T, Shi H, Wang Z, Wang C. Hypolipidemic effects of andrographolide and neoandrographolide in mice and rats. Phytother Res 2013; 27(4): 618-23.
[http://dx.doi.org/10.1002/ptr.4771] [PMID: 22744979]

[78]   Geetha A, Saranya P, Selvamathy SMKN. A biochemical study on the gastroprotective effect of andrographolide in rats induced with gastric ulcer. Indian J Pharm Sci 2011; 73(5): 550-7.
[http://dx.doi.org/10.4103/0250-474X.99012] [PMID: 22923868]

[79]   Nugroho A, Andrie M, Warditiani N, Siswanto E, Pramono S, Lukitaningsih E. Antidiabetic and antihiperlipidemic effect of *Andrographis paniculata* (Burm. f.) Nees and andrographolide in high-fructose-fat-fed rats. Indian J Pharmacol 2012; 44(3): 377-81.
[http://dx.doi.org/10.4103/0253-7613.96343] [PMID: 22701250]

[80]   Parichatikanond W, Suthisisang C, Dhepakson P, Herunsalee A. Study of anti-inflammatory activities of the pure compounds from *Andrographis paniculata* (Burm.f.) Nees and their effects on gene expression. Int Immunopharmacol 2010; 10(11): 1361-73.
[http://dx.doi.org/10.1016/j.intimp.2010.08.002] [PMID: 20728594]

[81]   Cai W, Li Y, Chen S, *et al.* 14-Deoxy-11,12-dehydroandrographolide exerts anti-influenza A virus activity and inhibits replication of H5N1 virus by restraining nuclear export of viral ribonucleoprotein complexes. Antiviral Res 2015; 118: 82-92.
[http://dx.doi.org/10.1016/j.antiviral.2015.03.008] [PMID: 25800824]

[82]   Lee S, Morita H, Tezuka Y. Preferentially cytotoxic constituents of *Andrographis paniculata* and their preferential cytotoxicity against human pancreatic cancer cell lines. Nat Prod Commun 2015; 10(7): 1934578X1501000704.
[http://dx.doi.org/10.1177/1934578X1501000704] [PMID: 26410998]

[83]   Tan HK, Muhammad TST, Tan ML. 14-Deoxy-11,12-didehydroandrographolide induces DDIT3-dependent endoplasmic reticulum stress-mediated autophagy in T-47D breast carcinoma cells. Toxicol Appl Pharmacol 2016; 300: 55-69.
[http://dx.doi.org/10.1016/j.taap.2016.03.017] [PMID: 27049118]

[84]   Awang K, Abdullah NH, Hadi AHA, Su Fong Y. Cardiovascular activity of labdane diterpenes from *Andrographis paniculata* in isolated rat hearts. J Biomed Biotechnol 2012; 2012: 1-5.
[http://dx.doi.org/10.1155/2012/876458] [PMID: 22536026]

[85]   Yoopan N, Thisoda P, Rangkadilok N, *et al.* Cardiovascular effects of 14-deoxy-11,-2-didehydroandrographolide and *Andrographis paniculata* extracts. Planta Med 2007; 73(6): 503-11.
[http://dx.doi.org/10.1055/s-2007-967181] [PMID: 17650544]

[86]   Chen CC, Lii CK, Lo CW, *et al.* 14-Deoxy-11,12-Didehydroandrographolide Ameliorates Glucose Intolerance Enhancing the LKB1/AMPKα/TBC1D1/GLUT4 Signaling Pathway and Inducing GLUT4 Expression in Myotubes and Skeletal Muscle of Obese Mice. Am J Chin Med 2021; 49(6): 1473-91.
[http://dx.doi.org/10.1142/S0192415X21500695] [PMID: 34240660]

[87]   Thisoda P, Rangkadilok N, Pholphana N, Worasuttayangkurn L, Ruchirawat S, Satayavivad J. Inhibitory effect of *Andrographis paniculata* extract and its active diterpenoids on platelet aggregation. Eur J Pharmacol 2006; 553(1-3): 39-45.
[http://dx.doi.org/10.1016/j.ejphar.2006.09.052] [PMID: 17081514]

[88]   Sule A, Ahmed QU, Latip J, *et al.* Antifungal activity of *Andrographis paniculata* extracts and active principles against skin pathogenic fungal strains *in vitro*. Pharm Biol 2012; 50(7): 850-6.
[http://dx.doi.org/10.3109/13880209.2011.641021] [PMID: 22587518]

[89]   Chandrasekaran CV, Thiyagarajan P, Deepak HB, Agarwal A. *In vitro* modulation of LPS/calcimycin induced inflammatory and allergic mediators by pure compounds of *Andrographis paniculata* (King of bitters) extract. Int Immunopharmacol 2011; 11(1): 79-84.
[http://dx.doi.org/10.1016/j.intimp.2010.10.009] [PMID: 21034865]

[90]   Reddy MVB, Kishore PH, Rao CV, Gunasekar D, Caux C, Bodo B. New 2'- oxygenated flavonoids from *Andrographis affinis*. J Nat Prod 2003; 66:295-297.

CHAPTER 5

Pharmacognostic Characterization of *Andrographis paniculata* (Burm. f.) Nees

Divya Kallingil Gopi[1,*], Nilesh Yadav Jadhav[2], Sunil Kumar Koppala Narayana[1], Narayanan Kannan[1], Phani Deepika Polampalli[3], Nemallapalli Yamini[4], Radha Rai[5], Chandrasekaran[5] and Vinod K. Nelson[6,*]

[1] *Department of Pharmacognosy, Siddha Central Research Institute (Central Council for Research in Siddha, Ministry of AYUSH, Government of India) Chennai 600106, Tamil Nadu, India*

[2] *Seva Shikshan Prasarak Mandal's Dr. N.J. Paulbudhe College of Pharmacy, Vasant Tekadi, Savedi, Ahmed Nagar, Maharashtra, India*

[3] *Department of Biotechnology, MNR College of Pharmacy, Sangareddy 502294, Telangana State, India*

[4] *Department of Pharmacology, JNTUA-OTRI, Jawaharlal Nehru Technological University, Antnatapur-515001, Andhra Pradesh, India*

[5] *Department of Pharmaceutical Chemistry, Krishna Teja Pharmacy College, Tirupati, Andhra Pradesh, India*

[6] *Centre for Global Health Research, Saveetha Medical College and Hospital, Saveetha Institute of Medical and Technical Sciences, Chennai 602105, Tamil Nadu, India*

Abstract: *Andrographis paniculata* (Burm. f.) Nees is a well-known medicinal plant of the genus *Andrographis* belonging to the family Acanthaceae. This species is widely distributed throughout tropical and sub-tropical Southeast Asia, including India. This herb finds its place not only in the traditional systems of medicine but is also registered under Indian Pharmacopoeia. *A. paniculata* is bestowed with high therapeutic value and is used for the treatment of various ailments. This herb is adulterated with other species like *Andrographis echioides* and *Swertia chirayita* due to the lack of constant supply and less availability of *A. paniculata*. The herbaceous species possess apparent macroscopic similarities, and it is a tedious job to identify the actual raw drug. This chapter will provide in-depth knowledge of the pharmacognostical characterization of *A. paniculata*. Detailed macroscopic evaluation will help in the identification of the species in the field, and the comprehensive microscopic evaluation with the help of a transverse section will help delineate the species from its adulterant. The powder microscopic study will help in the identification of this medicinal plant, even in its

---

* **Corresponding authors Divya Kallingil Gopi and Vinod K. Nelson:** Department of Pharmacognosy, Siddha Central Research Institute (Central Council for Research in Siddha, Ministry of AYUSH, Government of India) Chennai 600106, Tamil Nadu, India;
Centre for Global Health Research, Saveetha Medical College and Hospital, Saveetha Institute of Medical and Technical Sciences, Chennai 602105, Tamil Nadu, India; E-mail: minnu.kg@gmail.com; vinod.kumar457@gmail.com

powder form. The pharmacognostic standards put forward for the correct identification and authentication will prove to be a benchmark standard for this highly potent medicinal herb.

Keywords: Adulteration, Authentication, *Andrographis*, Andrographolide, Pharmacognosy.

INTRODUCTION

Andrographis paniculata (Burm. f.) Nees (AP) belongs to the family Acanthaceae. The other names of this plant are *Justicia latebrosa* Russell. ex Wall. and *Justicia paniculata* Burm.f [1]. *A. paniculata* is one of the biologically active medicinal plants broadly used in alternative medicinal systems in countries like India, China, and Sri Lanka [2]. The vernacular names of *A. paniculata* include Alui, Andrographids, Charita, Cherota, Kalmegh, Halviva, Sambilata, Sinta, and King of Bitters [3]. *A. paniculata* is an annual shrub with immense therapeutic value, and all parts of the plants are used to cure or prevent various diseases both in humans and animals [4]. *Andrographis paniculata* was traditionally used as an antipyretic agent, antibacterial agent, febrifuge, and bitter tonic and was used to treat gastrointestinal disorders, typhoid, and malaria [5]. This herb is used for curing influenza, swellings, itches, gonorrhea, general debility, dyspepsia, bronchitis, and snake bites. The decoction of leaves is the best medicine for infants for curing stomach ailments [6]. According to the Indian Pharmacopoeia, *A. paniculata* is the chief constituent of more than 25 Ayurvedic formulations, and because of its cold potency, *A. paniculata* is used to treat the common cold and fevers as a home remedy [7]. The recent literature points out that *Andrographis paniculata* possesses significant pharmacological activities, including anticancer, anti-inflammatory, antioxidant, hepatoprotective, antidiabetic, and cardioprotective activity [4]. Diterpene lactones are the important phytochemical derivatives of *A. paniculata* among such andrographolides held responsible for biological activity [8]. This plant has been subjected to a wide range of phytochemical, pharmacological, physiological, genetics, microbiological, and seed germination studies [7].

TRADITIONAL MEDICINE

AP has been used as a remedy to cure many diseases for centuries in Asian and European countries. In addition, it is also broadly used for healing purposes by various tribes and traditional practitioners as a folklore remedy in different parts of the world [9]. In Japan, Scandinavian countries, and traditional Thai medicine, it is commonly used to treat the common cold and fever [10]. In traditional Chinese Medicine, AP is widely used to cure diseases like snake bites, viral infections, dysentery, and respiratory infections like pneumonia and pharyngitis. In the Unani system of medicine, AP is used to treat inflammatory diseases, abdominal infection, scabies, and other skin infections [3].

PHARMACOGNOSTIC STUDIES

The systematic study of crude drugs obtained from natural sources like plants, animals, and minerals is termed pharmacognosy. The pharmacognostical approach deals with the nomenclature, collection, cultivation, habitat distribution, and macro and microscopic studies of the physical and chemical constituents of their therapeutic actions and adulterations of the genuine drug. AP can be grown in all types of soils and is found in diverse habitats like plains, hill slopes, farms, sea shores, and dry and wetlands [11]. *Andrographis* is represented by 26 species that are distributed throughout the Indian subcontinent, with South India showing the highest diversity [12]. These species are also distributed in the tropical and subtropical regions of Asia, the Caribbean Islands, Malaysia, Myanmar, and Thailand [12]. Sometimes, *A. paniculata* is substituted with ' Chirata ' (*Swertia chiravita)* in the market, but it is originally called Kalmegh in Ayurveda preparations, although it possesses anti-malarial properties [13].

The microscopic detailing of the stem showed the presence of glandular and non-glandular hairs, acicular crystals in the phloem region, and ectophloic siphonostele [14]. AP is an annual shrub with branches that grow 90 to 110 cm in height. The leaves are green, simple, opposite, lanceolate, and glabrous, with a short petiole measuring about 3 to 7 cm in length and 1 to 2.5 cm in width. The stems are dark green, reaching up to a height of 0.5 to 1 m and 2 to 6 mm in diameter, with incidence of longitudinal furrows and wings on the angles of young plants. It has many small seeds and is yellowish-brown in color [3]. The powdered microscopy of *A. paniculata* reveals the presence of leaf epidermis with diacytic stomata and lignified fibers with sharp cells. The plant appears grayish black to grayish brown under normal vision and light yellowish to grayish brown under ultraviolet light [3, 15].

PHARMACOGNOSTIC FEATURES OF *ANDROGRAPHIS PANICULATA*

Macroscopic Characteristics

Andrographis paniculata is a herbaceous plant with a quadrangular, woody, glabrous stem that appears green in color and moderately hard with numerous armed branches that are quadrangular. The lower part of the stem gives out adventitious roots, which are thin and slender. The roots are greyish brown in colorfrom the outside with starchy white inside. They appear cylindrical, curved, and tapering, measuring about 6 to 20 cm in length (Fig. **1**). The leaves (5 to 10 cm) are dark-green, simple, petiolate, acuminate apex, unicostate, margin entire, which re-curves at maturity. Petioles are greenish, glabrous, and slender, measuring up to 0.5 mm in length. Inflorescence is represented by axillary and terminal panicles possessing peduncles measuring 3 to 5 cm in length, and two persistent heteromorphic, hairy, green bracts are persistent. The flowers are bisexual, pentamerous, zygomorphic, calyx tubes possessing glandular hairs, corolla two-lipped, pinkish violet in color, hairy with posterior oblong lip hooded over the 3-lobed anterior lips. The gynoecium is represented by two carpels and a syncarpous superior ovary, hairy throughout, one terminal glabrous style, and a slightly bifid stigma. Fruit simple, dry, dehiscent capsule, a septum is visible in the center and measures 2 cm x 3mm in dimension and contains 6 to 12 seeds inside, which are flat, translucent, and golden brown in color [16, 17].

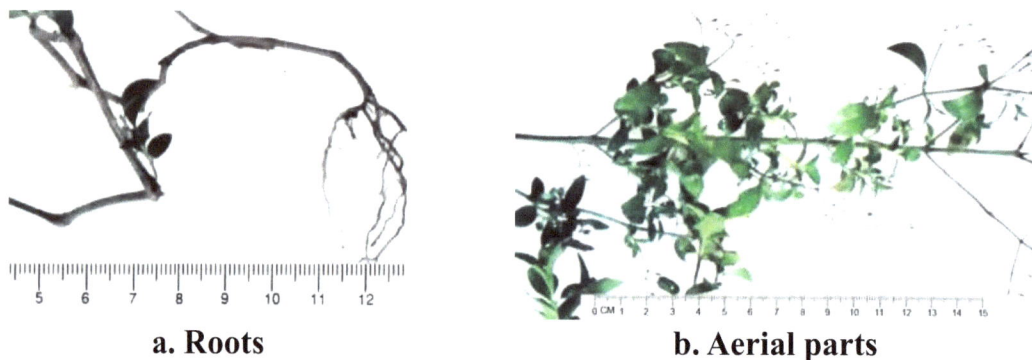

a. Roots   b. Aerial parts

Fig. (1). *Andrographis paniculata* plant.

Microscopy of *Andrographis paniculata* Root

The diagrammatic transverse sections of the root appear oval in outline, and the outermost covering layer consists of thin-walled compactly packed cells filled with brownish content followed by a narrow cortical region. Five to seven layers of rectangular, thin-walled cells are present, with narrow parenchyma and the cork aligned with sclereids as a ring, and the pit opening is about 2μm in diameter. The major wood portion consists of vessels that are circular, elliptical, or polygonal in shape, small in size, and arranged in radial rows of three or four in number. The diameter of the lumen of the vessel is approximately 10 to 42μm [4, 17]. A significant portion is occupied by central continuous radiating xylem elements. The cortex comprises 3 to 4 layers of radial elongated parenchymatous cells, and a phloem is present above the xylem composed of sieve elements and parenchyma. The xylem occupies most of the section, and the vessel elements are solitary and arranged in radial rows. Few tyloses are seen randomly, along with prismatic crystals of calcium oxalate (Fig. **2**).

TS of root

Outer region enlarged

Inner region enlarged

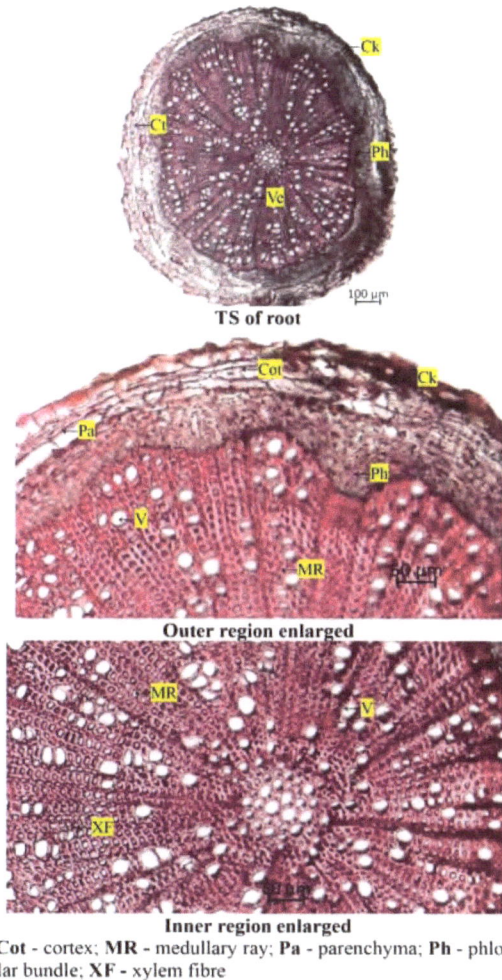

Ck - cork; Cot - cortex; MR - medullary ray; Pa - parenchyma; Ph - phloem; V - vessel;
VB - vascular bundle; XF - xylem fibre

Fig. (2). Transverse section of *Andrographis paniculata* root.

Microscopy of *Andrographis paniculata* Stem

The diagrammatic transverse section of the stem of *A. paniculata* appears quadrangular in outline, along with dense collenchyma winged projections on the four corners. The comprehensive observation of the section shows a single-layer epidermis covered with a thin cuticle and a few sessile glandular trichomes, and few of them are present in more giant cells to interrupt the continuity of the epidermis. The epidermis follows a single-layer of rectangular cells of parenchymatous hypodermis, and the cortex is narrowing heteromorphic with the outer cortex, which is made up of collenchymatous cells. Under the epidermis, 2-3 layers of collenchyma cells with secretary cavities are present. The cortex composed of approximately 6-7 layers of parenchyma along with chloroplasts was observed. Similarly, single sclereids in the cortex, along with thick-walled endodermis, consist of chloroplastids. The inner cortex is made up of chlorenchymatous cells with a distinct endodermis that surrounds the vascular region.

The majority of the section is occupied by a central parenchymatous pith encircled by continuous xylem fibers along with small size vessels, and the diameter of the vessel is roughly 15-40µm. The phloem is represented by narrow rows of thin-walled cells and traversed by few fibers. The xylem appears wide and composed of xylem vessels, tracheids, and xylem fibers, which are in uni- to multiseriate medullary rays traversing through the xylem, and a broad parenchymatous pith is present in the center (Fig. **3**). Medullary rays are evident and numerous in numbers, which are arranged uniseriate, biseriate medullary rays traversing through the xylem, and broad parenchymatous pith is present in the center. The cells of pith are filled with prismatic crystals of calcium oxalate.

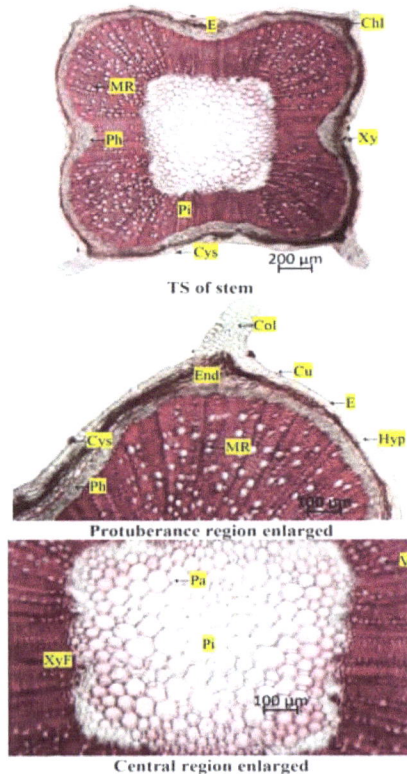

TS of stem

Protuberance region enlarged

Central region enlarged

Chl - chlorenchyma; Col-collenchyma; Cu-cuticle; Cys - cystolith; Hyp - hypodermis; MR - medullary ray; Pa- parenchyma; Ph- phloem; Pi - pith; V - vessel; VB- vascular bundle; Xy - xylem; XyF - xylem fibre

Fig. (3). Transverse section of *Andrographis paniculata* stem.

Microscopy of *Andrographis paniculata* Petiole

The petiole appears irregularly rectangular, with winged shape projections at all four corners. The high-magnified section shows a single-layered epidermis covered by distinct cuticles and a few simple trichomes. The upper side of these projections is longer, with two small meristeles, and these are absent in lower projections. A few layers of a chlorenchyma zone are present beneath the epidermis, followed by parenchymatous ground tissue. The ground tissue follows the composition of collenchymas and vascular with 15-17 layers arranged as an arc in the center. The vascular region is well-developed and arranged as an arc; the bundles are conjoint, collateral, and closed. Xylem fibers are arranged radially in 5-6 layers, along with a few phloem fibers. The endodermis is discontinued by surrounding the vascular bundles, and two rudimentary meristeles are seen in the upper winged region (Fig. **4**).

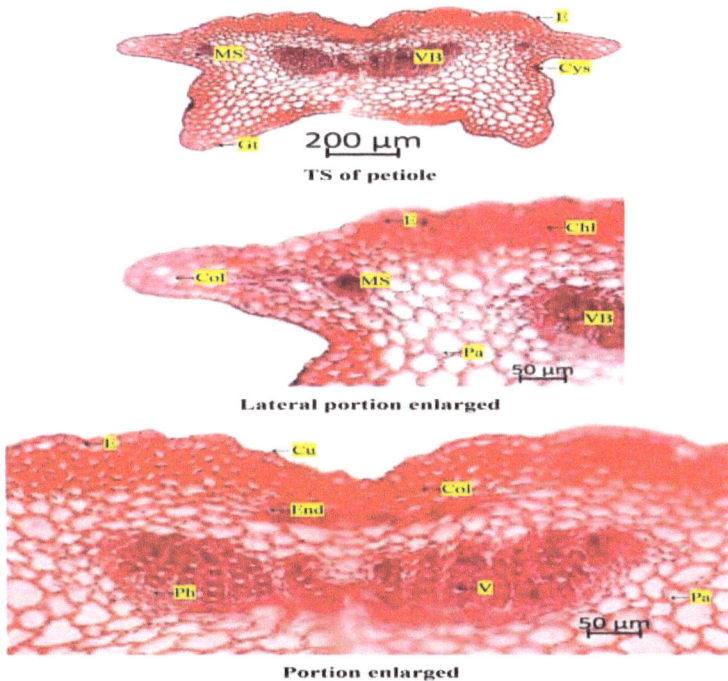

TS of petiole

Lateral portion enlarged

Portion enlarged

Chl - chlorenchyma; **Col** - collenchyma; **Cu** – cuticle; **Cys** – cystolith; **End** – endodermis; **E** – Epidermis; **GT** - ground tissue; **MS** - meristele; **Pa**- parenchyma; **Ph** - phloem; **Pi** - pith; **V** - vessel; **VB** - vascular bundle; **Xy** - xylem

Fig. (4). Transverse section of *Andrographis paniculata* petiole.

Microscopy of *Andrographis paniculata* Leaf

The shape of the transverse section of the midrib is characteristic and projected at two corners on the lower side, with a prominent ridge having a shallow groove in the middle on the adaxial side. The simple trichomes are seen toward the margin of the leaf on the lower epidermis, and just below it, two to three layers of collenchymatous cells are present. The ground tissue is collenchymatous, embedding the vascular bundles. The detailed TS shows the upper and lower epidermis covered by a thin cuticle, a few cystoliths, and stomata, followed by three to five layers of collenchymatous cells. The vascular bundles are arranged in an arc and embedded within the ground tissue. These bundles are conjoint, collateral and, closed and contain a narrow phloem region followed by a wider xylem region (Fig. **5**).

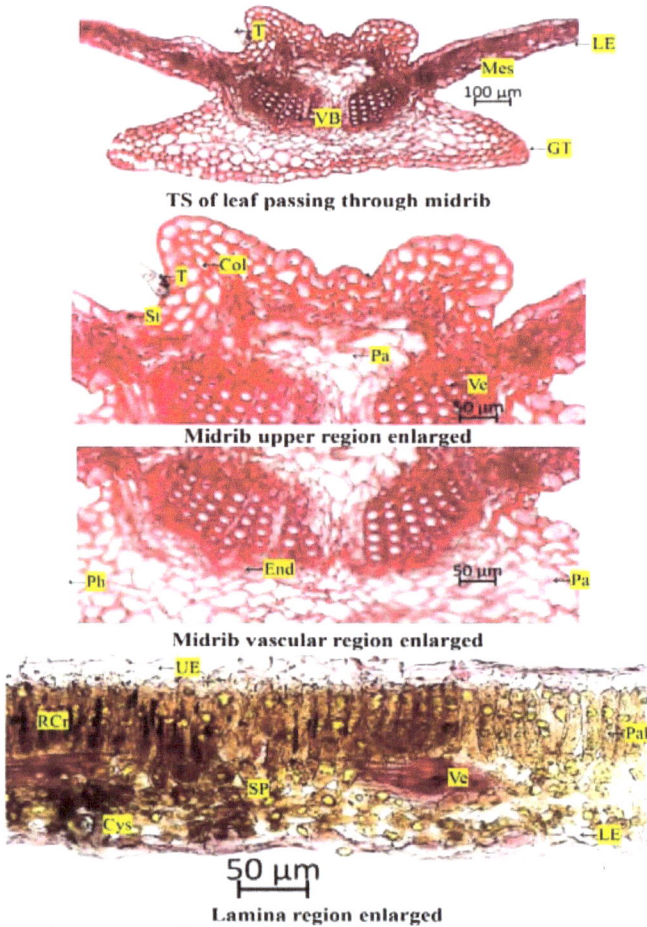

TS of leaf passing through midrib

Midrib upper region enlarged

Midrib vascular region enlarged

Lamina region enlarged

Chl- chlorenchyma; **Col-**collenchyma;**Cu-**cuticle;**Cys** - cystolith; **End** - endodermis; **GT** - ground tissue; **LE-**lower epidermis;**Mes-** mesophyll; **MR** - medullary ray; **Pa-** parenchyma;**Pal -** palisade parenchyma; **Ph-** phloem; **Pi** - pith; **RCr** - Rosette crystal; **SP** - spongy parenchyma; **UE** - upper epidermis; **V** - vessel; **VB-** vascular bundle; **Ve** - vein

Fig. (5). Transverse section of *Andrographis paniculata* leaf.

Powder Microscopy of *Andrographis paniculata* Whole Plant

The powder microscopic characteristics of the whole plant of *A. paniculata* are as follows. The powder was grayish green in color and showed cork fragments, parenchyma, pith parenchyma, pitted vessels, thick-walled vessels with narrow lumen, thin-walled fibers from the root; epidermal fragments with stomata, collenchyma cells, bordered pitted and spiral vessel, phloem fibers and thick-walled cells with broad lumen from stem; epidermal fragment with trichomes, upper epidermis, lower epidermis with diacytic stomata, mesophyll cells, cystolith and prismatic crystal from the leaf; anther fragment from the flower, sclereid from seed wall and starch grains from seed are also present (Fig. **6**).

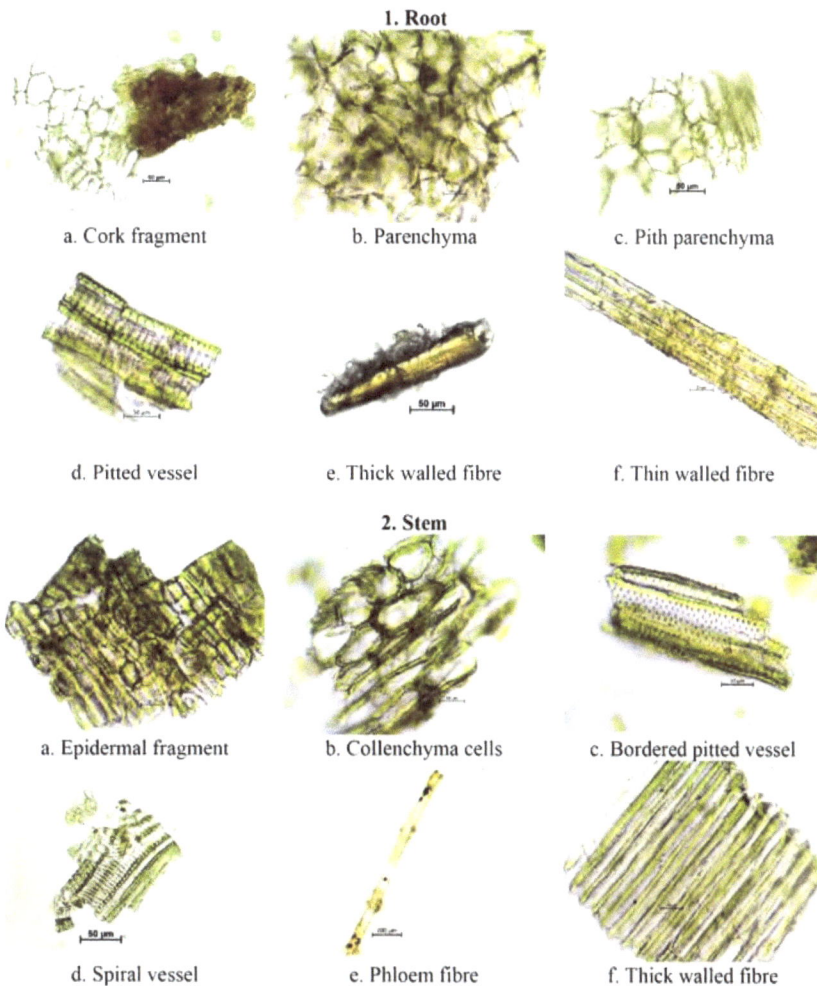

1. Root

a. Cork fragment   b. Parenchyma   c. Pith parenchyma

d. Pitted vessel   e. Thick walled fibre   f. Thin walled fibre

2. Stem

a. Epidermal fragment   b. Collenchyma cells   c. Bordered pitted vessel

d. Spiral vessel   e. Phloem fibre   f. Thick walled fibre

(Fig. 6) contd.....

3. Leaf

a. Epidermis with trichomes   b. Upper epidermis   c. Lower epidermis

d. Thik walled parenchyma   e. Epidermis with cystolyth   f. Prismatic crystals

4. Flower, fruit and seed

Anther fragment from flower   Sclereid from fruit wall   Starch grains from seed

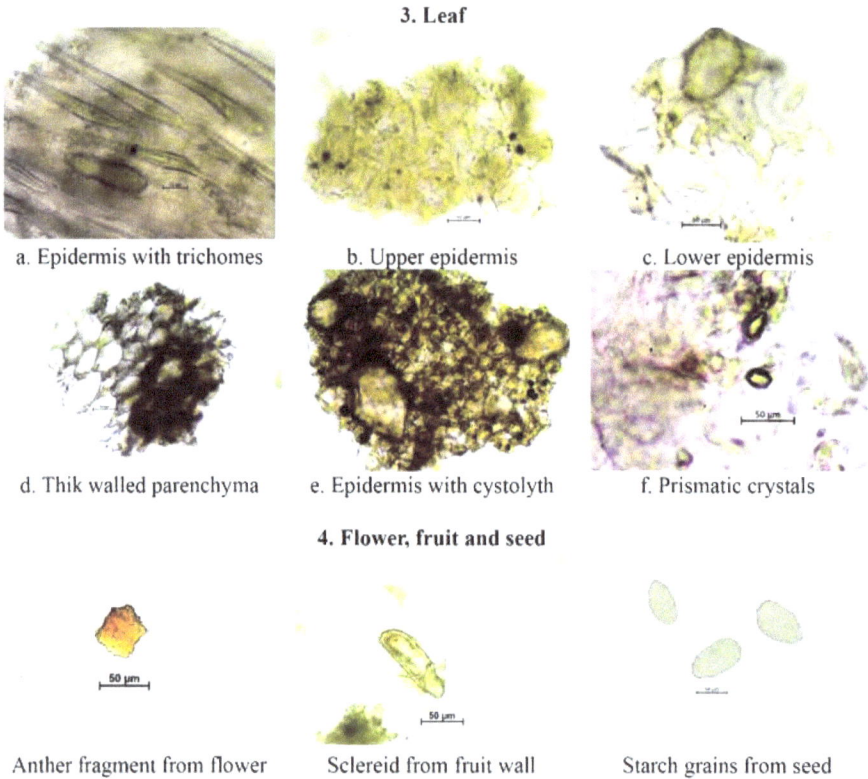

Fig. (6). Powder microscopy of *Andrographis paniculata*.

CONCLUSION

Demand for the usage of biologically active medicinal plants has increased globally. *A. paniculata* is one of the important medicinal plants with multiple pharmacological activities. The increased demand for medicinal herbs increases adulterated or substituted drugs, which sometimes cannot meet the therapeutic requirements. *Swertia chirayita* is used as an adulterant of *A. paniculata* since both species resemble similar morphology; however, the pharmacognostic characterization helps distinguish the adulterant and allows the safe use of authentic *A. paniculata* [18, 19]. Hence, programmed botanical and pharmacognostic studies help identify and supply the authenticated drug. This chapter provides complete botanical and pharmacognostic characterizations, including macro, micro, and powder microscopy of *A. paniculata*, to determine a proper and authenticated medicinal plant. This chapter will also provide useful information for quality control standardization parameters for crude drugs.

REFERENCES

[1] Dai Y, Chen SR, Chai L, Zhao J, Wang Y, Wang Y. Overview of pharmacological activities of *Andrographis paniculata* and its major compound andrographolide. Critical reviews in food science and nutrition 2019; 59: S17-s29.

[2] Raman S, Murugaiyah V, Parumasivam T. *Andrographis paniculata* dosage forms and advances in nanoparticulate delivery systems: An overview. Molecules 2022; 27(19): 6164.
[http://dx.doi.org/10.3390/molecules27196164] [PMID: 36234698]

[3] Hossain MS, Urbi Z, Sule A, Rahman KMH. *Andrographis paniculata* (Burm. f.) Wall. ex Nees: a review of ethnobotany, phytochemistry, and pharmacology. ScientificWorldJournal 2014; 2014: 1-28.
[http://dx.doi.org/10.1155/2014/274905] [PMID: 25950015]

[4] Sudhakaran MV. Botanical pharmacognosy of *Andrographis paniculata* (Burm. f.) Wall. ex Nees. Pharmacogn J 2012; 4(32): 1-10.
[http://dx.doi.org/10.5530/pj.2012.32.1]

[5] Mishra S, Sangwan N, Sangwan R. *Andrographis paniculata* (Kalmegh): A review. Pharmacogn Rev 2007; 1: 283-98.

[6] Scartezzini P, Speroni E. Review on some plants of Indian traditional medicine with antioxidant activity. J Ethnopharmacol 2000; 71(1-2): 23-43.
[http://dx.doi.org/10.1016/S0378-8741(00)00213-0] [PMID: 10904144]

[7] Varma A, Padh H, Shrivastava N. Andrographolide: a new plant-derived antineoplastic entity on horizon. Evid Based Complement Alternat Med 2011; 2011(1): 815390.
[http://dx.doi.org/10.1093/ecam/nep135] [PMID: 19752167]

[8] Sharma V, Sharma T, Kaul S, Kapoor KK, Dhar MK. Anticancer potential of labdane diterpenoid lactone "andrographolide" and its derivatives: a semi-synthetic approach. Phytochem Rev 2017; 16(3): 513-26.
[http://dx.doi.org/10.1007/s11101-016-9478-9]

[9] Silambarasan R, Sureshkumar J, Krupa J, Amalraj S, Ayyanar M. Traditional herbal medicines practiced by the ethnic people in Sathyamangalam forests of Western Ghats, India. Eur J Integr Med 2017; 16: 61-72.
[http://dx.doi.org/10.1016/j.eujim.2017.10.010]

[10] Jarukamjorn K, Nemoto N. Pharmacological Aspects of *Andrographis paniculata* on health and its major diterpenoid constituent andrographolide. J Health Sci 2008; 54(4): 370-81.
[http://dx.doi.org/10.1248/jhs.54.370]

[11] Bhattacharjya DK, Borah PC. Medicinal weeds of crop fields and role of women in rural health and hygiene in Nalbari district, Assam. Indian J Trad Knowl 2008;7.

[12] Neeraja C, Krishna PH, Reddy CS, Giri CC, Rao KV, Reddy VD. Distribution of *Andrographis* species in different districts of Andhra Pradesh. Proc Natl Acad Sci, India, Sect B Biol Sci 2015; 85(2): 601-6.
[http://dx.doi.org/10.1007/s40011-014-0364-1]

[13] Intharuksa A, Arunotayanun W, Yooin W, Sirisa-ard P. A Comprehensive review of *Andrographis paniculata* (Burm. f.) Nees and its constituents as potential lead compounds for COVID-19 drug discovery. Molecules 2022; 27(14): 4479.
[http://dx.doi.org/10.3390/molecules27144479] [PMID: 35889352]

[14] Raina AP, Gupta V, Sivaraj N, Dutta M. *Andrographis paniculata* (Burm. f.) Wall. ex Nees (kalmegh), a traditional hepatoprotective drug from India. Genet Resour Crop Evol 2013; 60(3): 1181-9.
[http://dx.doi.org/10.1007/s10722-012-9953-0]

[15] Lattoo S, Khan S, Dhar A, Choudhary DK, Gupta K, Sharma P. Genetics and mechanism of induced male sterility in *Andrographis paniculata* (Burm. L) Nees and its significance. Curr Sci 2006; 91: 515-

9.

[16] Niranjan A, Tewari S, Lehri A. Biological activities of Kalmegh (*Andrographis paniculata* Nees) and its active principles-A review. Indian J Nat Prod Resour 2010; 1: 125-35.

[17] Kumar RS, Reddy PR, Rao SG, Nethaji K. Botanical pharmacognosy on the leaves of medicinally important plant *Andrographis paniculata* (Nees) collected from the forest area of Medak District, Andhra Pradesh, India. Int J Pharm Sci Rev Res 2014; 25(2): 292-5.

[18] Sakuanrungsirikul S, Jetana A, Buddanoi P, Dithachaiyawong J. Intraspecific variability assessment of *Andrographis paniculata* collections using molecular markers. Acta Hortic 2008; (786): 283-6. [http://dx.doi.org/10.17660/ActaHortic.2008.786.34]

[19] Dharmadasa RM. Comparative pharmacognostic evaluation of *Munronia pinnata* (Wall.) Theob. (Meliaceae) and its substitute *Andrographis paniculata* (Burm.f.) Wall. ex Nees (Acanthaceae). World J Agric Res 2013; 1(5): 77-81.

CHAPTER 6

Pharmacology of Andrographolide and its Analogs: An Update

Vinod K. Nelson[1], Vinyas Mayasa[2], Lakshman Kumar Dogiparthi[3], Panga Shyam[4], Suryavanshu Roshini[4], Kona Karunya[5], Kola Venu[4], Vijetha Pendyala[6], Amit Upadhyay[7], Naveen Sharma[7], Jamal Basha Dudekula[7], Ravishankar Ram Mani[8,*] and Kranthi Kumar Kotha[9,*]

[1] *Centre for Global Health Research, Saveetha Medical College and Hospital, Saveetha Institute of Medical and Technical Sciences, Chennai 602105, Tamil Nadu, India*

[2] *Department of Pharmacology, GITAM School of Pharmacy, Gandhi Institute of Technology and Management Deemed to be University, Hyderabad, Telangana, India*

[3] *Department of Pharmacognosy, MB School of Pharmaceutical Sciences, Mohan Babu University, Tirupati, Andhra Pradesh, India*

[4] *Seva Shikshan Prasarak Mandal's Dr. N.J. Paulbudhe College of Pharmacy, Vasant Tekadi, Savedi, Ahmed Nagar, Maharashtra, India*

[5] *Department of Pharmacology, Bojjam Narasimhulu College of Pharmacy, Saidabad, Hyderabad, India*

[6] *Department of Pharmacognosy and Phytochemistry, Chebrolu Hanumaiah Institute of Pharmaceutical Sciences, Guntur, Pradesh, India*

[7] *Amity Institute of Pharmacy, Amity University Gwalior, Madhya Pradesh 474005, India*

[8] *Faculty of Pharmaceutical Sciences, UCSI University, Cheras, Kuala Lumpur 56000, Malaysia*

[9] *Department of Pharmaceutics, College of Pharmaceutical Sciences, Dayananda Sagar University, Bengaluru, Karnataka 560078, India*

Abstract: *Andrographis paniculata* (AP) is a traditional herb known as "king of bitters" and belongs to Acanthaceae. This plant is used traditionally to treat fever, sore throat, snake bites, and upper respiratory tract infections. The pharmacological effects exhibited by AP are actually due to the presence of several classes of phytocompounds. Among the numerous bioactive compounds generated by *Androgrpahis paniculata*, Andrographolide (AG) is the primary active phytochemical. This compound shows various biological functions, such as anti-inflammatory, anticancer, antimicrobial, neuroprotective, cardioprotective, and organ- and bone-protective activities. On the other hand, AG's structural analogs also showed various potent biological effects

* **Corresponding authors Ravishankar Ram Mani and Kranthi Kumar Kotha:** Faculty of Pharmaceutical Sciences, UCSI University, Cheras, Kuala Lumpur 56000, Malaysia; Department of Pharmaceutics, College of Pharmaceutical Sciences, Dayananda Sagar University, Bengaluru, Karnataka 560078, India; E-mails: Ravishankar@ucsiuniversity.edu.my; kranthikumarkotta@gmail.com

against different kinds of dreadful diseases. Hence, it is noteworthy to summarize the various pharmacological effects of AG and its analogs to help the researchers focus on this area. Therefore, in this chapter, we elaborated on various biological functions of AG and its derivatives; this review would be a standalone reference for AG's bio-actives and analogs.

Keywords: Andrographolide, Analogs, *Andrographis paniculata*, Bioactive compounds, Pharmacological activities.

INTRODUCTION

Andrographis paniculata (AP) is a traditional herbaceous medicinal plant placed under the family Acanthaceae. This plant is known as Kalmegh and King of Bitters because of its taste. Among the various species of this genus, *A. paniculata* is the primary and well-studied species. This plant species grows well on slopes, paths, and dams and in wet environments in different parts of Asian countries like India, China, Thailand, Malaysia, Myanmar, and Sri Lanka [1, 2]. From ancient times, this plant was traditionally used to treat diseases like jaundice, liver toxicity, cardiotoxicity, sore throat, and flu. Several studies also revealed that this plant extract can be used as a contraceptive in addition to its effects on various sexual disorders [3, 4]. In addition, for a very long time, the whole plant extract and the root extract of AP were recommended for treating various diseases. In earlier times, this plant extract was prescribed by various traditional medicine practitioners for treating diseases like pyrexia, fever, stomachache, intestinal problems, snake bites, dyspepsia, and aggravation [5]. The different kinds of pharmacological effects exhibited by *A. paniculata* extract were due to various classes of phytochemicals in the plant [6]. This plant mainly contains polyphenols, diterpenoids, alkaloids, and flavonoid compounds. Among the various bioactive compounds, andrographolide is the major phytocompound in terms of concentration and pharmacological properties [6]. This compound is highly bitter and belongs to the labdane diterpenoid class. On the other hand, the andrographolide analogs also show various health benefits in different kinds of disease conditions [3]. It was reported that 14-deoxy-11,12-didehydroan-ro-grapholide, an essential structural analog of andrographolide, possesses various pharmacological benefits like anti-infective, antiatherosclerotic, and immunomodulatory effects [7]. Besides, neoandrographolide also displays multiple biological functions, such as anti-inflammatory, antihepatotoxicity, and anti-infective [8]. In addition, 14-deoxyandrographolide also expresses promising pharmacological functions like hepatoprotective, cardioprotective, and immunomodulatory effects [9, 10]. Besides this, there are a few other minor structural analogs of andrographolide like andrograpanin, 3,19-isopropylidene andrographolide 14-deoxy-14,15-dehydroandrogr, andrographolide, and 14-acetyl andrographolide [4]. These compounds also show significant benefits on cardiovascular, liver, and cancer health [4]. Other than this structural analog of AG, there are a few different compounds belonging to the flavonoid class, such as 7-O-methyiwogonin, apigenin, insulin, and 3,4-caffeoylquinic acid, which also show various biological functions like cardioprotective and hepatoprotective [11]. Hence, studying the andrographolide and its analogs in detail is noteworthy. This chapter reviewed AG's most significant pharmacological functions and analogs in detail. In this way, this review will become a standalone reference for the research in this area.

Pharmacological Active Compounds of *Andrographis paniculata*

The bioactive compounds in the AP are extracted from several parts of the plant, like the leaf, stem, and root. Among the various available classes of compounds, the diterpenoid compounds (major) were isolated from a methanol fraction of ethanol or methanol extract of the whole plant, leaf, and stem [6, 12]. In the diterpenoids, andrographolide is available in high concentrations like 4%, 1.2%, and 6% in the whole plant, stem, and leaf extract (Shown in Fig. **1**) [13]. In addition, the other essential diterpenoids like neoandrographolide, isoandrographolide, 14-deoxy-11,12-didehydroandrographide, and deoxy andrographolide were also isolated from the methanol fraction of the extract of various parts of the plant (Shown in Fig. **1**) [13]. Similarly, the flavonoid bioactive compounds like 5-hydroxy-7,8,2'-trimethoxyflavone, 5-hydrox--7,8,2',3'-tetramethoxyflavone, 5-hydroxy-7,8-dimethoxyflavone, 5-hydrox--7,8,2',5'-tetramethoxyflavone, 2'-methyl ether, and 7-O-methyl wogonin were separated from ethyl acetate fraction of the methanol or ethanol extract of the whole plant (Shown in Fig. **1**).

Pharmacological Effects of Andrographolide and its Analogs

The extensive use of the *Andrographis paniculata* plant and its parts in various traditional medicines for treating different diseases led the researchers to focus further on this plant to validate its pharmacological efficacy. Hence, the scientists further investigated this plant and found that this plant provides significant health benefits by promoting various pharmacological functions like anticancer, antioxidant, antiangiogenic, antihepatotoxic, antibacterial, antiprotozoal, antiviral, and immunomodulatory effects. Due to the enormous health benefits provided by AP, it is noteworthy to study the medicinal values of the phytocompounds available in this plant [14].

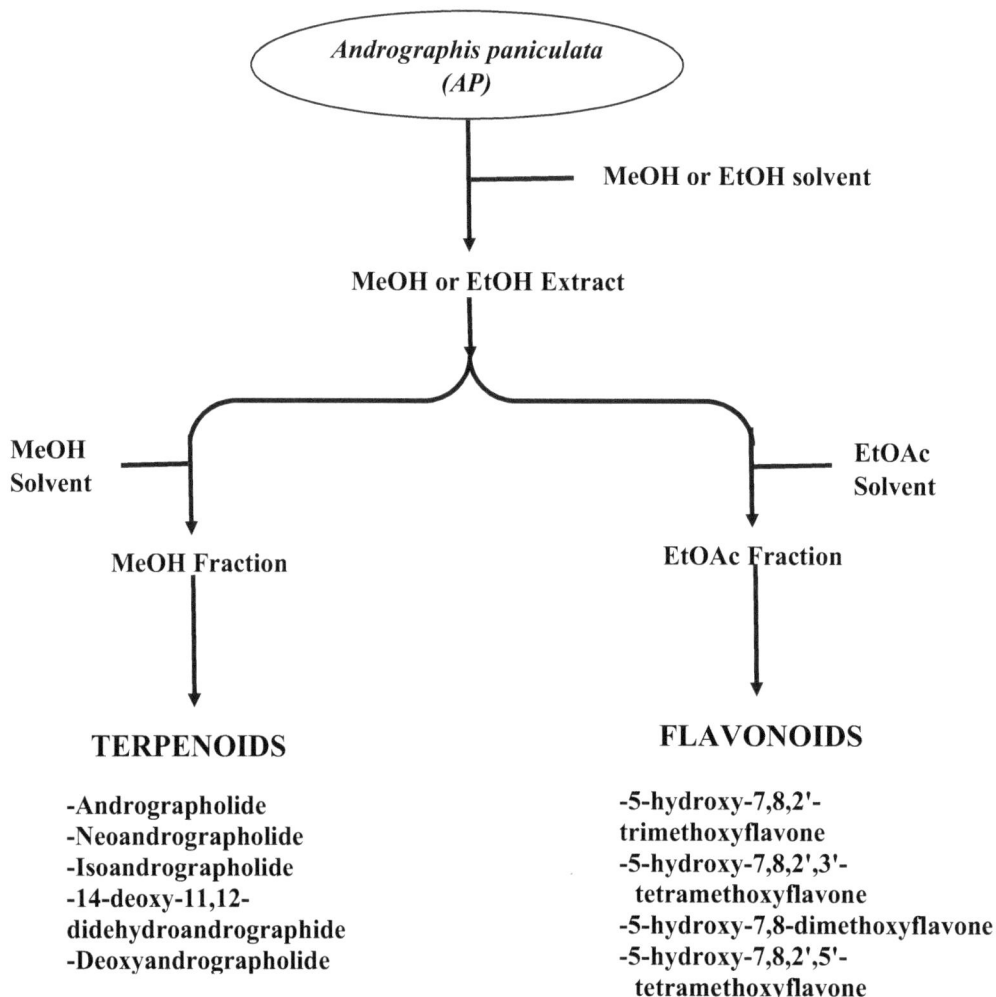

Fig. (1). Flowchart showing the extraction of various active compounds from AP extract.

Antimicrobial Activity

Several documented evidence revealed that *Andrographis paniculata* extract and its bioactive compounds display a prominent antimicrobial activity against different microorganisms like bacteria and fungi [15]. A study investigated water extracts of *A. paniculata*, AG, and arabinogalactan protein for their antibacterial activity against various bacteria [16]. This study tested the effect of samples separately and in combination. Finally, the obtained results revealed that the water extract and the arabinogalactan protein effectively inhibited the growth of *Pseudomonas aeruginosa, Escherichia coli*, and *Bacillus subtilis* bacteria. In contrast, the AG compound works well on only *Bacillus subtilis* [16]. However, all three samples significantly inhibited the growth of *Candida albicans* fungi. Besides, the AG structural analogs like andrographolides belonging to the class of noriridoides were also evaluated for their antibacterial effect against *Pseudomonas aeruginosa, B. subtilis, E. coli, Staphylococcus aureus,* and *Staphylococcus epidermidis* bacteria [17]. The results revealed that these analogs showed no significant antibacterial effect compared to standard compounds like gentamycin, ciprofloxacin, and chloramphenicol. In another study, Sule and his team investigated the three solvent extracts of AP on twelve skin infection-inducing bacteria strains. They found that these extracts inhibit the growth of all bacteria significantly [18]. In the same way, Nakanishi *et al.* estimated the antibacterial effect of methanol extract of *A. paniculata* on various bacterial strains like *Proteus vulgaris, Bacillus subtilis*, and *Escherichia coli*. This experiment results confirmed that the methanolic extract of *A. paniculata* successfully inhibited the growth of *P. vulgaris* and *B. subtilis* strains but not of *E. coli* [19]. Later, Mishra and his team studied the effect of ethanol extract of *A. paniculata* on *E.coli* and ten other Gram-negative and positive bacteria and found that the ethanol extract remarkably suppressed the growth of *E.coli* bacteria along with the different bacteria strains [19]. Furthermore, extracts of *A. paniculata* and phytocompounds like deoxy andrographolide, andrographolide, and neoandrographolide were also evaluated for their antimalarial activity. This study concluded that all the tested compounds and the extract have shown positive antimalarial activity in animal models by inhibiting the *Plasmodium berghei* NK65 protozoan growth. In a study, a group of scientists estimated the effect on the dengue vector and found that *A. paniculata* extract, along with compound AG, reduced the growth of *Aedes aegypti* mosquitoes. In the experiment, they found that the sample drastically decreased the larvae growth of the particular mosquitoes. Similarly, researchers also tested the plant's ethanol extract on the dengue-causing agent, and they found this extract is a promising anti-dengue agent and inhibits 75% of the growth [20]. In another study, both polar and non-polar extracts of the plant were explored for their antibacterial efficacy at different concentrations on skin infection-inducing strains like *Proteus mirabilis, Proteus vulgaris, Neisseria meningitis,* and *Pseudomonas aeruginosa* and six Gram positive strains *Staphylococcus epidermis, Streptococcus pyogenes, Micrococcus luteus, Bacillus anthracis, Staphylococcus aureus,* and *Staphylococcus saprophyticus*. The results revealed that both polarity extracts showed promising antibacterial effects by suppressing all the bacterial strains [20]. These studies finally concluded that AG and derivatives show potent antimicrobial activity.

Antiviral Activity

Several documented evidence revealed that *A. paniculata* and its derived compounds showed potent antiviral activity against various viruses. Previous studies on the effect of this extract on dengue virus displayed a noticeable anti-dengue effect. This study found that *A. paniculata* extract, along with the active component AG, reduced the viral generation and its corresponding infection. However, these samples did not inhibit the entry of the virus into the host cells or the growth of the host cells, such as HepG2 and Hela. Furthermore, the results also revealed that AG inhibits the virus growth by regulating heme oxygenase-1 enzyme (HO-1) [21]. Similarly, the antiviral effects of *A. paniculata* and its essential components were also checked for influenza A virus (IAV). This virus actually increases the cytokines load in the lungs, especially in the alveolar part, and induces inflammation, acute respiratory syndrome, and sometimes death. In this study, they studied the effect of the samples and found that AG inhibited the virus growth by altering the gene replication and functionally mature protein phases. In the same way, 14-deoxy-11,12-didehydroandrographolide inhibited the virus at the entry phase. On the other hand, 14-deoxy-11, 12-didehydroandrographolide, and AG significantly reduced a load of inflammatory markers like cytokines and chemokines, thereby improving the lung condition [22]. In addition, 14-deoxy-11,12-didehydroandrographolide also suppresses the highly pathogenic bird influenza virus H5N1 virus *via* decreasing nucleoprotein and mRNA synthesis. Besides, this compound also inhibited the nuclear export of viral ribonucleoprotein complexes at the replication stage [23]. In an investigation, researchers also studied the effect of AP and its compounds on human immunodeficiency virus (HIV). In this research, they found that 70% ethanol extract of *A. paniculata* and also its main phytochemical AG suppresses the core receptors like C-X-C receptor 4 (CXCR4) and C-C receptor 5 (CCR5), which are essential for binding of the virus to the CD4 receptor on the host cells. In addition, 14-deoxy-11,12-didehydroandrographolide (14-11, 12-DAG) also inhibits HIV entry into the host cells through binding of 14-11, 12-DAG to the gp120 protein of the virus. This gp120 protein is essential for HIV interacting with the host cell receptor CD4. This way, AP extract and its components AG and 14-11, 12- DAG inhibit the virus entry into the host cell and show significant anti-HIV activity. Similarly, andrographolide and its analogs also showed antiviral activity against herpes simplex virus (HSV), which causes conjunctivitis, retinal necrosis, and keratitis. This investigation found that AG and 14-deoxy androgapholide (14-DAG) successfully blocked the herpes virus entry and its production. Furthermore, these compounds inhibited the growth of another type of herpes virus, *i.e.*, Epstein-Barr virus (EBV), at its early stage of the lytic cycle by down-regulating the lytic proteins like Rta, Zta, and EA-D. In recent studies, *Andrographis paniculata* extract and its active compounds were evaluated for their effect on the severe acute respiratory syndrome coronavirus 2 (SARS-Co--2). In SARS-CoV-2 infection, the virus needs viral proteases like main protease (M^{pro}), 3C-like proteinases (3CLpro), and papain-like protease (PLpro). These non-structural proteins are essential for viral RNA replication and transcription. In addition, the interaction between virus spike glycoprotein and host cells receptor angiotensin-converting enzyme 2 (ACE2) is highly required to enter the virus into the host cells. In this investigation, both *in silico* and *in vitro* experiments revealed that andrographolide inhibits the main protease (M^{pro}) by binding with greater affinity. In addition, the other compounds of AP extract, like 14-deoxy-11, 12-didehydroandrographolide, neoandrographolide, and 14-deoxyandrographolide, were also reported to suppress papain-like protease (PL^{pro}). These phytocompounds show anticorona virus activity by affecting the replication and transcription of the SARS-CoV-2 RNA.

Anticancer Effect

Numerous studies revealed the anticancer potentials of *Andrographis paniculata* extract and its phytoconstituents [24]. In a study, Lee *et al*. studied the anticancer effect of *Andrographis paniculata* extract against pancreatic cancer cells. They found that 70% ethanol extract of *A. paniculata* shows cell-specific anticancer effects on PANC-1 and PSN-1 human pancreatic cells. In this investigation, they found that the andrographolide analog 14-deoxy-11,12-didehydroandrographolide exhibited a high anticancer effect on PANC-1 and PSN-1 cells. They also observed that 14-deoxy-11,12-didehydroandrographolide initiates apoptosis in pancreatic cancer cells [25]. AG also produced a significant anticancer effect on pancreatic cells like Panc-1 and AsPC-1 by inhibiting IL-6-linked p-JAK2 and p-STAT3 activation. In this study, they also found that AG, combined with gemcitabine drug, remarkably decreased the AsPC-1 cells generated tumor growth in mice models [26]. The other group studied the anticancer potentials of AG in the hepatocellular cancer (HCC) preclinical model. This study revealed that AG combined with 0PB-31121 protein showed promising antitumor effects against HCC tumors. However, this combination did not work well in clinical studies [27]. In addition, 19-O-triphenyl methyl andrographolide (RS-PP-050), an important analog of AG, also showed an anticancer effect *via* inhibiting T-cell factor/lymphocyte enhancing factor signaling molecules function in cancer cells with β-catenin up-regulation. In another investigation, a group of researchers found that AG successfully blocked the function of SOX9 and TCF-1 proteins, thereby inhibiting the growth of chondrosarcoma cells [28]. Later, in another investigation, the phytocompounds were isolated from the methanol extract's most active (DCM fraction) [29]. All the extracted compounds from the fraction were tested against various cancer cells. The results concluded that AG isolated from the DCM is extremely active, and it kills all types of cancer cells that were screened. However, other compounds like 14-deoxy-andrographolide and 14-deoxy-11, 12-didehydroandrographolide were active against a few cancer cell lines. A study by Singh *et al*. explained the anticancer potentials of the hydroalcoholic extract of the *Andrographis paniculata* plant toward ovary cancer cells, ovcar-5 [30]. This study found that this extract specifically inhibited the growth of ovarian cancer cells compared to other screened cancer cells. The same study also studied the combination of *A. paniculta* extract with hydro-alcoholic *Silybum marianum* extract on cancer cells [30]. However, this combination study did not produce any significant results. In the *A. paniculata* extract, andrographolide is the major compound, and it exhibited the most promising anticancer effect compared with other phytocompounds of the plant. This compound showed cytotoxic effects by promoting cell death mechanisms like apoptosis, necrosis, and autophagy. Earlier studies on the AG showed that this compound regulates intracellular ROS, which ultimately alters various signaling molecules like protein kinase C, macrophage-1 antigen (Mac-1), PI-3, mTOR, and PMA, encouraging cancer cell death. Similarly, Yuan *et al.* also studied the cytotoxic effect of AG on colon cancer cells. They found that AG inhibits angiogenesis by suppressing the phosphorylation of proteins like STAT3, JAK1, and JAK2. They also revealed that the above mechanism inhibits inflammatory markers like TNF-α-and IL-8. Conversely, andrographolide demonstrates anticancer effects in the HCT 116 colorectal cancer cell line *via* increasing IL-8. The activation of TNF-α linked IL-8 increased, and the effect was concentration-dependent and suppressed angiogenesis in the tumor microenvironment [31]. AG and its derivative's anticancer effect were also investigated on breast cancer [32]. In this study, two important andrographolide analogs like 3,19- (3-chloro-4-fluorobenzylidene) andrographolide (SRJ23) and 3,19-(2-bromobenzylidene) andrographolide (SRJ09) were tested on breast cancer cell lines MCF-7 [33]. The study revealed that these two compounds induce cell death *via* cell cycle arrest. They found that these derivatives increased the percentage of cells in the G1 phase, thereby increasing and decreasing the expression of p21 and CDK4, respectively [33]. AG also showed its potential by decreasing the growth of β-catenin overexpressed cells induced tumors in mice. This effect of AG is due to the synergistic action with the peptidomimetic drug CWP232291. AG also reduced the growth of nasopharyngeal cancer cells by targeting AMPK. Recent studies revealed that AG activates p-AMPK (AMP-activated protein kinase) and p-LKB1/STK11 (liver kinase B1 or serine/threonine kinase-11) and kills the nasopharyngeal cancer cells [34]. On the other hand, AG also triggers autophagic cell death in osteosarcoma cells like MG-63 and U-2OS *via* targeting AKT and MG-63 signaling molecules [35].

Antiatherosclerotic Activity

Andrographis paniculata extract and its bioactive compounds exhibit various pharmacological effects, including antiatherosclerotic activity [36]. A study conducted by Zhang and his team reported that hydroalcoholic extract of *A*.

paniculata significantly reduced blood pressure in different kinds of hypertensive rat models. In another study, different polarity solvent extracts of *A. paniculata* markedly decreased the average arterial blood pressure without affecting the heartbeat. In addition, 14-deoxyandrographolide, a crucial bioactive compound, also showed antiatherosclerotic activity by inducing a vasorelaxation effect in rat models [37]. On the other hand, 14-deoxy-11,12-didehydroandrographolide also reduced the arterial blood pressure and heartbeat in the right atria of anesthetized rats [38]. In another experiment, Yoopan and his team showed the muscle relaxant and hypotensive function of both *A. paniculata* extract and 14-deoxy-11,-2-didehydroandrographolide compound in rat model [39]. Furthermore, their investigation revealed that the antiatherosclerotic effect of these bioactive compounds was due to the activation of guanylyl cyclase and NOS, which helps release NO in the endothelial cells [39]. In another study, researchers found that prior administration of *A. paniculata* extract also induces cardioprotection by suppressing the level of inflammatory markers like COX-2 and NFκB [40]. They also identified that this plant extract exerts an effect by drastically decreasing cardiac hypertrophy biomarker proteins like atrial natriuretic peptide (ANP) and brain natriuretic peptide (BNP). They further confirmed that the cardioprotective activity of this plant extract is due to the suppression of inflammatory signaling molecules like IL-6, p-MRK5, and STAT3 that were elevated by the consumption of a high-fat diet. Zeng and his team also studied the cardioprotective effect on isoproterenol-induced cardiotoxicity in rabbits [41]. This study reported that AG reduces the high Ca^{+2} load-induced rapid depolarization in isolated rabbit left ventricular myocytes and left atrial myocytes [41]. In an *in vivo* study, they disclosed that AG induces a cardioprotective effect *via* decreasing Ca+2 and Na+ ion channels in rabbits [41].

Neuroprotective Activity

Neurodegenerative diseases (NDs) like Parkinson's, Alzheimer's, and Huntington's diseases are age-related diseases, claiming millions of lives every year. However, the available treatment options for various NDs only offer temporary relief from the symptoms but not a complete cure. Hence, there is an urgent need for an ideal and unique treatment that can completely reverse the disease. Medicinal plants and their isolated phytocompounds from ancient times contributed much to identifying novel drugs for various diseases. One such plant-derived compound is andrographolide, which has substantial pharmacological properties and benefits against various neurological disorders. Several documents explain its neuroprotection in various models. Multiple pharmacodynamics studies on AG revealed that AG passes through the blood-brain barrier and acts on the brain directly [42]. This property of AG can be used to develop a potential drug candidate for various NDs. In the earlier studies, Yang *et al.* reported that

AG was protective against cerebral ischemia. This study found that AG exhibits neuroprotection by altering the level of various signaling molecules like Nrf2-HO-1, p38 MAPK, Bax, and iNOS [43]. Similarly, AG also induced neuroprotection against glutamate-initiated neurotoxicity in HT22 mouse hippocampal neuronal cells. This study found that AG suppressed the apoptosis linked with Ca+2 influx, oxidative stress, and lipid peroxidation. In addition, this study also revealed that AG alters the level of Bcl-2, Bax, and AIF [44]. The other study also confirmed the role of AG on intracerebral hemorrhage (ICH), a severe CNS disorder that causes a high death rate in the world. In this study, the researchers found that administering 1 or 2 mg of AG for 72 h to ICH rats significantly improved the neuronal condition. This result is due to decreased water levels in the brain and neurodegeneration in the brain [45]. Further investigation of the brain sample revealed that the AG reduced the activation of inflammatory markers like TNF-α and IL-6 in the brain [46]. This compound also impacted surgery-induced cognitive impairment in different animal models. In the earlier studies, Ding and his group observed that the AG significantly improved the learning ability and impairment in hippocampal neuronal integrity in rats. This study also revealed that AG remarkably inhibited the levels of essential signaling molecules like NF-κB, p88, and ERK1/2, thereby producing cognitive improvement in rat models [46]. This compound also showed a promising neuroprotective effect on multiple sclerosis (MS) disease by inhibiting the immune response developed by thymus-associated antigens and reducing MS symptoms in EAE mice. In addition, AG also inhibited the T-cell activation and, ultimately, the myelin sheath [46].

Antiulcer Activity

Along with several pharmacological benefits, *A. paniculata* and its phytocompounds also show an antiulcer effect in various models. A study conducted by Saranya *et al.* observed that the organic solvent that extracts a high amount of AG shows a promising antiulcer and antioxidant effect. In this study, they found that a comparatively hydroalcoholic extract of *A. paniculata* shows a higher antioxidant and antiulcer effect than ethanol, ethyl acetate, and petroleum ether extract [47].

Hepatoprotective Activity

Hepatic diseases initiated through different kinds of sources will always remain a primary health concern in the entire world. Due to the lack of ideal drug candidates, the death rate of the disease is continuously rising. Hence, there is a massive requirement for a unique drug candidate that possesses minimal toxicity. Several studies revealed that various plants and herbs offer better controlling effects on various kinds of hepatic disorders, and they even exhibit minimal toxicity [48]. Moreover, *Andrographis paniculata* has a long history of usage in the Indian system of medicine as a better hepatostimulant and hepatoprotective agent. In addition, it has been used as an important ingredient in many herbal formulations recommended for liver disorders like chronic hepatitis B viral-related diseases [49, 50]. In the earlier study, they also found the effect of andrographolide, one of the major compounds of *A. paniculata* extract, in concanavalin A-induced liver toxicity. This study found that AG reduces toxicity *via* decreasing concanavalin A-mediated apoptosis in hepatic cells [51]. In another study, researchers found the effect of AG on acetaminophen-associated liver toxicity. In this investigation, they identified that AG significantly reduced the amount of bile secretion compared to the silymarin-treated mice. In the same way, AG hepatoprotective effect was also studied in ethanol-mediated liver toxicity in mice models. This study also found that AG, like silymarin, shows a more prominent hepatoprotective role in ethanol-induced toxicity [52]. In another study, *A. paniculata* extract was pre- and post-evaluated the effect against ethanol-induced liver toxicity in a rat model. This investigation found that an extract of *A. paniculata* has shown a noticeable impact on ethanol-mediated serum transaminase upregulation. In the same way, *A. paniculata* extract, along with the AG compound, reduced the CCl_4 and paracetamol-induced liver damage [52, 53]. Besides, AG co-administered with other derivatives like neoandrographolide and andrographiside significantly eliminated the tert-butylhydroperoxide (tBHP) and CCl_4-induced hepatic injury in rats [52].

Antidiabetic Activity

Several documented evidence suggested that *Andrographis paniculata* and other plant materials were used as a traditional medicine against diabetes. Hence, this plant was tested along with other plant materials like *Syzygium cumini* and *Caesalpinia sappan* for antidiabetic activity against high-fat diet-mediated diabetes in a rat model. In this study, they found that the fixed concentration of mixed plant extract significantly decreased the level of cholesterol and low-density lipoprotein (LDL) compared to diabetic control and the metformin group. However, the same extract showed no effect on the level of triglycerides as compared to the other groups [54]. In another study, Nugroho and his team evaluated the antidiabetic effect of *A. paniculata* isolated fraction and its active constituent andrographolide in a high fructose-induced type II diabetic rat model. In this experiment, they found that the extract and the andrographolide reduced the blood glucose, triglyceride, and LDL levels significantly compared with the control and the metformin group [55]. In a recent study, Suemanotham and his team demonstrated the antidiabetic and antihyperglycemic effects of *A. paniculata* extract on hyperglycemic dogs. This study analyzed the blood glucose level and inflammatory and oxidative stress markers in 41 dog samples. In the results, they noticed that the amount of biochemical parameters like alanine aminotransferase, alkaline phosphatase, blood urea nitrogen, and creatinine were brought to normal levels in the AP-treated group compared to the diabetic group. On the other hand, the inflammatory and oxidative markers also decreased in comparison with the diabetic model. Moreover, the *Andrographis paniculata* produced no other animal toxicity [56]. Ahmad *et al.* also studied the antidiabetic effect of ethanol extract of AP in a streptozotocin-induced diabetic rat model. In this study, different extracts were obtained by changing the percentage of ethanol solvent. These obtained extracts were investigated for their effect on the model. Finally, 95% and 50% ethanol in water extract showed a significant antidiabetic impact *via* reducing various biochemical parameters compared to the control group. The HPLC-UV analysis of these extracts revealed the presence of andrographolide in high concentrations [57].

Immunomodulatory Effect

Several studies speculated that *Andrographis paniculata* extract and andrographolide modulate the immune system. However, no clear mechanism explains how *A. paniculata* extract and its phytocompounds alter immunity. Nevertheless, in a study, Iruretagoyena and his team said that AG decreases both humoral and cellular immune responses. This investigation found that AG initiates the immune response *via* inhibiting T-cells activated by dendritic cells. This action is ultimately due to andrographolide-mediated downregulation of the NF-kB pathway, thereby increasing tolerance in mice towards autoimmune disorders like encephalomyelitis [58, 59]. On the other hand, AG also improved the immune response in the cyclophosphamide-mediated immune suppression model *via* increasing response towards antibodies, phagocytosis, and cellularity in organs like the spleen and thymus. In addition, this compound also inhibits macrophage activation by blocking M1/M2 polarization. Besides, the other study also revealed that a combination of AG derivatives like 14-deoxy andrographolide and 14-deoxy-11,12-didehydroandrographolide along with AG improved the immunity in the cyclophosphamide-induced immunosuppression activity in the spleen-of-mice [60]. In this activity, the mixture of the compounds showed enhanced phagocytosis and immunoglobulin formation. Moreover, *A. paniculata* extract, as well as AG compound, significantly improved immunity by raising the antibody level after the injection of the Salmonella vaccine. The combination also increased the level of INF-γ production in spleen cells in the [61] vaccinated model, which has concluded the effect of extract and AG on humoral and cellular immunity.

Antifertility Activity

Andrographis paniculata and its bioactive compounds also showed the antifertility effect [53]. Multiple studies on different kinds of animal models have proven the antifertility effect of the extract of this plant. In a study, the stem of *A. paniculata* showed a significant antifertility impact on male Wistar mice, but there was no effect on female mice [53]. In another study, this plant induced abortion in a pregnant rabbit, and it also suppressed the growth of human placental chorionic trophoblastic cells in an *in vitro* experiment. Furthermore, the administration of the 2g/kg bw/day of plant powder for at least 6 weeks successfully blocked the pregnancy even after mating with control male mice [5]. In the same way, oral feeding of the dried *A. paniculata* leaf material to the albino rats of male species significantly reduced spermatogenesis and size of Leydig cells [62]. In addition, this powdered leaf material also induces degenerative changes in seminal vesicles and ventral prostate [62]. The active compound AG also initiated the same effect in male Wistar albino rats by killing sperm cells at 50mg/kg bw after eight weeks of treatment [63].

CONCLUSION

Numerous studies revealed the multiple pharmacological benefits of andrographolide. Hence, in recent times, many researchers and plant scientists have shifted their focus to this plant for further investigation. Moreover, due to its substantial health benefits, various structural analogs have also been synthesized recently for further development in pharmacological activities. In this chapter, we summarized the various critical biological functions of andrographolide and its different kinds of structural analogs, such as antimicrobial, antiviral, hepatoprotective, antidiabetic, immunomodulatory, and antifertility activities. In this way, the current review will be a ready-made reference for research and scientists working in this area.

REFERENCES

[1]   Hossain MS, Urbi Z, Sule A, Rahman KMH. *Andrographis paniculata* (Burm. f.) Wall. ex Nees: a review of ethnobotany, phytochemistry, and pharmacology. ScientificWorldJournal 2014; 2014: 1-28.
[http://dx.doi.org/10.1155/2014/274905] [PMID: 25950015]

[2]   Dutta N, Ghosh S, Nelson VK, Sareng HR, Majumder C, Mandal SC, *et al.* Andrographolide upregulates protein quality control mechanisms in cells and mice through upregulation of mTORC1 function. Biochimica et Biophysica Acta General subjects. 2021; 1865(6): 129885.

[3]   Tian J, Li C, Meng J, *et al.* Pharmacological effects and safety of *Andrographis paniculata* (Burm.f.) Nees. J Food Sci 2022; 87(3): 1319-30.
[http://dx.doi.org/10.1111/1750-3841.16079] [PMID: 35166368]

[4]   Zhang H, Li S, Si Y, Xu H. Andrographolide and its derivatives: Current achievements and future perspectives. Eur J Med Chem 2021; 224: 113710.
[http://dx.doi.org/10.1016/j.ejmech.2021.113710] [PMID: 34315039]

[5]   Mussard E, Jousselin S, Cesaro A, Legrain B, Lespessailles E, Esteve E, *et al. Andrographis paniculata* and its bioactive diterpenoids protect dermal fibroblasts against inflammation and oxidative stress. Antioxidants (Basel, Switzerland). 2020; 9(5).

[6]   Chao WW, Lin BF. Isolation and identification of bioactive compounds in *Andrographis paniculata* (Chuanxinlian). Chin Med 2010; 5(1): 17.
[http://dx.doi.org/10.1186/1749-8546-5-17] [PMID: 20465823]

[7]   Guan SP, Kong LR, Cheng C, Lim JCW, Wong WSF. Protective role of 14-deoxy-11,-2-didehydroandrographolide, a noncytotoxic analogue of andrographolide, in allergic airway inflammation. J Nat Prod 2011; 74(6): 1484-90.
[http://dx.doi.org/10.1021/np2002572] [PMID: 21598983]

[8]   Liu Y, Liu Y, Zhang HL, *et al.* Amelioratory effect of neoandrographolide on myocardial ischemic-reperfusion injury by its anti-inflammatory and anti-apoptotic activities. Environ Toxicol 2021; 36(12): 2367-79.
[http://dx.doi.org/10.1002/tox.23350] [PMID: 34397165]

[9]   Mandal S, Nelson VK, Mukhopadhyay S, *et al.* 14-Deoxyandrographolide targets adenylate cyclase and prevents ethanol-induced liver injury through constitutive NOS dependent reduced redox signaling in rats. Food Chem Toxicol 2013; 59: 236-48.
[http://dx.doi.org/10.1016/j.fct.2013.05.056] [PMID: 23764359]

[10]   Roy DN, Mandal S, Sen G, Mukhopadhyay S, Biswas T. 14-Deoxyandrographolide desensitizes hepatocytes to tumour necrosis factor-alpha-induced apoptosis through calcium-dependent tumour necrosis factor receptor superfamily member 1A release *via* the NO/cGMP pathway. Br J Pharmacol 2010; 160(7): 1823-43.
[http://dx.doi.org/10.1111/j.1476-5381.2010.00836.x] [PMID: 20649583]

[11]   Zeng B, Wei A, Zhou Q, *et al.* Andrographolide: A review of its pharmacology, pharmacokinetics, toxicity and clinical trials and pharmaceutical researches. Phytother Res 2022; 36(1): 336-64.
[http://dx.doi.org/10.1002/ptr.7324] [PMID: 34818697]

[12]   Kumar S, Singh B, Bajpai V. *Andrographis paniculata* (Burm.f.) Nees: Traditional uses, phytochemistry, pharmacological properties and quality control/quality assurance. J Ethnopharmacol 2021; 275: 114054.
[http://dx.doi.org/10.1016/j.jep.2021.114054] [PMID: 33831465]

[13]   Mussard E, Cesaro A, Lespessailles E, Legrain B, Berteina-Raboin S, Toumi H. Andrographolide, a natural antioxidant: An update. Antioxidants (Basel, Switzerland). 2019; 8(12).

[14]   Okhuarobo A, Ehizogie Falodun J, Erharuyi O, Imieje V, Falodun A, Langer P. Harnessing the medicinal properties of *Andrographis paniculata* for diseases and beyond: a review of its phytochemistry and pharmacology. Asian Pac J Trop Dis 2014; 4(3): 213-22.
[http://dx.doi.org/10.1016/S2222-1808(14)60509-0]

[15]   Kamaruzzaman WMIWM, Fekeri MFM, Nasir NAM, *et al.* Anticorrosive and microbial inhibition performance of a coating loaded with *Andrographis paniculata* on Stainless Steel in Seawater. Molecules 2021; 26(11): 3379.
[http://dx.doi.org/10.3390/molecules26113379] [PMID: 34205014]

[16]   Singha PK, Roy S, Dey S. Protective activity of andrographolide and arabinogalactan proteins from *Andrographis paniculata* Nees. against ethanol-induced toxicity in mice. J Ethnopharmacol 2007; 111(1): 13-21.
[http://dx.doi.org/10.1016/j.jep.2006.10.026] [PMID: 17127022]

[17]   Zhang L, Bao M, Liu B, *et al.* Effect of Andrographolide and Its Analogs on bacterial infection: A review. Pharmacology 2020; 105(3-4): 123-34.
[http://dx.doi.org/10.1159/000503410] [PMID: 31694037]

[18]   Hossain S, Urbi Z, Karuniawati H, *et al. Andrographis paniculata* (Burm. f.) Wall. ex Nees: An

updated review of phytochemistry, antimicrobial pharmacology, and clinical safety and efficacy. Life (Basel) 2021; 11(4): 348.
[http://dx.doi.org/10.3390/life11040348] [PMID: 33923529]

[19] Nakanishi K, Sasaki S, Kiang AK, *et al.* Phytochemical survey of Malaysian plants preliminary chemical and pharmacological screening. Chem Pharm Bull (Tokyo) 1965; 13(7): 882-90.
[http://dx.doi.org/10.1248/cpb.13.882] [PMID: 5867816]

[20] Krishnasamy KK, Ramalingam S, Karupannan S, *et al.* Anti-dengue activity of *Andrographis paniculata* extracts and quantification of dengue viral inhibition by SYBR green reverse transcription polymerase chain reaction. Ayu 2018; 39(2): 87-91.
[http://dx.doi.org/10.4103/ayu.AYU_144_17] [PMID: 30783363]

[21] Tseng CK, Lin CK, Wu YH, *et al.* Human heme oxygenase 1 is a potential host cell factor against dengue virus replication. Sci Rep 2016; 6(1): 32176.
[http://dx.doi.org/10.1038/srep32176] [PMID: 27553177]

[22] Jiang M, Sheng F, Zhang Z, *et al. Andrographis paniculata* (Burm.f.) Nees and its major constituent andrographolide as potential antiviral agents. J Ethnopharmacol 2021; 272: 113954.
[http://dx.doi.org/10.1016/j.jep.2021.113954] [PMID: 33610706]

[23] Cai W, Li Y, Chen S, *et al.* 14-Deoxy-11,12-dehydroandrographolide exerts anti-influenza A virus activity and inhibits replication of H5N1 virus by restraining nuclear export of viral ribonucleoprotein complexes. Antiviral Res 2015; 118: 82-92.
[http://dx.doi.org/10.1016/j.antiviral.2015.03.008] [PMID: 25800824]

[24] Malik Z, Parveen R, Parveen B, *et al.* Anticancer potential of andrographolide from *Andrographis paniculata* (Burm.f.) Nees and its mechanisms of action. J Ethnopharmacol 2021; 272: 113936.
[http://dx.doi.org/10.1016/j.jep.2021.113936] [PMID: 33610710]

[25] Lee S, Morita H, Tezuka Y. Preferentially Cytotoxic Constituents of *Andrographis paniculata* and their preferential cytotoxicity against human pancreatic cancer cell lines. Nat Prod Commun 2015; 10(7): 1934578X1501000704.
[http://dx.doi.org/10.1177/1934578X1501000704] [PMID: 26410998]

[26] Bao GQ, Shen BY, Pan CP, Zhang YJ, Shi MM, Peng CH. Andrographolide causes apoptosis *via* inactivation of STAT3 and Akt and potentiates antitumor activity of gemcitabine in pancreatic cancer. Toxicol Lett 2013; 222(1): 23-35.
[http://dx.doi.org/10.1016/j.toxlet.2013.06.241] [PMID: 23845849]

[27] Farooqi AA, Attar R, Sabitaliyevich UY, *et al.* The prowess of andrographolide as a natural weapon in the war against cancer. Cancers (Basel) 2020; 12(8): 2159.
[http://dx.doi.org/10.3390/cancers12082159] [PMID: 32759728]

[28] Zhang HT, Yang J, Liang GH, *et al.* Andrographolide induces cell cycle arrest and apoptosis of chondrosarcoma by targeting TCF-1/SOX9 Axis. J Cell Biochem 2017; 118(12): 4575-86.
[http://dx.doi.org/10.1002/jcb.26122] [PMID: 28485543]

[29] Rajagopal S, Kumar RA, Deevi DS, Satyanarayana C, Rajagopalan R. Andrographolide, a potential cancer therapeutic agent isolated from *Andrographis paniculata*. J Exp Ther Oncol 2003; 3(3): 147-58.
[http://dx.doi.org/10.1046/j.1359-4117.2003.01090.x] [PMID: 14641821]

[30] Singh S, Mehta A, Baweja S, Ahirwal L, Mehta P. Mehta PJJoP, Toxicology. Anticancer activity of *Andrographis paniculata* and *Silybum marianum* on five human cancer cell lines. Journal of Pharmacology and Toxicology 2012; 8(1): 42-8.
[http://dx.doi.org/10.3923/jpt.2013.42.48]

[31] Yuan M, Meng W, Liao W, Lian S. Andrographolide Antagonizes TNF-α-Induced IL-8 *via* Inhibition of NADPH Oxidase/ROS/NF-κB and Src/MAPKs/AP-1 Axis in Human Colorectal Cancer HCT116 Cells. J Agric Food Chem 2018; 66(20): 5139-48.
[http://dx.doi.org/10.1021/acs.jafc.8b00810] [PMID: 29672044]

[32]   Varma A, Padh H, Shrivastava N. Andrographolide: a new plant-derived antineoplastic entity on horizon. Evid Based Complement Alternat Med 2011; 2011(1): 815390.
[http://dx.doi.org/10.1093/ecam/nep135] [PMID: 19752167]

[33]   Jada SR, Matthews C, Saad MS, *et al.* Benzylidene derivatives of andrographolide inhibit growth of breast and colon cancer cells *in vitro* by inducing G $_1$ arrest and apoptosis. Br J Pharmacol 2008; 155(5): 641-54.
[http://dx.doi.org/10.1038/bjp.2008.368] [PMID: 18806812]

[34]   Wu B, Chen X, Zhou Y, *et al.* Andrographolide inhibits proliferation and induces apoptosis of nasopharyngeal carcinoma cell line C666-1 through LKB1-AMPK-dependent signaling pathways. Pharmazie 2018; 73(10): 594-7.
[PMID: 30223924]

[35]   Liu Y, Zhang Y, Zou J, *et al.* Andrographolide induces autophagic cell death and inhibits invasion and metastasis of human osteosarcoma cells in an autophagy-dependent manner. Cell Physiol Biochem 2017; 44(4): 1396-410.
[http://dx.doi.org/10.1159/000485536] [PMID: 29197865]

[36]   Al Batran R, Al-Bayaty F, Al-Obaidi MMJ, Hussain SF, Mulok TZ. Evaluation of the effect of andrographolide on atherosclerotic rabbits induced by *Porphyromonas gingivalis*. BioMed Res Int 2014; 2014: 1-11.
[http://dx.doi.org/10.1155/2014/724718] [PMID: 25215291]

[37]   Burgos RA, Loyola M, Hidalgo MA, Labranche TP, Hancke JL. Effect of 14-deoxyandrographolide on calcium-mediated rat uterine smooth muscle contractility. Phytother Res 2003; 17(9): 1011-5.
[http://dx.doi.org/10.1002/ptr.1275] [PMID: 14595578]

[38]   Zhang C, Kuroyangi M, Tan BK. Cardiovascular activity of 14-deoxy-11,-2-didehydroandrographolide in the anaesthetised rat and isolated right atria. Pharmacol Res 1998; 38(6): 413-7.
[http://dx.doi.org/10.1006/phrs.1998.0373] [PMID: 9990649]

[39]   Yoopan N, Thisoda P, Rangkadilok N, *et al.* Cardiovascular effects of 14-deoxy-11,-2-didehydroandrographolide and *Andrographis paniculata* extracts. Planta Med 2007; 73(6): 503-11.
[http://dx.doi.org/10.1055/s-2007-967181] [PMID: 17650544]

[40]   Hsieh YL, Shibu MA, Lii CK, *et al. Andrographis paniculata* extract attenuates pathological cardiac hypertrophy and apoptosis in high-fat diet fed mice. J Ethnopharmacol 2016; 192: 170-7.
[http://dx.doi.org/10.1016/j.jep.2016.07.018] [PMID: 27401291]

[41]   Zeng M, Jiang W, Tian Y, *et al.* Andrographolide inhibits arrhythmias and is cardioprotective in rabbits. Oncotarget 2017; 8(37): 61226-38.
[http://dx.doi.org/10.18632/oncotarget.18051] [PMID: 28977859]

[42]   Khadka B, Lee JY, Park DH, Kim KT, Bae JS. The role of natural compounds and their nanocarriers in the treatment of cns inflammation. Biomolecules 2020; 10(10): 1401.
[http://dx.doi.org/10.3390/biom10101401] [PMID: 33019651]

[43]   Yang CH, Yen TL, Hsu CY, Thomas PA, Sheu JR, Jayakumar T. Multi-targeting andrographolide, a novel NF-κB Inhibitor, as a potential therapeutic agent for stroke. Int J Mol Sci 2017; 18(8): 1638.
[http://dx.doi.org/10.3390/ijms18081638]

[44]   Yang E-J, Song K-S. Andrographolide, a major component of *Andrographis paniculata* leaves, has the neuroprotective effects on glutamate-induced HT22 cell death. J Funct Foods 2014; 9: 162-72.
[http://dx.doi.org/10.1016/j.jff.2014.04.023]

[45]   Li X, Wang T, Zhang D, *et al.* Andrographolide ameliorates intracerebral hemorrhage induced secondary brain injury by inhibiting neuroinflammation induction. Neuropharmacology 2018; 141: 305-15.
[http://dx.doi.org/10.1016/j.neuropharm.2018.09.015] [PMID: 30218674]

[46]   Lu J, Ma Y, Wu J, *et al.* A review for the neuroprotective effects of andrographolide in the central nervous system. Biomed Pharmacother 2019; 117: 109078.
[http://dx.doi.org/10.1016/j.biopha.2019.109078] [PMID: 31181444]

[47]   Saranya P, Geetha A, Karthikeyan S, Selvamathy N. The antioxidant and H+K+ atpase inhibitory effect of *Andrographis paniculata* and andrographolide-*in vitro* and *in vivo* studies. Pharmacologyonline 2010; 1: 356-76.

[48]   Pullaiah CP, Nelson VK, Rayapu S, G v NK, Kedam T. Exploring cardioprotective potential of esculetin against isoproterenol induced myocardial toxicity in rats: *in vivo* and *in vitro* evidence. BMC Pharmacol Toxicol 2021; 22(1): 43.
[http://dx.doi.org/10.1186/s40360-021-00510-0] [PMID: 34266475]

[49]   Lam P, Cheung F, Tan H, Wang N, Yuen M, Feng Y. Hepatoprotective effects of Chinese medicinal herbs: A focus on anti-inflammatory and anti-oxidative activities. Int J Mol Sci 2016; 17(4): 465.
[http://dx.doi.org/10.3390/ijms17040465] [PMID: 27043533]

[50]   Tewari D, Mocan A, Parvanov ED, *et al.* Ethnopharmacological Approaches for Therapy of Jaundice: Part II. Highly Used Plant Species from Acanthaceae, Euphorbiaceae, Asteraceae, Combretaceae, and Fabaceae Families. Front Pharmacol 2017; 8: 519.
[http://dx.doi.org/10.3389/fphar.2017.00519] [PMID: 28848436]

[51]   Shi G, Zhang Z, Zhang R, *et al.* Protective effect of andrographolide against concanavalin A-induced liver injury. Naunyn Schmiedebergs Arch Pharmacol 2012; 385(1): 69-79.
[http://dx.doi.org/10.1007/s00210-011-0685-z] [PMID: 21947229]

[52]   Mondal M, Sarkar C, Saha S, *et al.* Hepatoprotective activity of andrographolide possibly through antioxidative defense mechanism in Sprague-Dawley rats. Toxicol Rep 2022; 9: 1013-22.
[http://dx.doi.org/10.1016/j.toxrep.2022.04.007] [PMID: 36518448]

[53]   Jayakumar T, Hsieh CY, Lee JJ, Sheu JR. Experimental and clinical pharmacology of *Andrographis paniculata* and its major bioactive phytoconstituent andrographolide. Evid Based Complement Alternat Med 2013; 2013: 1-16.
[http://dx.doi.org/10.1155/2013/846740] [PMID: 23634174]

[54]   Masaenah E, Elya B, Setiawan H, *et al.* Antidiabetic activity and acute toxicity of combined extract of *Andrographis paniculata*, *Syzygium cumini*, and *Caesalpinia sappan*. Heliyon 2021; 7(12): e08561.
[http://dx.doi.org/10.1016/j.heliyon.2021.e08561] [PMID: 34950791]

[55]   Nugroho A, Andrie M, Warditiani N, Siswanto E, Pramono S, Lukitaningsih E. Antidiabetic and antihiperlipidemic effect of *Andrographis paniculata* (Burm. f.) Nees and andrographolide in high-fructose-fat-fed rats. Indian J Pharmacol 2012; 44(3): 377-81.
[http://dx.doi.org/10.4103/0253-7613.96343] [PMID: 22701250]

[56]   Suemanotham N, Phochantachinda S, Chatchaisak D, *et al.* Antidiabetic effects of *Andrographis paniculata* supplementation on biochemical parameters, inflammatory responses, and oxidative stress in canine diabetes. Front Pharmacol 2023; 14: 1077228.
[http://dx.doi.org/10.3389/fphar.2023.1077228] [PMID: 36865924]

[57]   Ahmad M, Razak A, Akowuah GA, Asmawi Z, Zhari I. HPLC profile and antihyperglycemic effect of ethanol extracts of *Andrographis paniculata* in normal and streptozotocin-induced diabetic rats. J Nat Med 2007; 61(4): 422-9.
[http://dx.doi.org/10.1007/s11418-007-0157-4]

[58]   Iruretagoyena MI, Tobar JA, González PA, *et al.* Andrographolide interferes with T cell activation and reduces experimental autoimmune encephalomyelitis in the mouse. J Pharmacol Exp Ther 2005; 312(1): 366-72.
[http://dx.doi.org/10.1124/jpet.104.072512] [PMID: 15331658]

[59]   Iruretagoyena MI, Sepúlveda SE, Lezana JP, *et al.* Inhibition of nuclear factor-kappa B enhances the capacity of immature dendritic cells to induce antigen-specific tolerance in experimental autoimmune

encephalomyelitis. J Pharmacol Exp Ther 2006; 318(1): 59-67.
[http://dx.doi.org/10.1124/jpet.106.103259] [PMID: 16597709]

[60]   Naik S, Hule A. Evaluation of immunomodulatory activity of an extract of andrographolides from *Andographis paniculata*. Planta Med 2009; 75(8): 785-91.
[http://dx.doi.org/10.1055/s-0029-1185398] [PMID: 19263340]

[61]   Lee MJ, Rao YK, Chen K, Lee YC, Chung YS, Tzeng YM. Andrographolide and 14-deoxy-11,-2-didehydroandrographolide from *Andrographis paniculata* attenuate high glucose-induced fibrosis and apoptosis in murine renal mesangeal cell lines. J Ethnopharmacol 2010; 132(2): 497-505.
[http://dx.doi.org/10.1016/j.jep.2010.07.057] [PMID: 20813180]

[62]   Akbarsha MA, Murugaian P. Aspects of the male reproductive toxicity/male antifertility property of andrographolide in albino rats: effect on the testis and the cauda epididymidal spermatozoa. Phytother Res 2000; 14(6): 432-5.
[http://dx.doi.org/10.1002/1099-1573(200009)14:6<432::AID-PTR622>3.0.CO;2-I]   [PMID: 10960897]

[63]   Gupta S, Mishra KP, Kumar B, Singh SB, Ganju L. Andrographolide attenuates complete freund's adjuvant induced arthritis *via* suppression of inflammatory mediators and pro-inflammatory cytokines. J Ethnopharmacol 2020; 261: 113022.
[http://dx.doi.org/10.1016/j.jep.2020.113022] [PMID: 32569719]

CHAPTER 7

Andrographolide and its Structural Analogs in Parkinson's Disease

Ravilla Jyothsna Naidu[1], Juturu Mastanaiah[2], Sasikala Chinnappan[3], Boyina Hemanthkumar[4], Alagusundaram Muthumanickam[5], Goli Venkateswarlu[5], Arijit Chaudhuri[5] and Vinod K. Nelson[6,*]

[1] *Department of Pharmacology, Raghavendra Institute of Pharmaceutical Education and Research (RIPER) - Autonomous, Anantapur, Andhra Pradesh, India*

[2] *Department of Pharmacology, Balaji College of Pharmacy, Anantapur, Andhra Pradesh, India*

[3] *Faculty of Pharmaceutical Sciences, UCSI University, Cheras, Kuala Lumpur 56000, Malaysia*

[4] *University Institute of Pharma Sciences, Chandigarh University, Gharuan Mohali 140413, Punjab, India*

[5] *Department of Pharmaceutics, School of Pharmacy, ITM University, Gwalior, Madhya Pradesh, India*

[6] *Centre for Global Health Research, Saveetha Medical College and Hospital, Saveetha Institute of Medical and Technical Sciences, Chennai 602105, Tamil Nadu, India*

Abstract: Parkinson's disease (PD), a leading movement disorder, is instigated due to the progressive apoptosis of dopaminergic neurons in the substantia nigra pars compacta and due to exhausted levels of dopamine in the striatum of the brain. Currently, all treatments available for PD are palliative rather than curative. Researchers are still investigating the complex interplay of genetic and environmental factors that contribute to the development of PD. Natural product's renaissance is due to their ability to target multiple molecular pathways involved in the disease, as well as due to fewer side effects. A diterpenoid lactone compound, andrographolide, is found in the plant *Andrographis paniculata* and is commonly used in traditional medicine to treat various ailments. It has been discovered to have numerous biological activities, including antioxidant, anti-inflammation, anticancer, and neuroprotective effects. In preclinical studies, andrographolide has been shown to have neuroprotective effects in animal models of PD due to its high antioxidant potential, which can help reduce the impact of inflammation in the brain, and its ability to promote the survival and growth of dopaminergic cells. Several structural analogs of andrographolide have been studied for neuroprotective effects, including 14-deoxy-11-oxoandrographolide, 14-deoxy-11, 12-didehydroandrographolide (DDA), and 14-deoxy andrographolide (DA). Both DDA and DA are analogs of andrographolide that have been shown to have neuroprotective effects in animal models of PD disease. DDA is more potent than andrographolide in

* **Corresponding author Vinod K. Nelson:** Centre for Global Health Research, Saveetha Medical College and Hospital, Saveetha Institute of Medical and Technical Sciences, Chennai 602105, Tamil Nadu, India; E-mail: vinod.kumar457@gmail.com

S. Karuppusamy, Vinod K. Nelson & T. Pullaiah (Eds.)

terms of neuroprotection. The anti-inflammatory and antioxidant properties of 14-deoxy-11, 14-deoxy-11, 12-didehydroandrographolide-19-oic acid (DDAA), and 7--Methyl-andrographolide were found to be more potent than andrographolide. On the other hand, andrographolide derivatives, such as 14-deoxyandrographolide, andrographolide epoxide, and andrographolide sulfonates possess potent anti-inflammatory and anticancer properties. Given that andrographolide and its structural analogs and derivatives have substantial therapeutic potential and have been proven to be neuroprotective, we intend to highlight this promising compound's role in PD disease.

Keywords: Andrographolide, Dopaminergic neurons, Parkinson's disease, Structural analogs.

INTRODUCTION

Parkinson's disease (PD) is a progressive neurodegenerative disorder characterized by the degeneration of dopamine-producing neurons in the Substantia Nigra pars compacta (SNpc) region of the brain. The exact cause of PD is unknown, but it is believed to be a complex interplay of genetic and environmental factors. Other potential contributing factors include oxidative stress, neuroinflammation, and accumulation of alpha-synuclein, a protein that agglomerates in the brains of PD patients. The characteristics of PD include tremors that are most noticeable at rest and decrease with movement, the rigidity of the muscles, which causes stiffness and resistance to movement, bradykinesia that affects fine motor skills and overall mobility, and postural instability that can lead to falls. The symptoms of PD typically develop slowly over time and progress as the disease advances, leading to a decline in quality of life and decreased independence. Most cases are diagnosed in people over the age of 60, but it can happen at any age. Men are slightly more likely to develop PD than women. Family history also plays a role, with those who have a first-degree relative with the disease being at higher risk. Additionally, certain environmental factors, such as exposure to certain toxins or pesticides, may increase the risk of developing PD [1].

PD prevalence typically ranges from 100 to 300 per 100,000 people [2]. PD is still comparatively rare despite being the second-most prevalent neurodegenerative illness after Alzheimer's. However, the number of Parkinson's disease patients is expected to quadruple by 2030 as the population ages [3]. With age, the frequency of PD dramatically rises. It is uncommon before the age of 50, and both its incidence and prevalence increase steadily after that. According to a meta-analysis of prevalence studies, the prevalence increased from 107 per 100,000 people between the ages of 50 and 59 to 1087 per 100,000 people between the ages of 70 and 79 [2]. Males typically have PD at a rate of around 1.5 times that of females

[4 - 6]. This difference can be explained by X-linked genetic variables, more frequent occupational exposures in men, and neuroprotection from estrogens in women. Although the amount of the risk varied between studies, ranging from 1.26 to 3.79, most investigations discovered a considerably higher risk of mortality in PD cases compared with individuals free of illness of similar age and gender [7, 8]. According to inception cohorts that monitored incident PD cases, the estimated pooled mortality ratio was estimated to be 1.52 (95% CI: 1.23–1.88) with little heterogeneity, a 5% annual decline in survival for PD patients, and a mean median survival of 12.6 years from disease onset compared to 16.0 years in non-PD subjects. Longer follow-ups led to an increase in mortality ratios. There was no credible evidence that mortality declined after levodopa was introduced. Younger PD patients have a higher mortality risk than older PD patients when compared to age-matched PD-free controls [9, 10]. The severity of axial damage [11], the existence of dementia [12], and the decline in motor function all raise the risk of mortality. The three most significant causes of death in PD are heart disease, pneumonia, and stroke [13 - 17].

The current therapeutic strategy against PD primarily relies on restoring the optimum level of dopamine (DA) and its associated signaling pathways, for which levodopa or L-DOPA (L-3, 4-dihydroxyphenylalanine), a precursor of DA, is administered to PD patients [18]. L-DOPA provides an initial benefit by slowing disease progression; however, long-term benefits are unlikely [19]. Moreover, it is also administered in combination with carbidopa, a peripheral decarboxylase inhibitor. This helps alleviate the side effects of L-DOPA, mainly gastrointestinal and cardiovascular problems [18]. Another PD therapy strategy is using monoamine oxidase B (MAO-B) inhibitors. The activity of the MAO-B enzyme is increased on account of DA metabolism, which elevates oxidative stress and mitochondrial dysfunction [19]. Carbidopa decreases the amount of levodopa and prevents or lessens some of the side effects of levodopa medication, including nausea, vomiting, low blood pressure, and restlessness. Levodopa users should never stop taking it without first consulting a physician. Serious adverse effects from abruptly quitting the medication include becoming immobile or having trouble breathing. Levodopa is needed to improve symptoms. Unfortunately, all existing therapies are palliative rather than curative for PD.

Targeting Ionotropic Glutamate Receptors

It is not unusual that blockers of both classifications of metabotropic glutamate receptors have been investigated for neuroprotective potential, albeit with mixed results, given that both AMPA and NMDA receptors are found within the SNPC. Clinical trials have been conducted with NMDA (N-methyl-D-aspartate) receptor antagonists, including those that target receptors that contain the NR2B subunit.

Studies in the early 1990s initially recognized the advantages of NMDA receptor targeting. For instance, research by Crossman's group demonstrated that administering kynurenic acid and MK-801, two broad-spectrum NMDA antagonists, to MPTP-treated monkeys had antiparkinsonian effects, including a reduction in rigidity, tremor, and akinesia. Like this, when administered to the SNpr or entopeduncular nucleus (a rodent homolog of the internal pallidum), the NMDA antagonist CPP reversed reserpine-induced akinesia in rats. In rat and primate models, systemic administration of these agents alone had little impact [20, 21].

Talampanel (LY300164) and topiramate, which cause dephosphorylation and blockage of AMPA receptors, effectively reduced LID in the MPTP-treated primate. These were two AMPA antagonists that initially showed promise. Unfortunately, these findings did not hold up in clinical settings; three randomized, placebo-controlled trials found no LID reduction when the AMPA antagonist perampanel was given alongside L-DOPA. The potential of selective AMPA receptor antagonists, such as IEM-1460, which is effective in both rat and primate models of LID and appears to prevent the increases in striatal AMPA flip variant subunit expression associated with LID, is currently the focus of research.

Targeting Metabotropic Glutamate (mGlu) Receptors

The antagonists or negative allosteric modulators (NAMs) of this family are the subject of interest because the group I mGlu receptors, mGlu1 and mGlu5, are mostly postsynaptic and couple through Gq/11, leading to more significant neuronal excitation. Agonists or positive allosteric modulators (PAMs) of these receptors are preferred because group II receptors (mGlu2 and mGlu3 in the brain) and group III receptors (mGlu4, 7, and 8 in the brain) coupled with Gi/Go inhibit glutamate release when found on glutamatergic neuron terminals or produce neurotrophic agents when expressed on glia. In mouse models of PD, motor symptoms can be effectively alleviated by group I mGlu receptor antagonists, specifically mGlu5 NAMs like MPEP and MTEP [22].

Mitochondria as Targets in the Treatment of Parkinson's Disease

In the cell cytoplasm, mitochondria are found in groups as free-floating organelles. They are referred to as the cell's "powerhouse". The primary energy source mitochondria (ATP) produces is adenosine 50 triphosphate. They have a very complex structure and are very dynamic. Lipid and amino acid metabolism takes place in the mitochondria. Additionally, they keep the Kreb intermediate products of pyruvate oxidation [23, 24].

Mutations in these genes cause mitochondrial dysfunction, leading to neurodegeneration in PD. Therefore, restoring mitochondrial function will be an important therapeutic strategy for PD. Mitochondrial biogenesis is a promising target for PD. Mitochondria are responsible for producing ROS and antioxidants. They play an essential role in detoxification, apoptosis, and Ca^{2+} buffering, among other things. Therefore, mitochondria can be a potent target for developing new therapeutic strategies. PGC1a, sirtuins, and AMPK pathways are implicated in the mitochondrial biogenesis pathway and as a compensatory mechanism to adapt to mitochondrial defects in PD [20, 25].

The role of midbrain dopamine (DA) neurons in developing the unique nuclear receptor Nurr1 suggests that Nurr1 may be a target for Parkinson's disease. Studies conducted *in vitro* and *in vivo* have shown that Nurr1-activating substances and Nurr1 gene therapy enhance DA neurotransmission and shield DA neurons from the damaging effects of environmental pollutants or microglia-mediated neuroinflammation. Interactions with the retinoid X receptor, neurotropic factors produced by glial cell lines, cyclic AMP-responsive element binding protein, and the Wnt/B catenin pathway may benefit Nurr1-based therapy. A novel treatment method for PD entails testing these molecular processes in IPSC-derived neurons and animal models [23].

Another strategy for creating treatment plans for PD is to modify transcriptional circuits that control antioxidant enzymes or mitochondrial biogenesis. One such pathway is the Nrf2/ARE pathway. Triterpenoids, for example, have been shown to activate this system and provide neuroprotection against MPTP-induced toxicity. In animal models and *in vitro* investigations, the novel medication dimethyl fumarate (DMF) (Tecfidera) activates the Nrf2 pathway to produce anti-inflammatory and antioxidant pathways. It is a potential medicine for the treatment of PD and has been used successfully to treat multiple sclerosis.

Neuroinflammation in Parkinson's Disease

Microglia are inflammatory cells in the brain that serve as the defensive mechanism for neural tissue. Pó Del Ro Hortega initially identified microglia cells in brain tissue samples more than a century ago, using silver carbonate staining. He called microglia the "real third element", following astrocytes and neurons. His description of microglia as a diverse cell type with a range of morphologies, from highly ramified to ameboid-shaped cells, provided a first hint that there might be different subpopulations of microglia.

Alternative strategies that mainly target the transformation of microglia from a proinflammatory (M1) to an anti-inflammatory (M2) state have been proposed, considering these findings [26]. TNF-, IL-1, and IFN-, proinflammatory cytokines, can suppress the M1 state. This theory is supported by the finding that 6-OHDA-treated rats' nigra overexpressed dominant-negative TNF (DN-TNF), which prevented the loss of dopaminergic neurons. Altering the endocannabinoid system may be a different strategy to lessen pro-inflammatory microglial toxicity. Various CNS diseases, including AD and PD, have been reported to increase the expression of the cannabinoid receptor CB2 in glial cells.

Interestingly, while the abundance of CB2 is enhanced in activated PD microglia, an immunolabeling study on human postmortem nigral tissue revealed that CB2 levels are decreased in dopaminergic neurons from PD patients. This observation coincided with diminished tyrosine hydroxylase-containing neurons in the PD tissue. In line with these findings, giving the CB2 agonist caryophyllene to rotenone-challenged rats reduced proinflammatory cytokines' release, preventing dopaminergic neuron degeneration and glial cell activation. Clare Finlay and Duty [27] highlighted the therapeutic potential of targeting glutamate receptors and the role of glutamate in the pathophysiology of Parkinson's disease and examined the possibility of drugs acting at ionotropic or metabotropic glutamate receptors to alleviate its various symptoms based on preclinical and clinical data from past and ongoing studies.

In this context, new therapies for Parkinson's disease are desperately needed, and one of the best paths is to explore Mother Nature for her miraculous gifts that have been showering on humanity for eons.

Importance of Natural Products in Neurodegenerative Disorders

Natural products are crucial in discovering and developing drugs to treat various diseases. The current renaissance of natural products research has the potential to lead to the discovery of new and effective treatments for some of the world's most challenging diseases, such as neurodegenerative disorders [28, 83 - 88]. Plants have played an inevitable role from time immemorial as food, spices, and medicines and have been found to have many phytochemicals with various bioactivities [28, 89 - 94]. Natural product-based agents can lower the potential side effects and offer promising treatment and prevention. Of late, plenty of ethnopharmacological studies have been reported to claim the role of herbal preparations and functional foods in treating or preventing NDDs, which are superior to synthetic drugs. Although the exact molecular mechanism of action remains elusive, optimization of ROS production is a prime target of these natural plant products. The fact that many of the earliest drugs used to treat neurological disorders were derived from plants, including opiate and tropane alkaloids, galantamine, anticholinesterases like physostigmine, and Huperzine A, to name a few, illustrates the importance of plant-derived natural products for the treatment of neurological diseases. According to scientists [29], out of 26 plant-based drugs launched between 2000 and 2006, 7 are for neurological diseases (PD). They noted that 13 plant-derived medications for treating pain and neurological disorders were in various stages of clinical trials in 2006 [29]. Several naturally occurring substances with plant origins can be developed into PD medications.

Antioxidant properties, apoptosis prevention, DA-transporter function inhibition, microglial activation prevention, anti-inflammation, nitric oxide synthesis reduction, monoamine oxidase inhibition, and enhancement of trophic factors, such as brain-derived neurotrophic factor (BDNF) and glial cell line-derived neurotrophic factor (GDNF), are the main mechanisms of neuroprotection. Some additional features are demonstrated by some plant products, *e.g.*, modulation of endogenous transition metal homeostasis, upregulation of heme oxygenase, inhibition of prostaglandin production, regulation of cyclooxygenase-2 activity, and blockage of adenosine A2A receptors.

Until now, mitochondrial dysfunction and altered oxidative stress have been proposed as significant culprits in neuronal cell death. Therefore, therapeutic approaches that optimize reactive oxygen species (ROS) and ameliorate mitochondrial function are being thoroughly considered in the current scenario, and a pharmacological approach involving a natural extract from medicinal plants has been shown to impart a beneficial effect in PD [30].

Research during the last couple of decades has identified several plants that show medicinal properties against PD, like *Bacopa monnieri* [31], *Mucuna pruriens* [32, 33], *Withania somnifera, Curcuma longa* [34 - 36], *Gingko biloba, Camellia sinensis,* and *Andrographis paniculata,* which have been used as anti-PD medications due to their neuroprotective mechanisms that have been scientifically validated, *e.g.*, antiapoptotic, MAO inhibition, antioxidant, and neuroprotective potential in multiple models of the disease. The actions of these herbal extracts or chemicals can be employed to enhance the effectiveness of symptomatic medications already in use, like L-DOPA. They assist in lowering the dosage of these medications to be administered to patients. These natural compounds also have several pharmacological effects relevant to PD therapy, including attenuating behavioral impairments and limiting the death of dopaminergic cells, which is their most significant feature [37].

Andrographolide is a labdane diterpenoid isolated from the leaves and roots of *Andrographis paniculata*. It is a bitter herb commonly used in Siddha, Ayurvedic, and homeopathic medicines, as well as tribal medicines in India and some other countries like Java, Malaysia, Indonesia, the West Indies, Hong Kong, China,

Bangladesh, Pakistan, India, the Philippines, Vietnam, and the United States. The plant is chiefly found in plains throughout India [38].

Pharmacological Effects of Andrographolide

In modern pharmacology, andrographolide has been confirmed both experimentally and clinically to have a broad spectrum of pharmacological activities, including antiplatelet aggregation [39], immunomodulatory activity [40, 41], anticancer [42, 43], anti-inflammatory [44], antivirus [45], antibacterial, antimicrobial [46], antimalarial [47], anti-hepatitis [48, 49], hepatoprotective [50, 51], antioxidant [52], and sexual dysfunction [53]. Additionally, andrographolide effectively prevents the common cold. It significantly improves clinical symptoms such as sore throat, shivering, muscular aches, tiredness, headaches, sinus pain, and rhinitis [54, 55] and plays an essential role in SARS-CoV-2 [56]. It is also the main ingredient of Xiyanping injection, which has been used for decades in treating viral pneumonia, upper respiratory tract infections, and bronchitis in China [57]. Much experimental evidence *in vivo* or *in vitro* shows that *A. paniculata* has an excellent protective and preventive effect on liver-related diseases. *A. paniculata* is effective against viral hepatitis, liver injury, liver fibrosis, fatty liver, and liver cancer. *A. paniculata* inhibits the Nuclear Factor-B (NF-B) pathway and related inflammatory indicators, Tumor Necrosis Factor (TNF-), interleukin-1 (IL-1) interleukin-6 (IL-6), and cyclooxygenase-2 (COX-2), in a dose-dependent manner. As a potent activator of Nrf2, it mediates miRNAs to regulate related enzymes such as HO-1, TXN1, and GSH to reduce oxidative stress. miRNAs play an essential role in regulating tumors [58]. AP cell-dependently prevents further development of liver cancer by causing apoptosis, cell cycle prolongation, and autophagic death. In addition, the downregulation of vascular endothelial growth factor (VEGF) to inhibit angiogenesis can improve the mitigation of liver fibrosis and cancer. Taken together, AP intervenes and treats liver diseases through various signaling pathways. However, AP is rarely used in clinical settings due to its low solubility and bioavailability. Furthermore, andrographolide has amazing hypolipidemic effects in animal models, protecting the cardiovascular system without harming the liver, as well as lowering total cholesterol, triglycerides (TG), LDL, and HDL. *A. paniculata* refined extracts significantly reduced blood glucose, LDL, and TG levels [59].

AGP AND ITS STRUCTURAL ANALOG'S ROLE IN THE PD

AGP Reduces the Activation of NF-κB and Nrf2

The NF-kB transcription factor is one of the most important transcription factors for producing inflammatory mediators that affect microglia-mediated A toxicity. It was studied to see how it affected A (1-42)-induced neuroinflammation. The findings showed that, in comparison to the control groups, A (1–42) significantly decreased the inhibitory kappa (IκB) level and the nuclear NF-κB p65 subunit, indicating NF-κB pathway activation. The results showed that IκB and the nuclear NF-κB p65 subunit alterations were significantly suppressed by pre-treatment with 5 M AGP. As a result, the AGP treatment prevented the NF-κB activation by A (1-42) in BV-2 cells and primary microglia [60, 61].

Further research on the effects of AGP therapy on the Nrf2 protein was conducted in mouse hippocampus HT22 cells. Using a western blot, the expression model of nuclear Nrf2 was examined. In this instance, the AGP treatment (10 M) significantly increased nuclear Nrf2 by 3.4 times and Nrf2 by 2.6 times compared to control cells. Further supporting the translocation of Nrf2 from the cytoplasm to the nucleus was the upregulation of Nrf2 expression following the AGP treatment in both the cytoplasm and the nucleus. The Nrf2 inhibitor Kelch-like ECH-associated protein 1 (Keap1), which is a cytoplasmic protein and a key regulatory component in the oxidative stress signaling pathway [62].

AGP DECREASES THE PRODUCTION OF INFLAMMATORY MEDIATORS

According to the study, AGP therapy after LPS administration reduced TNF- at both the translational (24 and 48 h) and transcriptional levels. The ELISA and RT-PCR results, on the other hand, showed that AGP administration significantly boosted TGF expression at both the translational and transcriptional levels. AGP administration also reduced the translational and transcriptional levels of the IL-1 LPS deponent over 24 hours. Compared to the LPS-induced group, the mixed glial cells' expression of IL-10 increased after receiving AGP therapy. Additionally, the impact of AGP on macrophage inflammasome protein 1 (MIP1), a pro-inflammasome cytokine and another critical indicator of neuroinflammation, was assessed. The western blot test result revealed a significant downregulation of the MIP1 expression [63].

Notably, the prefrontal cortex's expression of iNOS and COX-2 was considerably lowered after taking AGP. According to the immunoblotting results, the level of iNOS in primary cells dramatically decreased compared to the LPS control group. The prefrontal cortex of the mature animal showed lower levels of LPS-induced iNOS mRNA expression. The central microglial culture displayed a considerable elevation of the other microglia phenotypic markers, such as arginase 1, according to the immunofluorescence data (Arg-1). Transforming growth factor beta (TGF-) and interleukin 10 (IL-10) have anti-inflammatory properties and protect neurons from inflammation and degeneration. Tests revealed significantly reduced levels of MIP1 expression. TNF-, another pro-inflammatory glial mediator, is essential in neurodegeneration.

AGP DECREASES TAU PHOSPHORYLATION IN AD MODELS

The tau protein, particularly in its phosphorylated form, is one of AD's most significant and early indicators. This led researchers to investigate the degree of AT8 tau epitope appearance around A plaques. However, since the tau phosphorylation was distributed throughout the cortex and hippocampus, AT8-positive cells in a ring-shaped region around amyloid plaques (r 100 mm) were investigated. The results showed an apparent reduction in AT8-positive neurons near amyloid deposits in young APPswe/PS-1 mice (7 months old). Additionally, the total number of AT8-positive cells in the circular regions near the A plaques rapidly decreased during AGP therapy [64].

AGP DECREASED AB40 AND AB42 PEPTIDES AND AB AGGREGATES IN AD MODELS

The A40 and A42 peptides in the degus' hippocampus were studied using the ELISA experiment to investigate the effects of AGP treatment on cognitive impairment in AD patients and animal models. The findings showed that the AGP treatment decreased the level of A42, which had been rising in old degus. Immunophenotyping, immunofluorescence, and ELISA tests showed that systemic LPS treatment raised the A level in the amygdala and prefrontal cortex compared to control groups. In this instance, AGP therapy significantly lowered the level of the precursor protein for amyloid (APP) in the prefrontal cortical region. After receiving AGP therapy, the prefrontal cortex's response to the LPS-induced elevations in A had significantly recovered. This study also looked at a variation in the hippocampus's caudate nucleus (DG) area, but no appreciable alterations were found [65].

AGP INHIBITS GSK-3B, PREVENTING LTD INDUCTION

An important enzyme called glycogen synthase kinase 3 beta (GSK-3) has been studied in relation to plasticity, memory, and neurodegenerative diseases. The latest studies revealed that transgenic AD models had increased GSK-3 activity. Therefore, immunoblotting was performed to determine how AGP affected GSK-3 activity in the cortex and hippocampus of 12-month-old APPswe/PS-1 mice. The findings revealed that while phosphorylation of an inactive form of GSK-3 increased, phosphorylation of tyrosine 216 (Tyr-216), the active form, reduced. These findings showed that AGP protected synaptic proteins and a specific enzyme in the neuropathology of AD [64].

Andrographolide has a Tmax of 1–2 h and a half-life of 6.6 h in humans, with about 55% of the molecule bound to plasma proteins [66]. In pursuing higher efficacy and lower toxicity, many andrographolide analogs have been isolated or synthesized to improve the therapeutic index for anti-inflammatory treatment. Some analogs that have been evaluated for anti-inflammatory potential are neoandrographolide [67] andrograpanin/14-deoxy andrographolide [68], 14-deoxy-11,12-didehydroandrographolide (DDAG) (Fig. **1**) [69], 14-deoxy-14,-5-dehydroandrographolide [70] 3,19-O-diacetylanhydroandrographolide, 19--acetylanhydroandrographolide, isoandrographolide [71], 3,19-dipalmitoyl--4-deoxy-11,12-didehydroandrographolide [72], andrographolide sulfonate [73] AL1/andrographolide-lipoic acid [74], 3,19-diacetyl-14-deoxy-1-,12-didehydroandrographolide (SRS27) [75], and andrographiside [76]. Among the mentioned andrographolide analogs, 14-deoxy-14,15-dehydroandrgr-apholide, 3,19-O-diacetylanhydro-andrographolide, and 19-O acetylanhydro-andrographolide have been found to have more potent inhibitory effects on NF-κB transactivation, and TNF-α, IL-6, MIP-2 and NO expressions as compared to andrographolide.

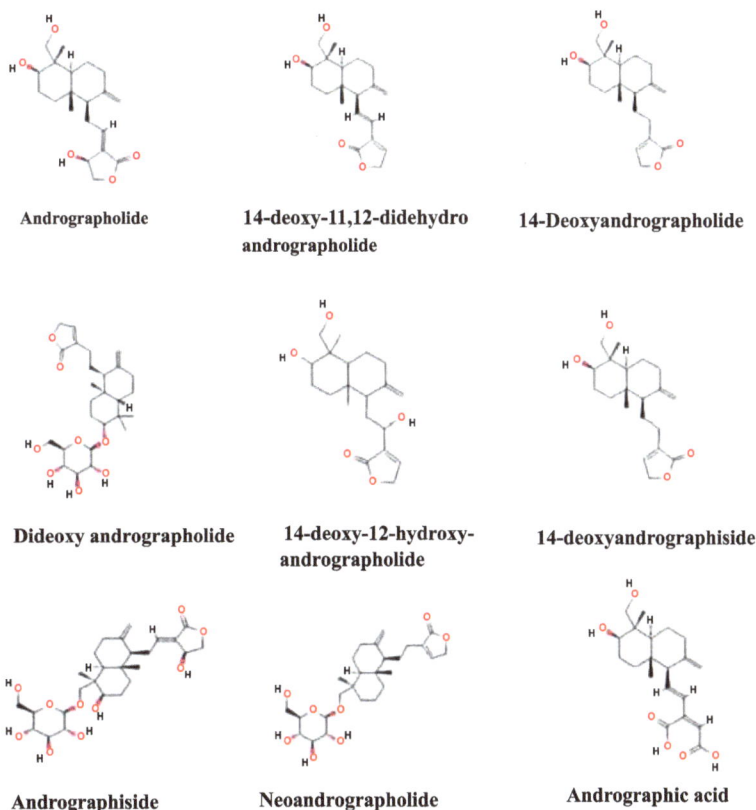

Andrographolide

14-deoxy-11,12-didehydro
andrographolide

14-Deoxyandrographolide

Dideoxy andrographolide

14-deoxy-12-hydroxy-
andrographolide

14-deoxyandrographiside

Andrographiside

Neoandrographolide

Andrographic acid

(Fig. 1) contd.....

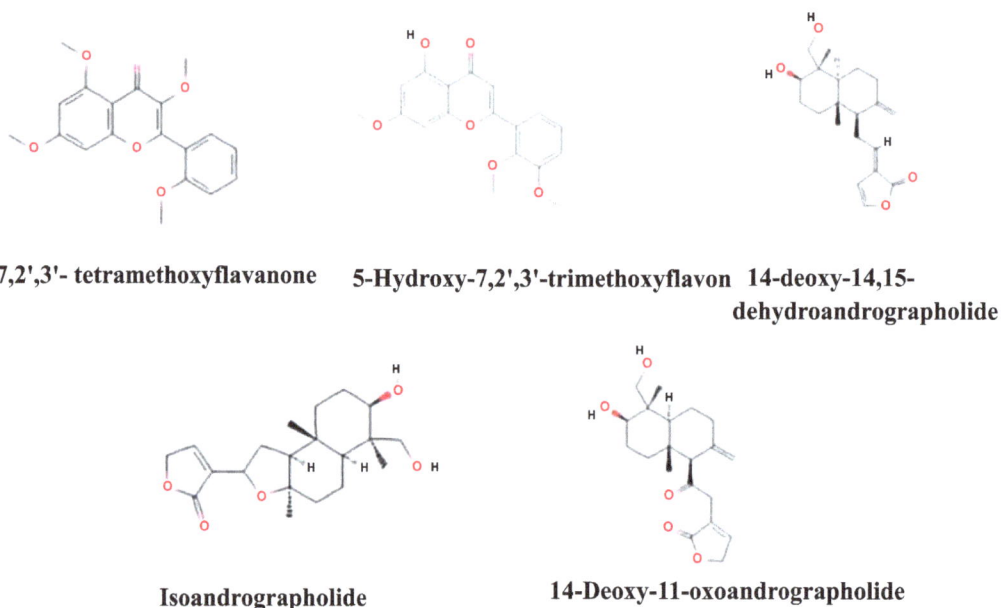

5,7,2',3'- tetramethoxyflavanone   5-Hydroxy-7,2',3'-trimethoxyflavon   14-deoxy-14,15-dehydroandrographolide

Isoandrographolide   14-Deoxy-11-oxoandrographolide

Fig. (1). Chemical structures of andrographolide and its analogs.

Additionally, the results of Wang *et al.* [77] have shown that andrographolide inhibits microglial activation to lessen inflammation-mediated dopaminergic neurotoxicity in mesencephalic neuroglia cultures. Studies by Habtemariam [78] revealed that TNF-induced intercellular adhesion molecule-1 (ICAM-1) expression could be reduced by incubating endothelial cells with non-toxic doses of andrographolide (0.16–16.7 g/mL). Andrographolide also prevented TNF-α induced endothelial-monocyte adhesion at comparable dose ranges in a concentration-dependent manner. Due to its anti-inflammatory properties, this diterpene lactone has also been used to treat cardiovascular disorders and upper respiratory tract infections. For example, Bao *et al.* [79] described that persistent activation of NF-κB has been associated with the development of asthma. Andrographolide has been demonstrated to inhibit NF-κB activity at the level of inhibitory κB kinase-Bactivation. AL-1, andrographolide-lipoic acid conjugate, is a dual-functional agent with both anti-oxidative and anti-inflammatory activities and has been evaluated for treating PD. α-lipoic acid is a potent antioxidant and has been reported to protect against 6-hydroxydopamine-induced neurotoxicity and rotenone-induced damage in nigral dopaminergic neurons in rat models. AL-1 was found to protect against 1-methyl-4-phenylpyridinium (MPP+)-induced neurotoxicity *in vitro* . In an MPP+/1-methyl-4-phenyl-1,2,3,6-tetrahydropyridine (MPTP) mouse model of PD, AL-1 prevented the loss of tyrosine hydroxylase (TH)-positive neurons, minimized impairment in behavior, and enhanced dopamine and 3,4-dihydroxyphenylacetic acid levels. Besides, the levels of NO and MDA were significantly reduced, while the SOD level was upregulated. Immunoblotting assay showed that AL-1 markedly reduced the level of phosphorylated NK-κB p65, providing a molecular mechanism for neuroprotection in PD [79]. Additionally, recent research has suggested that andrographolide may reduce inflammation by modifying neutrophil and macrophage activity. Studies have shown that andrographolide prevents microglial activation, reducing inflammation-mediated dopaminergic neurotoxicity in mesencephalic neuroglia cultures. Additionally, their findings suggested that andrographolide might be clinically useful for the treatment of neurodegenerative illnesses linked to inflammation, such as Parkinson's disease. Studies [80] have revealed for the first time that OVA-induced inflammation, cell recruitment into BAL fluid, IL-4, IL-5, and IL-13, eotaxin production, serum IgE synthesis, pulmonary eosinophilia, mucus hypersecretion, mast cell degranulation, and AhR in a mouse asthma model were all significantly decreased by the naturally occurring non-cytotoxic analog of andrographolide, 14-deoxy-11,12 didehydroandrographolide [81]. In lipopolysaccharide-stimulated macrophages, andrographolide was observed to decrease NF-κB and activation protein binding activity. Additionally, it inhibits the activation of NF-κB and STAT3 by interfering with the expression of SOCS1 and SOCS3 signaling, suppressing the pro-inflammatory genes iNOS and COX-2 [82]. Several of the actions of *A. paniculata* extract described in conventional medicine may be significantly influenced by this function of analogs.

CONCLUSION

There are already several synthetic medications available for the treatment of PD that offer momentary symptom alleviation. Long-term use of these medications can have negative repercussions. Some PD patients may even become resistant to medication. Therefore, testing new bioactive compounds with fewer side effects is necessary to address this significant issue. The phytotherapy may help halt the progression of PD. Generally, andrographolide is a labdane diterpenoid isolated from the leaves and roots of *Andrographis paniculata*. This bitter plant has several beneficial characteristics that can help prevent neurodegeneration. The thorough material in this chapter also concludes regarding the probable function of medicinal herbs and andrographolide in combating the development, progression, and protection against related complications during aging. However, before using these molecules in clinical settings, several of their pharmacokinetic properties need to be investigated. The acute and long-term toxicity must be evaluated in several PD models, along with metabolite synthesis, route of elimination, and their interaction with other commonly used medications, to propose fresh approaches for the treatment of PD and other age-related neurodegenerative illnesses.

REFERENCES

[1] Cha Y, Park TY, Leblanc P, Kim KS. Current status and future perspectives on stem cell-based therapies for Parkinson's disease. J Mov Disord 2023; 16(1): 22-41.
[http://dx.doi.org/10.14802/jmd.22141] [PMID: 36628428]

[2] Pringsheim T, Jette N, Frolkis A, Steeves TDL. The prevalence of Parkinson's disease: A systematic review and meta-analysis. Mov Disord 2014; 29(13): 1583-90.
[http://dx.doi.org/10.1002/mds.25945] [PMID: 24976103]

[3] Dorsey ER, Constantinescu R, Thompson JP, *et al.* Projected number of people with Parkinson disease in the most populous nations, 2005 through 2030. Neurology 2007; 68(5): 384-6.
[http://dx.doi.org/10.1212/01.wnl.0000247740.47667.03] [PMID: 17082464]

[4] Wooten GF, Currie LJ, Bovbjerg VE, Lee JK, Patrie J. Are men at greater risk for Parkinson's disease than women? J Neurol Neurosurg Psychiatry 2004; 75(4): 637-9.
[http://dx.doi.org/10.1136/jnnp.2003.020982] [PMID: 15026515]

[5] Elbaz A, Bower JH, Maraganore DM, *et al.* Risk tables for parkinsonism and Parkinson's disease. J Clin Epidemiol 2002; 55(1): 25-31.
[http://dx.doi.org/10.1016/S0895-4356(01)00425-5] [PMID: 11781119]

[6] Taylor KSM, Cook JA, Counsell CE. Heterogeneity in male to female risk for Parkinson's disease. J Neurol Neurosurg Psychiatry 2007; 78(8): 905-6.
[http://dx.doi.org/10.1136/jnnp.2006.104695] [PMID: 17635983]

[7] Macleod AD, Taylor KSM, Counsell CE. Mortality in Parkinson's disease: A systematic review and meta-analysis. Mov Disord 2014; 29(13): 1615-22.
[http://dx.doi.org/10.1002/mds.25898] [PMID: 24821648]

[8] Elbaz A, Bower JH, Peterson BJ, *et al.* Survival study of Parkinson disease in Olmsted county, Minnesota. Arch Neurol 2003; 60(1): 91-6.
[http://dx.doi.org/10.1001/archneur.60.1.91] [PMID: 12533094]

[9] Hobson P, Meara J, Ishihara-Paul L. The estimated life expectancy in a community cohort of Parkinson's disease patients with and without dementia, compared with the UK population. J Neurol Neurosurg Psychiatry 2010; 81(10): 1093-8.
[http://dx.doi.org/10.1136/jnnp.2009.198689] [PMID: 20571039]

[10] Posada IJ, Benito-León J, Louis ED, *et al.* Mortality from Parkinson's disease: A population-based prospective study (NEDICES). Mov Disord 2011; 26(14): 2522-9.
[http://dx.doi.org/10.1002/mds.23921] [PMID: 21915906]

[11] Levy G, Tang MX, Louis ED, *et al.* The association of incident dementia with mortality in PD. Neurology 2002; 59(11): 1708-13.
[http://dx.doi.org/10.1212/01.WNL.0000036610.36834.E0] [PMID: 12473757]

[12] Ishihara LS, Cheesbrough A, Brayne C, Schrag A. Estimated life expectancy of Parkinson's patients compared with the UK population. J Neurol Neurosurg Psychiatry. 2007;78(12):1304-9.
[http://dx.doi.org/10.1136/jnnp.2006.100107] [PMID: 17400591]

[13] Auyeung M, Tsoi TH, Mok V, *et al.* Ten year survival and outcomes in a prospective cohort of new onset Chinese Parkinson's disease patients. J Neurol Neurosurg Psychiatry 2012; 83(6): 607-11.
[http://dx.doi.org/10.1136/jnnp-2011-301590] [PMID: 22362919]

[14] Driver JA, Smith A, Buring JE, Gaziano JM, Kurth T, Logroscino G. Prospective cohort study of type 2 diabetes and the risk of Parkinson's disease. Diabetes Care 2008; 31(10): 2003-5.
[http://dx.doi.org/10.2337/dc08-0688] [PMID: 18599528]

[15] Duarte J, García Olmos LM, Mendoza A, Clavería LE. The natural history of Parkinson's disease in the province of Segovia: mortality in a longitudinal study (20-year follow-up). Acta Neurol Scand 2013; 127(5): 295-300.
[http://dx.doi.org/10.1111/ane.12003] [PMID: 22957805]

[16]   Pennington S, Snell K, Lee M, Walker R. The cause of death in idiopathic Parkinson's disease. Parkinsonism Relat Disord 2010; 16(7): 434-7.
[http://dx.doi.org/10.1016/j.parkreldis.2010.04.010] [PMID: 20570207]

[17]   Schootman M, Schootman M, Kung N, Evanoff BA, Perlmutter JS, Racette BA. Predictors of survival in patients with Parkinson disease. Arch Neurol 2012; 69(5): 601-7.
[http://dx.doi.org/10.1001/archneurol.2011.2370] [PMID: 22213411]

[18]   Yuan H, Zhang ZW, Liang LW, *et al.* Treatment strategies for Parkinson's disease. Neurosci Bull 2010; 26(1): 66-76.
[http://dx.doi.org/10.1007/s12264-010-0302-z] [PMID: 20101274]

[19]   LeWitt PA, Fahn S. Levodopa therapy for Parkinson disease. Neurology 2016; 86(14_supplement_1) (Suppl. 1): S3-S12.
[http://dx.doi.org/10.1212/WNL.0000000000002509] [PMID: 27044648]

[20]   Finlay C, Duty S. Therapeutic potential of targeting glutamate receptors in Parkinson's disease. J Neural Transm (Vienna) 2014; 121(8): 861-80.
[http://dx.doi.org/10.1007/s00702-014-1176-4] [PMID: 24557498]

[21]   Klockgether T, Turski L. NMDA antagonists potentiate antiparkinsonian actions of L -dopa in monoamine-depleted rats. Ann Neurol 1990; 28(4): 539-46.
[http://dx.doi.org/10.1002/ana.410280411] [PMID: 2252365]

[22]   Conn PJ, Battaglia G, Marino MJ, Nicoletti F. Metabotropic glutamate receptors in the basal ganglia motor circuit. Nat Rev Neurosci 2005; 6(10): 787-98.
[http://dx.doi.org/10.1038/nrn1763] [PMID: 16276355]

[23]   Bose A, Beal MF. Mitochondrial dysfunction in Parkinson's disease. J Neurochem 2016; 139(S1) (Suppl. 1): 216-31.
[http://dx.doi.org/10.1111/jnc.13731] [PMID: 27546335]

[24]   Dong J, Li S, Mo JL, Cai HB, Le WD. Nurr1-based therapies for Parkinson's disease. CNS Neurosci Ther 2016; 22(5): 351-9.
[http://dx.doi.org/10.1111/cns.12536] [PMID: 27012974]

[25]   Tang FL, Liu W, Hu JX, *et al.* VPS35 deficiency or mutation causes dopaminergic neuronal loss by impairing mitochondrial fusion and function. Cell Rep 2015; 12(10): 1631-43.
[http://dx.doi.org/10.1016/j.celrep.2015.08.001] [PMID: 26321632]

[26]   Badanjak K, Fixemer S, Smajić S, Skupin A, Grünewald A. The contribution of microglia to neuroinflammation in Parkinson's disease. Int J Mol Sci 2021; 22(9): 4676.
[http://dx.doi.org/10.3390/ijms22094676] [PMID: 33925154]

[27]   Franco R. Neurotransmitter receptor heteromers in neurodegenerative diseases and neural plasticity. J Neural Transm (Vienna) 2009; 116(8): 983-987

[28]   Newman DJ, Cragg GM. Natural products as sources of new drugs over the 30 years from 1981 to 2010. J Nat Prod 2012; 75(3): 311-35.
[http://dx.doi.org/10.1021/np200906s] [PMID: 22316239]

[29]   Saklani A, Kutty SK. Plant-derived compounds in clinical trials. Drug discovery today. 2008; 13(3-4):161-71.36.
[http://dx.doi.org/10.1016/j.drudis.2007.10.010]

[30]   Sarrafchi A, Bahmani M, Shirzad H, Rafieian-Kopaei M. Oxidative stress and Parkinson's disease: New hopes in treatment with herbal antioxidants. Curr Pharm Des 2015; 22(2): 238-46.
[http://dx.doi.org/10.2174/1381612822666151112151653] [PMID: 26561062]

[31]   Jadiya P, Khan A, Sammi SR, Kaur S, Mir SS, Nazir A. Anti-Parkinsonian effects of *Bacopa monnieri:* Insights from transgenic and pharmacological *Caenorhabditis elegans* models of Parkinson's disease. Biochem Biophys Res Commun 2011; 413(4): 605-10.

[http://dx.doi.org/10.1016/j.bbrc.2011.09.010] [PMID: 21925152]

[32]   Kasture S, Pontis S, Pinna A, *et al.* Assessment of symptomatic and neuroprotective efficacy of *Mucuna pruriens* seed extract in rodent model of Parkinson's disease. Neurotox Res 2009; 15(2): 111-22.
[http://dx.doi.org/10.1007/s12640-009-9011-7] [PMID: 19384573]

[33]   Yadav SK, Rai SN, Singh SP. *Mucuna pruriens* reduces inducible nitric oxide synthase expression in Parkinsonian mice model. J Chem Neuroanat 2017; 80: 1-10.
[http://dx.doi.org/10.1016/j.jchemneu.2016.11.009] [PMID: 27919828]

[34]   van der Merwe C, van Dyk HC, Engelbrecht L, *et al.* Curcumin rescues a PINK1 knock down SH-SY5Y cellular model of Parkinson's disease from mitochondrial dysfunction and cell death. Mol Neurobiol 2017; 54(4): 2752-62.
[http://dx.doi.org/10.1007/s12035-016-9843-0] [PMID: 27003823]

[35]   Zbarsky V, Datla KP, Parkar S, Rai DK, Aruoma OI, Dexter DT. Neuroprotective properties of the natural phenolic antioxidants curcumin and naringenin but not quercetin and fisetin in a 6-OHDA model of Parkinson's disease. Free Radic Res 2005; 39(10): 1119-25.
[http://dx.doi.org/10.1080/10715760500233113] [PMID: 16298737]

[36]   Khuwaja G, Khan MM, Ishrat T, *et al.* Neuroprotective effects of curcumin on 6-hydroxydopamin--induced Parkinsonism in rats: Behavioral, neurochemical and immunohistochemical studies. Brain Res 2011; 1368: 254-63.
[http://dx.doi.org/10.1016/j.brainres.2010.10.023] [PMID: 20951685]

[37]   Nagashayana N, Sankarankutty P, Nampoothiri MRV, Mohan PK, Mohanakumar KP. Association of l-DOPA with recovery following Ayurveda medication in Parkinson's disease. J Neurol Sci 2000; 176(2): 124-7.
[http://dx.doi.org/10.1016/S0022-510X(00)00329-4] [PMID: 10930594]

[38]   Jayakumar T, Hsieh CY, Lee JJ, Sheu JR. Experimental and clinical pharmacology of *Andrographis paniculata* and its major bioactive phytoconstituent andrographolide. Evidence-Based Complementary and Alternative Medicine. 2013; 2013.

[39]   Wu TS, Chern HUEI-JEN, Damu AG, *et al.* Flavonoids and *ent* -labdane diterpenoids from *Andrographis paniculata* and their antiplatelet aggregatory and vasorelaxing effects. J Asian Nat Prod Res 2008; 10(1): 17-24.
[http://dx.doi.org/10.1080/10286020701273627] [PMID: 18058376]

[40]   Naik S, Hule A. Evaluation of immunomodulatory activity of an extract of andrographolides from *Andographis paniculata.* Planta Med 2009; 75(8): 785-91.
[http://dx.doi.org/10.1055/s-0029-1185398] [PMID: 19263340]

[41]   Xu Y, Chen A, Fry S, Barrow RA, Marshall RL, Mukkur TKS. Modulation of immune response in mice immunised with an inactivated Salmonella vaccine and gavaged with *Andrographis paniculata* extract or andrographolide. Int Immunopharmacol 2007; 7(4): 515-23.
[http://dx.doi.org/10.1016/j.intimp.2006.12.008] [PMID: 17321475]

[42]   Rajagopal S, Kumar RA, Deevi DS, Satyanarayana C, Rajagopalan R. Andrographolide, a potential cancer therapeutic agent isolated from *Andrographis paniculata.* J Exp Ther Oncol 2003; 3(3): 147-58.
[http://dx.doi.org/10.1046/j.1359-4117.2003.01090.x] [PMID: 14641821]

[43]   Ajaya Kumar R, Sridevi K, Vijaya Kumar N, Nanduri S, Rajagopal S. Anticancer and immunostimulatory compounds from *Andrographis paniculata.* J Ethnopharmacol 2004; 92(2-3): 291-5.
[http://dx.doi.org/10.1016/j.jep.2004.03.004] [PMID: 15138014]

[44]   Sheeja K, Shihab PK, Kuttan G. Antioxidant and anti-inflammatory activities of the plant *Andrographis paniculata* Nees. Immunopharmacol Immunotoxicol 2006; 28(1): 129-40.
[http://dx.doi.org/10.1080/08923970600626007] [PMID: 16684672]

[45]   Wiart C, Kumar K, Yusof MY, Hamimah H, Fauzi ZM, Sulaiman M. Antiviral properties of ent-labdene diterpenes of *Andrographis paniculata* nees, inhibitors of herpes simplex virus type 1. Phytother Res 2005; 19(12): 1069-70.
[http://dx.doi.org/10.1002/ptr.1765] [PMID: 16372376]

[46]   Dai Y, Chen SR, Chai L, Zhao J, Wang Y, Wang Y. Overview of pharmacological activities of *Andrographis paniculata* and its major compound andrographolide. Critical reviews in food science and nutrition. 2019; 59(sup1):S17-29.

[47]   Misra P, Pal NL, Guru PY, Katiyar JC, Srivastava V, Tandon JS. Antimalarial Activity of *Andrographis paniculata* (Kalmegh) against *Plasmodium berghei* NK 65 in *Mastomys natalensis*. International Journal of Pharmacognosy 1992; 30(4): 263-74.
[http://dx.doi.org/10.3109/13880209209054010]

[48]   Tan BK, Zhang AC. *Andrographis paniculata* and the cardiovascular system. Herbal and Traditional Medicine. CRC Press 2004; pp. 399-415.

[49]   Sharma A, Singh RT, Sehgal V, Handa SS. Antihepatotoxic activity of some plants used in herbal formulations. Fitoterapia 1991; 62(2): 131-8.

[50]   Kapil A, Koul IB, Banerjee SK, Gupta BD. Antihepatotoxic effects of major diterpenoid constituents of *Andrographis paniculata*. Biochem Pharmacol 1993; 46(1): 182-5.
[http://dx.doi.org/10.1016/0006-2952(93)90364-3] [PMID: 8347130]

[51]   Kamdem RE, Sang S, Ho CT. Mechanism of the superoxide scavenging activity of neoandrographolide - a natural product from *Andrographis paniculata* Nees. J Agric Food Chem 2002; 50(16): 4662-5.
[http://dx.doi.org/10.1021/jf025556f] [PMID: 12137494]

[52]   Singh RP, Banerjee S, Rao AR. Modulatory influence of *Andrographis paniculata* on mouse hepatic and extrahepatic carcinogen metabolizing enzymes and antioxidant status. Phytother Res 2001; 15(5): 382-90.
[http://dx.doi.org/10.1002/ptr.730] [PMID: 11507728]

[53]   Akbarsha MA, Murugaian P. Aspects of the male reproductive toxicity/male antifertility property of andrographolide in albino rats: effect on the testis and the cauda epididymidal spermatozoa. Phytother Res 2000; 14(6): 432-5.
[http://dx.doi.org/10.1002/1099-1573(200009)14:6<432::AID-PTR622>3.0.CO;2-I]   [PMID: 10960897]

[54]   Hancke J, Burgos R, Caceres D, Wikman G. A double-blind study with a new monodrug Kan Jang: Decrease of symptoms and improvement in the recovery from common colds. Phytother Res 1995; 9(8): 559-62.
[http://dx.doi.org/10.1002/ptr.2650090804]

[55]   Cáceres DD, Hancke JL, Burgos RA, Wikman GK. Prevention of common colds with *Andrographis paniculata* dried extract. A Pilot double blind trial. Phytomedicine 1997; 4(2): 101-4.
[http://dx.doi.org/10.1016/S0944-7113(97)80051-7] [PMID: 23195395]

[56]   Sa-ngiamsuntorn K, Suksatu A, Pewkliang Y, *et al.* Anti-SARS-CoV-2 activity of *Andrographis paniculata* extract and its major component andrographolide in human lung epithelial cells and cytotoxicity evaluation in major organ cell representatives. J Nat Prod 2021; 84(4): 1261-70.
[http://dx.doi.org/10.1021/acs.jnatprod.0c01324] [PMID: 33844528]

[57]   Zhang XY, Lv L, Zhou YL, *et al.* Efficacy and safety of Xiyanping injection in the treatment of COVID -19: A multicenter, prospective, open-label and randomized controlled trial. Phytother Res 2021; 35(8): 4401-10.
[http://dx.doi.org/10.1002/ptr.7141] [PMID: 33979464]

[58]   Khan NH, Mir M, Ngowi EE, *et al.* Nanomedicine: A Promising way to manage Alzheimer's disease. Front Bioeng Biotechnol 2021; 9: 630055.

[http://dx.doi.org/10.3389/fbioe.2021.630055] [PMID: 33996777]

[59]   Zeng B, Wei A, Zhou Q, *et al.* Andrographolide: A review of its pharmacology, pharmacokinetics, toxicity and clinical trials and pharmaceutical researches. Phytother Res 2022; 36(1): 336-64.
[http://dx.doi.org/10.1002/ptr.7324] [PMID: 34818697]

[60]   Abedi Z, Basri H, Hassan Z, Mat LNI, Khaza'ai H, Mohamad NA. A review of the neuroprotective effects of andrographolide in Alzheimer's disease. Advances in Traditional Medicine 2021; 21(2): 253-66.
[http://dx.doi.org/10.1007/s13596-021-00573-8]

[61]   Das S, Mishra KP, Ganju L, Singh SB. Andrographolide - A promising therapeutic agent, negatively regulates glial cell derived neurodegeneration of prefrontal cortex, hippocampus and working memory impairment. J Neuroimmunol 2017; 313: 161-75.
[http://dx.doi.org/10.1016/j.jneuroim.2017.11.003] [PMID: 29146293]

[62]   Yang D, Zhang W, Song L, Guo F. Andrographolide protects against cigarette smoke-induced lung inflammation through activation of heme oxygenase-1. J Biochem Mol Toxicol 2013; 27(5): 259-65.
[http://dx.doi.org/10.1002/jbt.21483] [PMID: 23629921]

[63]   Liu C, Liang MC, Soong TW. Nitric oxide, iron and neurodegeneration. Front Neurosci 2019; 13: 114.
[http://dx.doi.org/10.3389/fnins.2019.00114] [PMID: 30833886]

[64]   Collingridge GL, Peineau S, Howland JG, Wang YT. Long-term depression in the CNS. Nat Rev Neurosci 2010; 11(7): 459-73.
[http://dx.doi.org/10.1038/nrn2867] [PMID: 20559335]

[65]   Wang L, Cao F, Zhu L, *et al.* Andrographolide impairs alpha-naphthylisothiocyanate-induced cholestatic liver injury in vivo. J Nat Med 2019; 73(2): 388-96.
[http://dx.doi.org/10.1007/s11418-018-01275-3] [PMID: 30617707]

[66]   Panossian A, Hovhannisyan A, Mamikonyan G, *et al.* Pharmacokinetic and oral bioavailability of andrographolide from *Andrographis paniculata* fixed combination Kan Jang in rats and human. Phytomedicine 2000; 7(5): 351-64.
[http://dx.doi.org/10.1016/S0944-7113(00)80054-9] [PMID: 11081986]

[67]   Kumar G, Singh D, Tali JA, Dheer D, Shankar R. Andrographolide: Chemical modification and its effect on biological activities. Bioorg Chem. 2020; 95:103511.
[http://dx.doi.org/10.1016/j.bioorg.2019.103511] [PMID: 31884143]

[68]   Chandrasekaran CV, Thiyagarajan P, Deepak HB, Agarwal A. *In vitro* modulation of LPS/calcimycin induced inflammatory and allergic mediators by pure compounds of *Andrographis paniculata* (King of bitters) extract. Int Immunopharmacol 2011; 11(1): 79-84.
[http://dx.doi.org/10.1016/j.intimp.2010.10.009] [PMID: 21034865]

[69]   Tzeng YM, Lee YC, Cheng WT, *et al.* Effects of andrographolide and 14-deoxy-11,-2-didehydroandrographolide on cultured primary astrocytes and PC12 cells. Life Sci 2012; 90(7-8): 257-66.
[http://dx.doi.org/10.1016/j.lfs.2011.11.004] [PMID: 22154981]

[70]   Chao WW, Kuo YH, Lin BF. Anti-inflammatory activity of new compounds from *Andrographis paniculata* by NF-kappaB transactivation inhibition. J Agric Food Chem 2010; 58(4): 2505-12.
[http://dx.doi.org/10.1021/jf903629j] [PMID: 20085279]

[71]   Suebsasana S, Pongnaratorn P, Sattayasai J, Arkaravichien T, Tiamkao S, Aromdee C. Analgesic, antipyretic, anti-inflammatory and toxic effects of andrographolide derivatives in experimental animals. Arch Pharm Res 2009; 32(9): 1191-200.
[http://dx.doi.org/10.1007/s12272-009-1902-x] [PMID: 19784573]

[72]   Guo W, Liu W, Chen G, *et al.* Water-soluble andrographolide sulfonate exerts anti-sepsis action in mice through down-regulating p38 MAPK, STAT3 and NF-κB pathways. Int Immunopharmacol 2012; 14(4): 613-9.

[http://dx.doi.org/10.1016/j.intimp.2012.09.002] [PMID: 23036579]

[73]   Yang Y, Yan H, Jing M, *et al*. Andrographolide derivative AL-1 ameliorates TNBS-induced colitis in mice: involvement of NF-κB and PPAR-γ signaling pathways. Sci Rep 2016; 6(1): 29716.
[http://dx.doi.org/10.1038/srep29716] [PMID: 27435110]

[74]   Lim JCW, Goh FY, Sagineedu SR, *et al*. A semisynthetic diterpenoid lactone inhibits NF-κB signalling to ameliorate inflammation and airway hyperresponsiveness in a mouse asthma model. Toxicol Appl Pharmacol 2016; 302: 10-22.
[http://dx.doi.org/10.1016/j.taap.2016.04.004] [PMID: 27089844]

[75]   Zhang H, Li S, Si Y, Xu H. Andrographolide and its derivatives: Current achievements and future perspectives. Eur J Med Chem. 2021; 224:113710.
[http://dx.doi.org/10.1016/j.ejmech.2021.113710] [PMID: 34315039]

[76]   Toppo E, Al-Dhabi N, Sankar C, *et al*. Hepatoprotective effect of selected isoandrographolide derivatives on steatotic HepG2 cells and High Fat Diet fed rats. Eur J Pharmacol 2021; 899: 174056

[77]   Wang T, Liu B, Zhang W, Wilson B, Hong JS. Andrographolide reduces inflammation-mediated dopaminergic neurodegeneration in mesencephalic neuron-glia cultures by inhibiting microglial activation. J Pharmacol Exp Ther 2004; 308(3): 975-83.
[http://dx.doi.org/10.1124/jpet.103.059683] [PMID: 14718612]

[78]   Habtemariam S. Andrographolide inhibits the tumour necrosis factor-α-induced upregulation of ICAM-1 expression and endothelial-monocyte adhesion. Phytother Res 1998; 12(1): 37-40.
[http://dx.doi.org/10.1002/(SICI)1099-1573(19980201)12:1<37::AID-PTR186>3.0.CO;2-N]

[79]   Bao Z, Guan S, Cheng C, *et al*. A novel antiinflammatory role for andrographolide in asthma *via* inhibition of the nuclear factor-kappaB pathway. Am J Respir Crit Care Med 2009; 179(8): 657-65.
[http://dx.doi.org/10.1164/rccm.200809-1516OC] [PMID: 19201922]

[80]   Guan SP, Kong LR, Cheng C, Lim JCW, Wong WSF. Protective role of 14-deoxy-11,-2-didehydroandrographolide, a noncytotoxic analogue of andrographolide, in allergic airway inflammation. J Nat Prod 2011; 74(6): 1484-90.
[http://dx.doi.org/10.1021/np2002572] [PMID: 21598983]

[81]   Lee YC, Lin HH, Hsu CH, Wang CJ, Chiang TA, Chen JH. Inhibitory effects of andrographolide on migration and invasion in human non-small cell lung cancer A549 cells *via* down-regulation of PI3K/Akt signaling pathway. Eur J Pharmacol 2010; 632(1-3): 23-32.
[http://dx.doi.org/10.1016/j.ejphar.2010.01.009] [PMID: 20097193]

[82]   Lee KC, Chang HH, Chung YH, Lee TY. Andrographolide acts as an anti-inflammatory agent in LPS-stimulated RAW264.7 macrophages by inhibiting STAT3-mediated suppression of the NF-κB pathway. J Ethnopharmacol 2011; 135(3): 678-84.
[http://dx.doi.org/10.1016/j.jep.2011.03.068] [PMID: 21497192]

[83]   Ghosh S, Hazra J, Pal K, Nelson VK, Pal M. Prostate cancer: Therapeutic prospect with herbal medicine. Current Research in Pharmacology and Drug Discovery 2021; 2: 100034.
[http://dx.doi.org/10.1016/j.crphar.2021.100034] [PMID: 34909665]

[84]   Nelson VK, Paul S, Roychoudhury S, *et al*. Heat shock factors in protein quality control and spermatogenesis. Adv Exp Med Biol 2022; 1391: 181-99.
[http://dx.doi.org/10.1007/978-3-031-12966-7_11] [PMID: 36472823]

[85]   Nelson VK, Pullaiah CP, Saleem TS M, *et al*. Natural products as the modulators of oxidative stress: An herbal approach in the management of prostate cancer. Adv Exp Med Biol 2022; 1391: 161-79.
[http://dx.doi.org/10.1007/978-3-031-12966-7_10] [PMID: 36472822]

[86]   Dutta N, Pemmaraju DB, Ghosh S, *et al*. Alkaloid-rich fraction of *Ervatamia coronaria* sensitizes colorectal cancer through modulating AMPK and mTOR signalling pathways. J Ethnopharmacol 2022; 283: 114666.
[http://dx.doi.org/10.1016/j.jep.2021.114666] [PMID: 34592338]

[87]   Dutta N, Ghosh S, Nelson VK, *et al.* Andrographolide upregulates protein quality control mechanisms in cell and mouse through upregulation of mTORC1 function. Biochim Biophys Acta, Gen Subj 2021; 1865(6): 129885.
[http://dx.doi.org/10.1016/j.bbagen.2021.129885] [PMID: 33639218]

[88]   Badavenkatappa gari S, Nelson VK, Peraman R. *Tinospora sinensis* (Lour.) Merr alkaloid rich extract induces colon cancer cell death *via* ROS mediated, mTOR dependent apoptosis pathway: "an *in-vitro* study". BMC Complementary Medicine and Therapies 2023; 23(1): 33.
[http://dx.doi.org/10.1186/s12906-023-03849-5] [PMID: 36737760]

[89]   De S, Paul S, Manna A, *et al.* Phenolic phytochemicals for prevention and treatment of colorectal cancer: A critical evaluation of *in vivo* studies. Cancers (Basel) 2023; 15(3): 993.
[http://dx.doi.org/10.3390/cancers15030993] [PMID: 36765950]

[90]   Pullaiah CP, Nelson VK, Rayapu S, G v NK, Kedam T. Exploring cardioprotective potential of esculetin against isoproterenol induced myocardial toxicity in rats: *in vivo* and *in vitro* evidence. BMC Pharmacol Toxicol 2021; 22(1): 43.
[http://dx.doi.org/10.1186/s40360-021-00510-0] [PMID: 34266475]

[91]   Nelson V, Sahoo NK, Sahu M, Sudhan H, Pullaiah CP, Muralikrishna KS. *In vitro* anticancer activity of *Eclipta alba* whole plant extract on colon cancer cell HCT-116. BMC Complementary Medicine and Therapies 2020; 20(1): 355.
[http://dx.doi.org/10.1186/s12906-020-03118-9] [PMID: 33225921]

[92]   Singh BK, Vatsa N, Nelson VK, *et al.* Azadiradione restores protein quality control and ameliorates the disease pathogenesis in a mouse model of Huntington's disease. Mol Neurobiol 2018; 55(8): 6337-46.
[http://dx.doi.org/10.1007/s12035-017-0853-3] [PMID: 29294248]

[93]   Nelson VK, Ali A, Dutta N, *et al.* Azadiradione ameliorates polyglutamine expansion disease in *Drosophila* by potentiating DNA binding activity of heat shock factor 1. Oncotarget 2016; 7(48): 78281-96.
[http://dx.doi.org/10.18632/oncotarget.12930] [PMID: 27835876]

[94]   Mandal S, Nelson VK, Mukhopadhyay S, *et al.* 14-Deoxyandrographolide targets adenylate cyclase and prevents ethanol-induced liver injury through constitutive NOS dependent reduced redox signaling in rats. Food Chem Toxicol 2013; 59: 236-48.
[http://dx.doi.org/10.1016/j.fct.2013.05.056] [PMID: 23764359]

CHAPTER 8

Neuroprotective Potential of Andrographolide (AG) and its Structural Analogs in Alzheimer's Disease

Beere Vishnusai[1], **Alugubelli Gopi Reddy**[2], **Sasikala Chinnappan**[3], **Jayaraman Rajangam**[4], **Angala Parameswari Sundaramoorthy**[5], **Vijeta Bhattacharya**[6], **Namrata Mishra**[6], **Vinyas Mayasa**[7] and **Vinod K. Nelson**[8,*]

[1] *Department of Pharmacology and Toxicology, National Institute of Pharmaceutical Education and Research, Hajipur, Bihar, India*

[2] *Department of Pharmaceutical Chemistry, Sana College of Pharmacy, Kodad, Suryapet Dist, Telangana, India*

[3] *Faculty of Pharmaceutical Sciences, UCSI University, Cheras, Kuala Lumpur56000, Malaysia*

[4] *AMITY Institute of Pharmacy, AMITY University, Lucknow Campus, Uttar Pradesh-226010, India*

[5] *Department of Pharmaceutical Analysis, Ratnam Institute of Pharmacy, Pidathapolur, Nellore, Andhra Pradesh, India*

[6] *Department of Pharmaceutics, School of Pharmacy, ITM University, Gwalior, Madhya Pradesh, India*

[7] *GITAM School of Pharmacy, Gandhi Institute of Technology and Management Deemed to be University, Rudraram, Telangana-502329, India*

[8] *Centre for Global Health Research, Saveetha Medical College and Hospital, Saveetha Institute of Medical and Technical Sciences, Chennai 602105, Tamil Nadu, India*

Abstract: Alzheimer's disease (AD) is a brain disorder that usually has a chronic or progressive nature and results in a reduction in cognitive function that is more than what would be expected from the typical effects of the biological aging process, which is a significant cause of dementia. Even though tau and amyloid-β (Aβ) have been identified as the main components in the formation of tangles and plaques, respectively, there is still little known about the causes of Alzheimer's disease, and no effective treatments are available. It affects an estimated 40 million people worldwide, most of whom are over 60, and is expected to double every 20 years, at least until 2050. Most current efforts at therapeutic intervention are based on the hypothesized pathogenic mechanisms for AD. These include amyloids, inflammatory mediators, excitotoxicity, steroid hormone deficiencies, loss of cholinergic function, dietary fac-

Corresponding author Vinod K. Nelson: Centre for Global Health Research, Saveetha Medical College and Hospital, Saveetha Institute of Medical and Technical Sciences, Chennai 602105, Tamil Nadu, India;
E-mail: vinod.kumar457@gmail.com

S. Karuppusamy, Vinod K. Nelson & T. Pullaiah (Eds.)

tors, oxidative stress, band g-secretase effectors, *etc.* Still, these therapies were neither completely effective nor safe for prolonged usage to check this problem. Various natural products have been tested. One such natural product is andrographolide (AG), which has several potential therapeutic benefits, including anti-inflammatory, immunomodulatory, and antiangiogenic properties. It is traditionally used for the treatment of various ailments. AG and its derivatives were found to be effective in the reduction of synaptic proteins associated with Alzheimer's disease by overturning the microglia-mediated growth of pro-inflammatory cytokines, and the research has shown that these compounds decrease amyloid beta aggregation and suppress the neuro-inflammatory response and synaptic dysfunction. In the current review, the therapeutic potential of andrographolide and its analogs is outlined, and its mechanism of action against this disease is examined to explore the possibility of AG for the prevention and treatment of AD.

Keywords: Alzheimer's disease, Andrographolide, Amyloid beta, Dementia, Neurodegenerative disorder.

INTRODUCTION

Dementia is a disorder that typically has a persistent or progressive nature and results in a fall in cognitive capability (*i.e.*, the capacity for mental processing) further than what might be predicted from the usual effects of the biological aging process. Memory, thinking, direction, comprehension, computation, language, learning capacity, and judgment are all impacted. Consciousness is not affected. The impairment of cognitive function is frequently accompanied by fluctuations in mood, emotional stability, patterns of behavior, or motivation, but they can also happen before it [1]. One of the primary healthcare challenges of the 21st century is Alzheimer's disease, which is the leading cause of dementia. Three main groups of symptoms make up the chronic, progressive neurodegenerative disorder known as Alzheimer's disease. Memory loss, difficulty speaking and understanding, and executive dysfunction are all included in the first category of cognitive dysfunction. The second category includes behavioral and mental health issues, such as agitation, hallucinations, depression, and delusions, which are collectively referred to as non-cognitive symptoms; the third category consists of people who have trouble performing daily activities of living (considered "basic" for getting dressed and eating by themselves, *etc.*) [2].

In December 2013, the G8 declared that dementia should receive international attention and expressed their hope that a treatment or a cure would be readily accessible by 2025 [3]. Since tau and amyloid β (Aβ) were discovered to be the core elements of plaques and tangles, there has been significant progress in our understanding of molecular pathogenetic events; however, little is known about the causes of AD, and there is no cure. Aβ plaques and NFTs are the disease's two primary pathological markers. As per the amyloid cascade hypothesis, brain dysfunction and neuronal death are brought on by the buildup of amyloid beta (Aβ) [4]. Furthermore, although the presence of Alzheimer's pathological changes is a requirement for diagnosis and is sufficient in some patients to cause symptoms, patients who develop symptoms after the age of 75 may have multiple causes [3].

Dementia affects an estimated 40 million people worldwide, most of whom are over 60, and is expected to replicate every 20 years, at least until 2050 [5]. AD is the 6th most common cause of mortality in the USA and the 5th most common cause of death for people over 65. Even though deaths from other leading causes have dropped significantly in recent years, the proportion of deaths related to AD has increased sharply. Heart disease, stroke, and prostate cancer deaths as a percentage of all deaths decreased between 2000 and 2008, while AD deaths as a percentage of all deaths increased by 66% [6].

In developing countries with young populations, the projected increase in dementia prevalence is significantly higher than in Western Europe and the USA, where the population is already far older. There are few accurate projections of the incidence of early-onset dementia and Alzheimer's disease (before age 65). Dementia affects fewer than one in 4000 people before they turn fifty, with AD accounting for about 30% of cases [7]. Around 800,000 people with AD live alone (1 in 7), and up to 50% of them lack a caregiver. Dementia patients who live alone are more likely to experience risks such as poor self-care, untreated medical conditions, malnutrition, falls, wandering off unattended, and accidental deaths than those who live with others [6].

Most current efforts at therapeutic intervention are based on the hypothesized pathogenic mechanisms for AD. These include the amyloid cascade, inflammatory mediators [NSAIDs], excitotoxicity (memantine), steroid hormone deficiencies, loss of cholinergic function, dietary factors, oxidative stress (antioxidant therapy), and band g-secretase effectors [8].

It has been discovered that cognitive dysfunction and the loss of cholinergic function are closely related. Inhibition of cholinesterase, postsynaptic cholinergic excitation with muscarinic agonists, precursors of choline, and stimulation of presynaptic cholinergic receptors with nicotinic agonists are some of the therapeutics that have been studied over the past 20 years [9].

It has been known since 1986 that nerve growth factor (NGF) infused into the rat brain stops basal frontal brain cholinergic neuron destruction, both naturally and after injury [10]. However, because the NGF protein cannot cross the blood-brain barrier (BBB), it has a short half-life and a significant impact on biological signals; it has proven difficult to deliver these neurotrophins effectively in the clinical setting [11]. Oxidative stress is a crucial pathogenic process connected to aging and AD, according to a wealth of research. Therefore, antioxidants may lessen cognitive impairment in AD or slow the condition's progression [12].

Simvastatin has been demonstrated to reduce cerebral Aβ levels *in vivo* [13], and just recently, a study that showed a neuropathological change associated with statin use (a reduction in the burden of neurofibrillary tangles at autopsy) was published [14]. However, recent extensive prospective cohort studies and two significant randomized placebo-controlled experiments of statins for the prevention of CHD failed to demonstrate any evidence of a protective effect against cognitive impairment [15, 16]. Estrogen modifies the impact of nerve growth factors, raises blood supply to the brain, avoids cholinergic neuron atrophy, reduces oxidative stress, and more [17].

Since there is no effective treatment for AD as of now, present approved drug treatments have focused entirely on managing symptoms and delaying the progression of the illness. AD is a progressive neurodegenerative disorder. Natural products can provide various options to lessen disease progression and symptoms. Natural products have once again been recognized as a source of innovative medicines due to the prominence of secondary metabolites as an essential and distinctive compound. A novel therapeutic strategy for treating AD uses natural products. The ability of natural substances to treat various diseases and other conditions associated with aging and AD has also been demonstrated [18].

The prevention and treatment of AD require the use of neuroprotective strategies with a variety of mechanisms of action. Compositions or derivatives of natural products with a range of bioactive components and neuroprotective properties are preferred in the hunt for new anti-AD medications. If more thorough and practical quality control guidelines are created to ensure the safety and efficacy of these therapies, as well as novel approaches and ways to promote the CNS access of these neuroprotective substances, such as the inclusion of nanotechnology in the transport of natural products, then natural product therapy can play a crucial role in the prevention and treatment of AD [19]. The lack of effective medications or treatments for AD has given researchers a fresh outlook on developing new and effective medicines from natural sources.

Andrographolide is a natural compound with a bitter taste found in the areal parts of the plant *Andrographis paniculata*. Chemically, it is a bicyclic diterpenoid lactone; it has a variety of pharmacological uses. Treatments of fever, tuberculosis, common cold, upper respiratory tract infection (URTI), inflammation, tonsillitis, pharyngitis, laryngitis, hepatic impairment, *etc.*, are some traditional uses [22].

Since the discovery of AG, significant efforts have been made to identify novel, highly potent analogs with various biological functions by chemical modifications. Several new andrographolide pharmacological effects, numerous new analogs with outstanding biological profiles, and varied modes of action have been discovered, which is encouraging [24]. Only andrographolide and a handful of its derivatives were studied in clinical trials; as a result, the majority of the findings for AG and its derivatives were restricted to *in vitro* and *in vivo* [animal] investigations. For instance, AGs impressive anticancer properties have prompted some clinical investigations to assess its possible use in chemotherapy [25]. In addition to their anticancer properties, andrographolide and its derivatives as a drug will include further research into their well-known and extensively studied anti-fibrosis and anti-inflammation potential [21] and their alluring anti-virus effect in clinical trials [23].

The recovery followed the treatment with Andrographolide (AG) in numerous neurotoxicity studies and various AD model systems, which is evidence of the neuroprotective effect of AG. Aging and environmental toxins cause cognitive decline, which is associated with diminished synaptic activity and an increase in primary AD symptoms [20]. Through a variety of mechanisms, from antioxidation to anti-neuroinflammation, andrographolide affects CNS disorders like cerebral ischemia and multiple sclerosis in a preventative and therapeutic manner. AG's anti-inflammatory and antioxidative effects may be linked since it has been widely reported that the induction of Nrf2-mediated anti-oxidative response mediates the anti-inflammatory potential of AG in a wide range of cell types, including epithelial cells and PC12 cells [26]. This is due to the discovery that the NF-KB is a moderator in generating mediators indicative of high levels of oxidative stress, such as NO and ROS [27].

The neuroprotective effects of andrographolide in the CNS may also be mediated by a variety of additional mechanisms, including inhibition of damage to the cerebral endothelial cells, the restoration of BBB integrity and synaptic function, promotion of VSMC apoptosis, VSMC proliferation, and hippocampal neurogenesis, as well as suppression of platelet activation and aggregation and inhibition of Aβ aggregation [20].

Risk Factors involved in Alzheimer's Disease

Over 20 risk factors, including age, hereditary, aluminum exposure, brain trauma (TBI), and co-morbid conditions like cardiovascular diseases and infection, were discovered in early studies of Alzheimer's disease (AD). In light of recent research, we discuss these risk factors, identify those deemed necessary, and discuss how they affect AD prevention and treatment [28, 29]. According to more recent research, different risk factors were also identified, and some of the factors that Henderson [30] discussed have seen increased support. Therefore, in a recent study, over sixty environmental risk factors were linked to AD and categorized into several groups. It is still challenging to understand how many seemingly unrelated risk factors can cause AD [31].

The etiology of AD has been the subject of numerous theories over the years, which can be categorized into two main groups. The lymphatic system hypothesis, cholinergic hypothesis, vascular dysfunction hypothesis, metal ion hypothesis, and inflammation hypothesis are a few theories that explain potential causes of AD. Second, some theories, such as the mitochondrial cascade, amyloid cascade, hypothesis of tau propagation, and calcium homeostasis hypothesis, place more emphasis on the pathological events that occur after AD has begun [32]. However, no one theory has received widespread acceptance, and it is now generally accepted that several risk factors are probably at play. Some of these risk factors are discussed below:

Age

Numerous epidemiological studies concur that age is among the most significant risk factors for cognitive impairment and AD among the different demographic factors like age, gender, race, and social class [33]. The prevalence of AD rises with age, reaching an estimated 19% in people aged 75 to 84 [34] and 30–35%, possibly even 50%, in people over 85 [35]. Given that many of the biological changes linked to Alzheimer's disease are similar to those present in normal aging, except for severity, AD may be an accelerated condition of normal aging. Thus, there is an age-related reduction in brain size and mass, expansion of ventricles, and decline of synapses and dendrites in particular areas alongside immunoreactive senile plaques [SP] and NFTs in the brain of cognitively normal individuals [36].

Genetic Factors

There was constant evidence that first-level relatives of these patients had a higher risk of dementia themselves, despite challenges in analyzing initial findings of familial cases, such as biased recollection by relatives and the precise disorders that were present [30]. In a previous study, Heyman *et al.* emphasized that the genetic link's strength differed among individuals [37]. Early-onset familial AD is typically brought on by autosomal dominant genetic variations in the APP, presenilin 1 and 2 genes. About 2-5% of AD cases are this type [38].

Regarding genetic influences, the apoE4 allele of apolipoprotein E [APOE] may play a role in this risk. The pathology of this mental disorder is also influenced by other genes [39]. The only genetic component that has been proven to play a role in both the early-onset and late-onset forms of AD is the apoE4 allele. Although it makes people more vulnerable to AD, this factor is neither required nor sufficient for the disease to manifest. With age, the risk associated with having the apoE4 allele decreases. Generally speaking, this risk may be responsible for 15–20% of AD cases [40].

Vascular Risk Factors

Several connections between Alzheimer's disease and cardiovascular diseases [CVDs] have been found in numerous studies [42]. The vascular system's health is essential for normal brain function, and aging-related changes to the vasculature cause problems with autoregulation, BBB leakage, neovascular coupling, and decreased vascular tone [41]. Vascular risk factors, such as smoking, overweight, and elevated levels of total cholesterol, as well as vascular morbidity, such as high blood pressure, type 2 diabetes, and asymptomatic cerebral infarction, are associated with a higher risk of dementia, including AD.

Patients who had experienced a stroke and clinically quiet cerebral infarction confirmed by MRI were found to have a significantly increased risk of dementia and AD [48]. Neuropathological studies show that dementia syndrome frequently exhibits clinically coexisting lesions in cerebral vasculature, coronary artery disease, and neurodegenerative changes in the brain [49].

Alcohol Consumption and Smoking

It is common knowledge that excessive drinking leads to alcohol dementia. Furthermore, it was discovered that middle-aged heavy drinkers, particularly those who carried the apoE4 allele, had a later-life risk of dementia and AD that was more than three times higher [43]. On the other hand, light and medium-range drinkers had a lower risk of dementia and development of AD.

Alcohol harms the brain in heavy users; even light to medium-range alcohol intake has been connected to shrinkage and volume loss in the brain [44].

Various analytical studies have discovered a markedly elevated risk of AD related to smoking, particularly in people who do not carry the apoE4 allele [45]. With RR=1.79 and 95% CI 1.43–2.23, meta-analyses concluded that smoking was related to a higher risk of developing AD [46, 47].

Nutritional Factors

A daily dose of antioxidants, like Vit C and Vit E, in the diet or through dietary supplements was linked to a lower risk of AD, according to several studies [50]. However, some studies discovered a detrimental impact [51]. Despite vascular risk factors, additional analyses revealed that the Mediterranean diet was linked to a lower risk of AD [52]. It was also noted that while a diet high in omega-3 fatty acids, such as fish, may protect against dementia, a diet high in saturated fats, LDL, and VLDL cholesterol increases the risk of AD [53].

Infectious Agents

It has been hypothesized that infectious agents may play a role in AD and pose a risk. The infection of the herpes simplex virus (HSV), to which immunoglobulins may be noticed in the cerebral spinal fluid (CSF) in AD, was suggested in one of the earliest studies to suggest that infection may be a risk factor for AD, may induce abnormal protein formation leading to NFT [54]. A virus invasion can also cause microglia and pericytes to become activated, leading to the deposition of Aβ [55].

Observations of significant structural and biochemical changes in the AD brain's olfactory-related regions, particularly the olfactory bulb and entorhinal cortex, lend further credence to this theory [56]. However, more recent research has examined the DNA of AD patients' brains and peripheral blood leucocytes for cytomegalovirus (CMV), human herpes virus 6 (HHV-6), Epstein-Barr virus (EBS), with the results indicating that HHV-6 and CMV may be risk factors for cognitive impairment and the development of AD [57].

Diabetes

Numerous long-term research has discovered an elevated risk of both neurodegenerative and vascular dementia in diabetics [58, 59]. A systematic review supported this risk [60]. The onset of AD and other dementias may be significantly influenced by the existence of diabetes in middle age or by diabetes that has persisted for a more extended period [61]. Additionally, pre-diabetes, impaired glucose tolerance, and other borderline conditions are linked to an increased risk of AD and different types of dementia in geriatrics [62]. Comorbidities associated with diabetes, such as hypertension and dyslipidemia, may help to explain this relationship [63] partially.

Traumatic Brain Injury

TBI may damage the BBB, allowing plasma proteins to leak out and making the immune system more sensitive to brain antigens that are typically kept separate. After that, several studies revealed a link between head trauma and AD. APP is found in neuronal cells and dystrophic neurites surrounding Aβ deposits in head injury survivors, like AD [64]. It was later discovered that few neurons in the medial temporal lobe (MTL) release high amounts of APP and that TBI increased the number of APP-immunoreactive neurons in these regions [65]. As a result, the elevated expression of APP in cases of head trauma may be an acute-phase reaction to neuronal injury [66], As a result, increased APP expression in cases of head trauma may be an acute-phase expression to neuronal damage, with excessive APP expression resulting in the deposition of Aβ.

The identification of chronic traumatic encephalopathy (CTE), a neurodegenerative condition believed to be directly related to recurrent head trauma, further emphasizes the connection between TBI and AD [67]. Clinically, the symptoms of CTE are similar to those of AD and also include motor symptoms, behavioral changes, mood disturbances, and impairment of memory and executive function [68].

AD is a serious public health issue. Since its etiology is still unknown, it is essential to research any potential risk factors that might impact how it develops. Genetic factors are the most significant in early diagnosis and practical primary or secondary prevention applications.

Current Treatment Strategies and Side Effects

These findings have been the focus of newly emerging therapies with potential disease-modifying effects. Only N-methyl-D-aspartate (NMDA) receptor antagonists and cholinesterase inhibitors (ChEIs) are currently recognized as effective treatments for AD. Even though these drugs are used frequently and for more extended periods, there are many disagreements regarding the clinical importance of their therapeutic effect and the cost-effectiveness that results from it.

Acetylcholinesterase Inhibitors (AChE)

The nucleus basalis of Meynert, a distinct population of basal frontal cortex neurons, provides a significant portion of the cerebral cortex's cholinergic innervation [69]. Additionally, it has been discovered that cognitive dysfunction and the loss of cholinergic function are closely related. Numerous therapeutics that target cholinesterase inhibition, postsynaptic cholinergic stimulation with muscarinic agonists, choline precursors, and presynaptic cholinergic stimulation with nicotinic agonists have been studied over the past 20 years [70].

Tacrine

Tacrine, the first ChEI approved for AD, works by inhibiting both acetylcholinesterase and butyrylcholinesterase, even though the therapeutic efficacy of butyrylcholinesterase inhibitory activity has yet to be established. Compared to other commercially available drugs, tacrine is more likely to cause gastrointestinal side effects. It also has a unique impact that causes a small group of patients to experience significant liver toxicity. Due to tacrine's brief half-life, q.i.d. dosing is necessary. Due to these factors, tacrine is now rarely used. However, its introduction demonstrated that ChEIs could deliver beneficial therapy to patients and their families [71].

Donepezil

A cholinergic drug derived from piperidine called donepezil is a non-competitive, central reversible inhibitor of ACE, the enzyme that breaks down acetylcholine. Additionally, donepezil also affects the pathogenesis of AD at the molecular and cellular levels by inhibiting different aspects of glutamate-induced excitotoxicity, reducing the early stimulation of inflammatory cytokines, inducing a neuroprotective isoform of AChE, and decreasing the effects of oxidative stress [72].

The dosage is usually increased from 5 to 10 mg daily after about a month [73]. A 10 mg/day dose of donepezil has been found to improve cognitive ability, fundamental daily living skills, and physician global impression levels, but not behavior or quality of life [74]. Additionally, studies investigating the efficacy of dose levels up to 23 mg/day have not revealed appreciable variations from a dose of 10 mg/day [75]. None of these doses investigated, however, has been able to stop AD's development [76]. On the other hand, this medication has mild side effects that primarily affect the nervous system or gastrointestinal tract and has good patient tolerance [77].

Galantamine

Galantamine is a tertiary isoquinoline alkaloid, a selective, competitive, and reversible acetylcholinesterase inhibitor. Additionally, it activates acetylcholine's natural effect on nicotinic receptors [78]. The medication is administered orally in different doses, either as an extended-release capsule or a quick-release solution [twice daily]. The recommended starting dose for treatment is 8 mg/day, which is increased to 16 mg/day BID after 4–8 weeks as a maintenance dose [79].

According to a recent meta-analysis by Li *et al.*, this medication is the best option for treating AD because it not only works to control behavioral symptoms but also enhances cognitive function, daily living skills, and clinicians' assessments of patients' overall health [80]. Even though this medication has a good safety and tolerability profile, some side effects can occur during use, including convulsions, extreme nausea, vomiting, irregular breathing, stomach cramps, muscle weakness, confusion, and irritation of the eyes [81].

N-Methyl D-Aspartate [NMDA] Antagonists

The major excitatory amino acid in the human brain is glutamate. In most hippocampal pathways, as well as corticocortical association fibers, it is essential for synaptic transmission [82]. Excessive glutamate receptor activation under pathologic circumstances causes cell death, hence the word "excitotoxicity." There is strong evidence that the excitotoxic component of AD's pathologic cascade exists. Numerous substances, including ones that control NMDA and AMPA/kainate receptors, have been created as modulators of various glutamate receptor subtypes. Agents regulating NMDA receptor signal transmission have been explored more thoroughly than AMPA receptor modulators, which have only been the subject of pilot studies [82 - 84].

Memantine

Memantine is a non-competitive, voltage-dependent NMDA receptor antagonist with moderate affinity. It counteracts the neuronal dysfunctional effects of pathologically high glutamate tonic levels. Both the manifestation of symptoms and the development of AD into neurodegenerative dementia are influenced by the dysfunction of glutamate-mediated synaptic transmission, especially at the NMDA receptors [85].

It comes in 10 mg tablets, 2 mg/mL solution, and slow-release capsules of various doses, with a starting dose of 5 mg daily for the 1st week [86]. Memantine may permit typical glutamatergic neurotransmission in physiological settings while preventing excitotoxicity in environments with long-term glutamatergic stimulation. Memantine enhances rats' cognitive function and protects against A-induced neurotoxicity [87]. Dizziness, headache, confusion, diarrhea, and constipation are the side effects to be aware of, though less frequently experienced side effects include fatigue, hypertension, pain, weight gain, hallucinations, confusion, abdominal pain, aggressive behavior, vomiting, urinary incontinence [88].

On the other hand, the FDA has also approved the use of memantine and donepezil together for the symptomatic management of mild to severe AD [89].

However, the European Medicines Agency has not approved Acrescent®, a different medication based on the hydrochlorides of memantine and donepezil, because there is insufficient proof of its efficacy in this pathology [90]. This drug cocktail stops the toxic effects of too much glutamate and the degradation of acetylcholine levels in the brain. Donepezil + Memantine is more effective than placebo at alleviating cognition as measured by the SIB scale and ADAS-Cog, daily activities, global assessment, and neuropsychiatric symptoms. Still, it is less tolerable than a single therapy or treatment with a placebo, according to scientific evidence [91].

Statins

Simvastatin has been demonstrated to decrease cerebral Ab levels in vivo, and only recently was the first study showing a neuropathological change associated with statin use (reduced NFT burden at post-mortem examination) published [92]. Although later research of a larger sample population from the Adult Changes in Thought (ACT) Study found a protective effect in subjects who started statin consumption before age 80, the ACT analysis also demonstrated a significant beneficial impact of statins against AD [93]. Numerous early epidemiologic studies concurred with these findings, showing that statin use significantly lowers the risk of AD [94]. The consistency of the findings across studies indicates that statins may delay the advancement of neurodegeneration but might not be able to reverse it once dementia already occurred [92].

Several other drugs are being tested for their therapeutic efficacy and safety at different levels of research, such as anti-amyloid medications that try to either lower the production of amyloid beta, boost its clearance, or lessen protein aggregation. Inhibiting tau phosphorylation and aggregation has been the focus of anti-tau therapies [95].

Importance of Medicinal Plants and Phytocompounds in AD

Currently, one of the most potent treatments for a variety of ailments, including cancer, diabetes mellitus, and neurological conditions like AD, is natural/herbal treatment [96]. Due to their effectiveness and lack of side effects, natural products have recently become very popular as supplements or alternative medicines [97]. Natural product mixtures or extracts may be more effective than individual natural compounds since they can simultaneously target multiple targets. Given the intricate pathophysiology of AD, this may be a cutting-edge treatment option [98].

When focusing on the combinations and extracts of natural compounds, the neuroprotective effects that have been identified are frequently acknowledged as being attained through anti-oxidative and/or anti-neuroinflammatory responses, preventing the aggregation of A and tau protein, and boosting cholinergic signaling. It is conceivable that natural compounds acting on various pathological targets could delay or even prevent the onset and advancement of AD [99].

Natural products display various effects such as anti-cholinesterase, antioxidant, anti-inflammatory, and neuroprotective properties, which are promising for the therapy of neurological diseases [100]. Vit C and Vit E, luteolin, resveratrol, quercetin, curcumin, huperzine A, melatonin, rosmarinic acid, *etc.*, were among others, have been used by AD patients and have demonstrated positive results [96].

Antioxidant - Neuroprotective Activity

Reactive nitrogen (RNS) and Reactive oxygen species (ROS) are strong oxidizing molecules that contain both non-radical and radical oxygen species. A variety of physiological processes that take place inside the human body, including controlling the cell cycle, activation of receptors and enzymes, as well as regulating inflammation, gene expression, signal transduction, and phagocytosis, are thought to depend on maintaining a milder level of these oxidative species [101]. The human body can neutralize and eliminate these oxidative species, ensuring that their levels stay within the standard accepted level. But when there is a lack of balance between the generation/abundance of these oxidizing agents and their elimination/neutralization, the overly high levels of RNS and ROS can cause oxidative stress, which can cause severe pathological damage [102].

Antioxidants are substances that can interact with free radicals and change them into harmless forms. Numerous studies have linked oxidative stress to the beginning and progression of AD, and antioxidants are effective at reducing oxidative stress's negative effects [103]. Antioxidants are divided into two categories based on how frequently they occur in nature: natural antioxidants and artificial antioxidants, with most of the synthetic compounds coming from natural sources. The most commonly known natural antioxidants include the vitamins A, C, and E and flavonoids, which are all crucial in protecting an organism from ROS-caused damage.

Six measured carotenoids and other antioxidants like retinol and -tocopherol have been discovered to have significantly lesser serum levels in AD patients. Additionally, as a neuroprotective defense mechanism in AD patients, antioxidants like vitamins and carotenoids may confer a decrease in oxidative damage [110]. Carotenoids can be added to the diet to reduce AD symptoms in animal models [111]. The latest clinical study further supported the advantages of consuming carotenoids such as lutein and zeaxanthin in reducing the incidence of

AD. Numerous epidemiological research have also linked a diet high in carotenes to a reduced risk of neurodegenerative disorders, such as AD [112].

Anti-neuroinflammatory Activity

An essential characteristic of AD pathology linked to neuroinflammation is the deposit of Aβ in the brain. A high level of ROS, elevated microglial activation, the generation of cytokines, and NF-KB all contribute to the neuroinflammatory process in AD. In particular, the stimulation of immune cells such as microglia triggers the synthesis and release of inflammatory cytokines, such as IL-1β, TNF-α, IFN-γ which in turn prompts nearby astrocytes to produce Aβ 42 oligomers [104]. More microglial cells may gather at the site of the extracellular insoluble Aβ aggregates to form microglia clusters. AD patients' serum, brain, and CSF were discovered in high concentrations [105].

Natural products can avert and improve neurodegeneration in Alzheimer's disease [AD] with fewer side effects than synthetic drugs, thanks to their anti-inflammatory and antioxidant properties [107]. The anti-neuroinflammatory potential of some natural products has been attributed to a variety of mechanisms, including the inhibition of microglia stimulation, the decline of pro-inflammatory cytokine accumulation from activated microglia, the inhibition of NF-KB, and the stimulation of p38 MAPK. These natural substances' capacity to activate Nrf2 and possess antioxidant qualities is also partially attributable to their anti-neuroinflammatory activity [106].

Alkaloids, terpenes, polyphenols, carotenoids, and marine products are some of the major structural categories of natural products with anti-neuroinflammatory activity. Cryptolepine, an alkaloid derived from the plant *Cryptolepis sanguinolenta*, is an example of an alkaloid compound with anti-neuroinflammatory properties. According to studies, Cryptolepine inhibits the activation of NF-B and p38 MAPK in the microglia, thereby lowering levels of TNF, IL-6, IL-1, Nitric oxide, and PGE2 in Lipopolysaccharide microglia [108]. It has been well-documented that flavonoids and polyphenols have anti-inflammatory properties. Kaempferol, apigenin, tiliroside, quercetin, punicalagin, mangiferin, epigallocatechin-3-gallate [EGCG], resveratrol, urolithin A, curcumin, and numerous other compounds are examples of this structural group. They primarily inhibit the activation of the NF-KB and p38 MAPK pathways while decreasing the production of pro-inflammatory mediators [109].

To develop new anti-AD medications, natural substance mixtures or extracts that contain a variety of bioactive substances and have a range of neuroprotective effects are preferred. Natural product therapy can play a crucial part in the prevention and treatment of AD if more comprehensive and practical quality control guidelines are developed to guarantee the safety and effectiveness of these treatments, as well as novel approaches and ways to help enhance the CNS access of these neuroprotective compounds, such as the inclusion of nanotechnology in the delivery of natural products.

Andrographolide and its Analogs in Treatment of Alzheimer's Disease

Researchers are working to create new medications with superior therapeutic efficacies. In some recent studies, andrographolide has demonstrated therapeutic potential in various AD models [113, 114]. For instance, it has been shown that long-term treatment with andrographolide (4 mg/kg, 3 months) suppresses the decline in spatial learning and memory function in Octodon degus, a type of South American rodent that produces pathology similar to Alzheimer's in later life [113].

Mitochondrial Dysfunction in APP/PS1

In the brain of AD patients, abnormal mitochondrial dysfunction leads to synaptic dysfunction, oxidative stress, and neuron death as one of the earliest and most prominent features in vulnerable neurons [115]. Transmission electron microscopy was used to identify mitochondrial swelling in APP/PS1 mice. The opening of the mitochondrial permeation transition pores promotes the swelling of the mitochondria (mPTP). By interacting with CypD, Aβ oligomers encourage an open and irreversible shape of mitochondrial mPTP. The mPTP opening penetrates the inner membrane of the mitochondria, increases the exchanges between the mitochondrial matrix and the cytoplasm, and causes mitochondrial perturbations, including the collapse of the membrane potential of the mitochondria, the secretion of pro-apoptotic factors, the generation of ROS, and calcium deregulation [116].

Treatment with andrographolide sulfonate reduced swelling in the mitochondria and restored the balance between oxidation and redox. While the precise mechanism still requires further research, andrographolide sulfonate can improve cognitive deficits in APP/PS1 mice by reducing mitochondrial dysfunction and preserving the ultrastructure of mitochondria [117].

Recovery of Synaptic Functions in AD

The main characteristic of cognitive and memory decline was revealed when protein and synaptic function in the AD brain were disrupted and altered in transgenic AD models [118]. In contrast to the young degus, a noticeable decline in postsynaptic proteins was seen in the aged degus. Additionally, 2 mg/kg AGP and 4 mg/kg AGP wholly and partially improved the GluN2A subunit of the N-methyl-D-aspartate (NMDA) receptor. In contrast, the opposite effect was seen for postsynaptic density 95 (PSD-95) [119]. The regulatory effects of AGP on pre-synaptic and postsynaptic proteins [120], reduction of NFκB, microglia inflammatory response [123], and Nrf2 activity [121, 122] may be responsible for its overall neuroprotective actions and improvement of cognitive and spatial memory in various natural models of AD.

Reduction of the Activation of NF-κB and Nrf2

One of the most crucial transcription factors for the expression of proinflammatory cytokines, which affects microglia-mediated Aβ toxicity, is the NF-κB [124]. The anti-inflammatory impact of AGP on p-NFκB activation in LPS-induced mice was investigated in an *in vitro* and *in vivo* study. The findings showed that, in comparison to control groups, LPS-induced adult brains, as well as mixed primary glial, had significantly more nuclear translocation of p-NFκ--p65. According to additional research, AGP significantly reduced the glial p-NFκB-p65 compared to the LPS control group [118].

CONCLUSION

This chapter outlines the diverse pharmacological effects of andrographolide and how it works to treat Alzheimer's disease. The lack of effective therapies for AD has given researchers a fresh outlook on developing new and effective medicines from natural ingredients. The recovery that followed treatment with AGP in numerous neurotoxicity studies and various AD model systems is evidence of the neuroprotective potential of AG.

Aging and environmental toxins cause cognitive decline, which is associated with diminished synaptic activity and an increase in primary AD symptoms. The following are the most significant effects of AG on neuroprotection: Postsynaptic protein protection, reduced NF-B and Nrf2 activation, the return of learning ability and spatial memory, reduction of phosphorylated tau protein, and Aβ aggregate maturation.

Research should, therefore, concentrate on the pharmacological properties of andrographolide and its analogs, as well as its detailed mechanisms in preventing and treating disorders affecting the central nervous system. Researchers should further assess the antidepressant-like activity of AG, thus promoting its development in the treatment of PD and depression.

REFERENCES

[1]   Available from: https://www.who.int/news-room/fact sheets/detail/dementia#:~:text=Alzheimer's%20disease%20is%20the%20most,dependency%20among%20older%20people%20globally

[2]   Roman GC. Brain infarction and the clinical expression of Alzheimer disease. JAMA 1997; 278(20): 113-4.
[http://dx.doi.org/10.1001/jama.1997.03550020045023]

[3]   Scheltens P, Blennow K, Breteler MMB, *et al.* Alzheimer's disease. Lancet 2016; 388(10043): 505-17.
[http://dx.doi.org/10.1016/S0140-6736(15)01124-1] [PMID: 26921134]

[4]   Hardy J. Has the amyloid cascade hypothesis for Alzheimer's disease been proved? Curr Alzheimer Res 2006; 3(1): 71-3.
[http://dx.doi.org/10.2174/156720506775697098] [PMID: 16472206]

[5]   Prince M, Bryce R, Albanese E, Wimo A, Ribeiro W, Ferri CP. The global prevalence of dementia: A systematic review and metaanalysis. Alzheimers Dement 2013; 9(1): 63-75.e2.
[http://dx.doi.org/10.1016/j.jalz.2012.11.007] [PMID: 23305823]

[6]   Thies W, Bleiler L. 2012 Alzheimer's disease facts and figures Alzheimer's Association ⸰. Alzheimers Dement 2012; 8(2): 131-68.
[http://dx.doi.org/10.1016/j.jalz.2012.02.001] [PMID: 22404854]

[7]   Lambert MA, Bickel H, Prince M, *et al.* Estimating the burden of early onset dementia; systematic review of disease prevalence. Eur J Neurol 2014; 21(4): 563-9.
[http://dx.doi.org/10.1111/ene.12325] [PMID: 24418291]

[8]   Shah RS, Lee HG, Xiongwei Z, Perry G, Smith MA, Castellani RJ. Current approaches in the treatment of Alzheimer's disease. Biomed Pharmacother 2008; 62(4): 199-207.
[http://dx.doi.org/10.1016/j.biopha.2008.02.005] [PMID: 18407457]

[9]   Hebert LE, Scherr PA, Bienias JL, Bennett DA, Evans DA. Alzheimer disease in the US population: prevalence estimates using the 2000 census. Arch Neurol 2003; 60(8): 1119-22.
[http://dx.doi.org/10.1001/archneur.60.8.1119] [PMID: 12925369]

[10]   Fischer W, Wictorin K, Björklund A, Williams LR, Varon S, Gage FH. Amelioration of cholinergic neuron atrophy and spatial memory impairment in aged rats by nerve growth factor. Nature 1987; 329(6134): 65-8.
[http://dx.doi.org/10.1038/329065a0] [PMID: 3627243]

[11]   Eriksdotter Jönhagen M, Nordberg A, Amberla K, *et al.* Intracerebroventricular infusion of nerve growth factor in three patients with Alzheimer's disease. Dement Geriatr Cogn Disord 1998; 9(5): 246-57.
[http://dx.doi.org/10.1159/000017069] [PMID: 9701676]

[12]   Nunomura A, Perry G, Pappolla MA, *et al.* RNA oxidation is a prominent feature of vulnerable neurons in Alzheimer's disease. J Neurosci 1999; 19(6): 1959-64.
[http://dx.doi.org/10.1523/JNEUROSCI.19-06-01959.1999] [PMID: 10066249]

[13]   Fassbender K, Simons M, Bergmann C, *et al.* Simvastatin strongly reduces levels of Alzheimer's disease β-amyloid peptides Aβ42 and Aβ40 *in vitro* and *in vivo.* Proc Natl Acad Sci USA 2001; 98(10): 5856-61.
[http://dx.doi.org/10.1073/pnas.081620098] [PMID: 11296263]

[14]   Li G, Larson EB, Sonnen JA, *et al.* Statin therapy is associated with reduced neuropathologic changes of Alzheimer disease. Neurology 2007; 69(9): 878-85.
[http://dx.doi.org/10.1212/01.wnl.0000277657.95487.1c] [PMID: 17724290]

[15]   Rea TD, Breitner JC, Psaty BM, *et al.* Statin use and the risk of incident dementia: the Cardiovascular Health Study. Arch Neurol 2005; 62(7): 1047-51.
[http://dx.doi.org/10.1001/archneur.62.7.1047] [PMID: 16009757]

[16]   Zandi PP, Sparks DL, Khachaturian AS, *et al.* Do statins reduce risk of incident dementia and Alzheimer disease? The Cache County Study. Arch Gen Psychiatry 2005; 62(2): 217-24.
[http://dx.doi.org/10.1001/archpsyc.62.2.217] [PMID: 15699299]

[17] Goutte C, Tsunozaki M, Hale VA, Priess JR. APH-1 is a multipass membrane protein essential for the Notch signaling pathway in *Caenorhabditis elegans* embryos. Proc Natl Acad Sci USA 2002; 99(2): 775-9.
[http://dx.doi.org/10.1073/pnas.022523499] [PMID: 11792846]

[18] Noori T, Dehpour AR, Sureda A, Sobarzo-Sanchez E, Shirooie S. Role of natural products for the treatment of Alzheimer's disease. Eur J Pharmacol 2021; 898: 173974.
[http://dx.doi.org/10.1016/j.ejphar.2021.173974] [PMID: 33652057]

[19] Chen X, Drew J, Berney W, Lei W. Neuroprotective natural products for Alzheimer's disease. Cells 2021; 10(6): 1309.
[http://dx.doi.org/10.3390/cells10061309] [PMID: 34070275]

[20] Lu J, Ma Y, Wu J, *et al.* A review for the neuroprotective effects of andrographolide in the central nervous system. Biomed Pharmacother 2019; 117: 109078.
[http://dx.doi.org/10.1016/j.biopha.2019.109078] [PMID: 31181444]

[21] Lee KC, Chang HH, Chung YH, Lee TY. Andrographolide acts as an anti-inflammatory agent in LPS-stimulated RAW264.7 macrophages by inhibiting STAT3-mediated suppression of the NF-κB pathway. J Ethnopharmacol 2011; 135(3): 678-84.
[http://dx.doi.org/10.1016/j.jep.2011.03.068] [PMID: 21497192]

[22] Maiti K, Gantait A, Kakali M, Saha BP, Mukherjee PK. Therapeutic potentials of andrographolide from *Andrographis paniculata*: a review. J Nat Rem 2006; 1-3.

[23] Hao M, Lv M, Xu H. Andrographolide: synthetic methods and biological activities. Mini Rev Med Chem 2020; 20(16): 1633-52.
[http://dx.doi.org/10.2174/1389557520666200429100326] [PMID: 32348215]

[24] Mishra SK, Tripathi S, Shukla A, Oh SH, Kim HM. Andrographolide and analogs in cancer prevention. Front Biosci (Elite Ed) 2015; 7(2): 255-66.
[PMID: 25553378]

[25] Devendar P, Nayak VL, Yadav DK, *et al.* Synthesis and evaluation of anticancer activity of novel andrographolide derivatives. MedChemComm 2015; 6(5): 898-904.
[http://dx.doi.org/10.1039/C4MD00566J]

[26] Tan WSD, Liao W, Peh HY, *et al.* Andrographolide simultaneously augments Nrf2 antioxidant defense and facilitates autophagic flux blockade in cigarette smoke-exposed human bronchial epithelial cells. Toxicol Appl Pharmacol 2018; 360: 120-30.
[http://dx.doi.org/10.1016/j.taap.2018.10.005] [PMID: 30291937]

[27] Anrather J, Racchumi G, Iadecola C. NF-kappaB regulates phagocytic NADPH oxidase by inducing the expression of gp91phox. J Biol Chem 2006; 281(9): 5657-67.
[http://dx.doi.org/10.1074/jbc.M506172200] [PMID: 16407283]

[28] Heyman A, e WE, Hurwitz BJ, *et al.* Alzheimer's disease: Genetic aspects and associated clinical disorders. Ann Neurol 1983; 14(5): 507-15.
[http://dx.doi.org/10.1002/ana.410140503] [PMID: 6228188]

[29] Heyman A, Wilkinson WE, Stafford JA, Helms MJ, Sigmon AH, Weinberg T. Alzheimer's disease: A study of epidemiological aspects. Ann Neurol 1984; 15(4): 335-41.
[http://dx.doi.org/10.1002/ana.410150406] [PMID: 6742780]

[30] Henderson AS. The risk factors for Alzheimer's disease: a review and a hypothesis. Acta Psychiatr Scand 1988; 78(3): 257-75.
[http://dx.doi.org/10.1111/j.1600-0447.1988.tb06336.x] [PMID: 3057813]

[31] Killin LOJ, Starr JM, Shiue IJ, Russ TC. Environmental risk factors for dementia: a systematic review. BMC Geriatr 2016; 16(1): 175.
[http://dx.doi.org/10.1186/s12877-016-0342-y] [PMID: 27729011]

[32]   Decourt B, D'Souza GX, Shi J, Ritter A, Suazo J, Sabbagh MN. The cause of Alzheimer's disease: The theory of multipathology convergence to chronic neuronal stress. Aging Dis 2022; 13(1): 37-60.
[http://dx.doi.org/10.14336/AD.2021.0529] [PMID: 35111361]

[33]   Doruk H, Naharci MI, Bozoglu E, Isik AT, Kilic S. The relationship between body mass index and incidental mild cognitive impairment, Alzheimer's disease, and Vascular Dementia in elderly. J Nutr Health Aging 2010; 14(10): 834-8.
[http://dx.doi.org/10.1007/s12603-010-0113-y] [PMID: 21125201]

[34]   Knopman DS. An overview of common non-alzheimer dementias. Clin Geriatr Med 2001; 17(2): 281-301.
[http://dx.doi.org/10.1016/S0749-0690(05)70069-0] [PMID: 11375136]

[35]   Ferri CP, Prince M, Brayne C, *et al.* Global prevalence of dementia: a Delphi consensus study. Lancet 2005; 366(9503): 2112-7.
[http://dx.doi.org/10.1016/S0140-6736(05)67889-0] [PMID: 16360788]

[36]   Rossor M, Mountjoy CQ. Post-mortem neurochemical changes in Alzheimer's disease compared with normal ageing. Can J Neurol Sci 1986; 13(S4) (Suppl.): 499-502.
[http://dx.doi.org/10.1017/S0317167100037203] [PMID: 2878713]

[37]   Bird TD. Genetic aspects of Alzheimer disease. Genet Med. 2008 Apr;10(4):231-9
[http://dx.doi.org/10.1097/GIM.0b013e31816b64dc] [PMID: 18414205]

[38]   Blennow K, de Leon MJ, Zetterberg H. Alzheimer's disease. Lancet 2006; 368(9533): 387-403.
[http://dx.doi.org/10.1016/S0140-6736(06)69113-7] [PMID: 16876668]

[39]   Huang W, Qiu C, von Strauss E, Winblad B, Fratiglioni L. APOE genotype, family history of dementia, and Alzheimer disease risk: a 6-year follow-up study. Arch Neurol 2004; 61(12): 1930-4.
[http://dx.doi.org/10.1001/archneur.61.12.1930] [PMID: 15596614]

[40]   Qiu C, Kivipelto M, Agüero-Torres H, Winblad B, Fratiglioni L. Risk and protective effects of the APOE gene towards Alzheimer's disease in the Kungsholmen project: variation by age and sex. J Neurol Neurosurg Psychiatry 2004; 75(6): 828-33.
[http://dx.doi.org/10.1136/jnnp.2003.021493] [PMID: 15145993]

[41]   Kalaria RN. Vascular basis for brain degeneration: faltering controls and risk factors for dementia. Nutr Rev 2010; 68(Suppl 2) (Suppl. 2): S74-87.
[http://dx.doi.org/10.1111/j.1753-4887.2010.00352.x] [PMID: 21091952]

[42]   Liu G, Yao L, Liu J, *et al.* Cardiovascular disease contributes to Alzheimer's disease: evidence from large-scale genome-wide association studies. Neurobiol Aging 2014; 35(4): 786-92.
[http://dx.doi.org/10.1016/j.neurobiolaging.2013.10.084] [PMID: 24231519]

[43]   Huang W, Qiu C, Winblad B, Fratiglioni L. Alcohol consumption and incidence of dementia in a community sample aged 75 years and older. J Clin Epidemiol 2002; 55(10): 959-64.
[http://dx.doi.org/10.1016/S0895-4356(02)00462-6] [PMID: 12464371]

[44]   Paul CA, Au R, Fredman L, *et al.* Association of alcohol consumption with brain volume in the Framingham study. Arch Neurol 2008; 65(10): 1363-7.
[http://dx.doi.org/10.1001/archneur.65.10.1363] [PMID: 18852353]

[45]   Ott A, Slooter AJC, Hofman A, *et al.* Smoking and risk of dementia and Alzheimer's disease in a population-based cohort study: the Rotterdam Study. Lancet 1998; 351(9119): 1840-3.
[http://dx.doi.org/10.1016/S0140-6736(97)07541-7] [PMID: 9652667]

[46]   Anstey KJ, von Sanden C, Salim A, O'Kearney R. Smoking as a risk factor for dementia and cognitive decline: a meta-analysis of prospective studies. Am J Epidemiol 2007; 166(4): 367-78.
[http://dx.doi.org/10.1093/aje/kwm116] [PMID: 17573335]

[47]   Peters R, Poulter R, Warner J, Beckett N, Burch L, Bulpitt C. Smoking, dementia and cognitive decline in the elderly, a systematic review. BMC Geriatr 2008; 8(1): 36.

[http://dx.doi.org/10.1186/1471-2318-8-36] [PMID: 19105840]

[48]   Vermeer SE, Prins ND, den Heijer T, Hofman A, Koudstaal PJ, Breteler MMB. Silent brain infarcts and the risk of dementia and cognitive decline. N Engl J Med 2003; 348(13): 1215-22.
       [http://dx.doi.org/10.1056/NEJMoa022066] [PMID: 12660385]

[49]   Esiri MM, Nagy Z, Smith MZ, Barnetson L, Smith AD. Cerebrovascular disease and threshold for dementia in the early stages of Alzheimer's disease. Lancet 1999; 354(9182): 919-20.
       [http://dx.doi.org/10.1016/S0140-6736(99)02355-7] [PMID: 10489957]

[50]   Barberger-Gateau P, Raffaitin C, Letenneur L, *et al.* Dietary patterns and risk of dementia. Neurology 2007; 69(20): 1921-30.
       [http://dx.doi.org/10.1212/01.wnl.0000278116.37320.52] [PMID: 17998483]

[51]   Gray SL, Anderson ML, Crane PK, *et al.* Antioxidant vitamin supplement use and risk of dementia or Alzheimer's disease in older adults. J Am Geriatr Soc 2008; 56(2): 291-5.
       [http://dx.doi.org/10.1111/j.1532-5415.2007.01531.x] [PMID: 18047492]

[52]   Laitinen MH, Ngandu T, Rovio S, *et al.* Fat intake at midlife and risk of dementia and Alzheimer's disease: a population-based study. Dement Geriatr Cogn Disord 2006; 22(1): 99-107.
       [http://dx.doi.org/10.1159/000093478] [PMID: 16710090]

[53]   Huang TL, Zandi PP, Tucker KL, *et al.* Benefits of fatty fish on dementia risk are stronger for those without *APOE* ε4. Neurology 2005; 65(9): 1409-14.
       [http://dx.doi.org/10.1212/01.wnl.0000183148.34197.2e] [PMID: 16275829]

[54]   Libíková H, Pogády J, Wiedermann V, Breier S. Search for herpetic antibodies in the cerebrospinal fluid in senile dementia and mental retardation. Acta Virol 1975; 19(6): 493-5.
       [PMID: 1996]

[55]   Wisniewski HM, Moretz RC, Lossinsky AS. Evidence for induction of localized amyloid deposits and neuritic plaques by an infectious agent. Ann Neurol 1981; 10(6): 517-22.
       [http://dx.doi.org/10.1002/ana.410100605] [PMID: 7198888]

[56]   Doty RL, Reyes PF, Gregor T. Presence of both odor identification and detection deficits in alzheimer's disease. Brain Res Bull 1987; 18(5): 597-600.
       [http://dx.doi.org/10.1016/0361-9230(87)90129-8] [PMID: 3607528]

[57]   Carbone I, Lazzarotto T, Ianni M, *et al.* Herpes virus in Alzheimer's disease: relation to progression of the disease. Neurobiol Aging 2014; 35(1): 122-9.
       [http://dx.doi.org/10.1016/j.neurobiolaging.2013.06.024] [PMID: 23916950]

[58]   Arvanitakis Z, Wilson RS, Bienias JL, Evans DA, Bennett DA. Diabetes mellitus and risk of Alzheimer disease and decline in cognitive function. Arch Neurol 2004; 61(5): 661-6.
       [http://dx.doi.org/10.1001/archneur.61.5.661] [PMID: 15148141]

[59]   Akomolafe A, Beiser A, Meigs JB, *et al.* Diabetes mellitus and risk of developing Alzheimer disease: results from the Framingham Study. Arch Neurol 2006; 63(11): 1551-5.
       [http://dx.doi.org/10.1001/archneur.63.11.1551] [PMID: 17101823]

[60]   Biessels GJ, Staekenborg S, Brunner E, Brayne C, Scheltens P. Risk of dementia in diabetes mellitus: a systematic review. Lancet Neurol 2006; 5(1): 64-74.
       [http://dx.doi.org/10.1016/S1474-4422(05)70284-2] [PMID: 16361024]

[61]   Roberts RO, Geda YE, Knopman DS, *et al.* Association of duration and severity of diabetes mellitus with mild cognitive impairment. Arch Neurol 2008; 65(8): 1066-73.
       [http://dx.doi.org/10.1001/archneur.65.8.1066] [PMID: 18695056]

[62]   Xu W, Qiu C, Winblad B, Fratiglioni L. The effect of borderline diabetes on the risk of dementia and Alzheimer's disease. Diabetes 2007; 56(1): 211-6.
       [http://dx.doi.org/10.2337/db06-0879] [PMID: 17192484]

[63]   Korf ESC, White LR, Scheltens P, Launer LJ. Brain aging in very old men with type 2 diabetes: the

Honolulu-Asia Aging Study. Diabetes Care 2006; 29(10): 2268-74.
[http://dx.doi.org/10.2337/dc06-0243] [PMID: 17003305]

[64] Gentleman SM, Nash MJ, Sweeting CJ, Graham DI, Roberts GW. β-Amyloid precursor protein (βAPP) as a marker for axonal injury after head injury. Neurosci Lett 1993; 160(2): 139-44.
[http://dx.doi.org/10.1016/0304-3940(93)90398-5] [PMID: 8247344]

[65] McKenzie JE, Gentleman SM, Roberts GW, Graham DI, Royston MC. Increased numbers of βAPP-immunoreactive neurones in the entorhinal cortex after head injury. Neuroreport 1994; 6(1): 161-4.
[http://dx.doi.org/10.1097/00001756-199412300-00041] [PMID: 7703405]

[66] Roberts BR, Ryan TM, Bush AI, Masters CL, Duce JA. The role of metallobiology and amyloid☐β peptides in Alzheimer's disease. J Neurochem 2012; 120(s1) (Suppl. 1): 149-66.
[http://dx.doi.org/10.1111/j.1471-4159.2011.07500.x] [PMID: 22121980]

[67] Geddes JF, Vowles GH, Nicoll JAR, Révész T. Neuronal cytoskeletal changes are an early consequence of repetitive head injury. Acta Neuropathol 1999; 98(2): 171-8.
[http://dx.doi.org/10.1007/s004010051066] [PMID: 10442557]

[68] Stern RA, Daneshvar DH, Baugh CM, *et al.* Clinical presentation of chronic traumatic encephalopathy. Neurology 2013; 81(13): 1122-9.
[http://dx.doi.org/10.1212/WNL.0b013e3182a55f7f] [PMID: 23966253]

[69] Farlow MR, Evans RM. Pharmacologic treatment of cognition in Alzheimer's dementia. Neurology 1998; 51(1_suppl_1) (Suppl. 1): S36-44.
[http://dx.doi.org/10.1212/WNL.51.1_Suppl_1.S36] [PMID: 9674761]

[70] Hebert LE, Scherr PA, Bienias JL, Bennett DA, Evans DA. Alzheimer disease in the US population: prevalence estimates using the 2000 census. Arch Neurol 2003; 60(8): 1119-22.
[http://dx.doi.org/10.1001/archneur.60.8.1119] [PMID: 12925369]

[71] Qizilbash N, Schneider LS. Practical recommendations and opinions on therapies for cognitive symptoms and prognosis modification Evidence-based dementia practice. London: Blackwell 2002; pp. 560-88.

[72] Jacobson SA, Sabbagh MN. Donepezil: potential neuroprotective and disease-modifying effects. Expert Opin Drug Metab Toxicol 2008; 4(10): 1363-9.
[http://dx.doi.org/10.1517/17425255.4.10.1363] [PMID: 18798705]

[73] Schneider LS, Tariot PN. Cognitive enhancers and treatments for Alzheimer's disease. Psychiatry 2003; •••: 2096-108.

[74] Homma A, Imai Y, Tago H, *et al.* Donepezil treatment of patients with severe Alzheimer's disease in a Japanese population: results from a 24-week, double-blind, placebo-controlled, randomized trial. Dement Geriatr Cogn Disord 2008; 25(5): 399-407.
[http://dx.doi.org/10.1159/000122961] [PMID: 18391486]

[75] Homma A, Atarashi H, Kubota N, Nakai K, Takase T. Efficacy and safety of sustained release donepezil high dose *versus* immediate release donepezil standard dose in Japanese patients with severe Alzheimer's disease: a randomized, double-blind trial. J Alzheimers Dis 2016; 52(1): 345-57.
[http://dx.doi.org/10.3233/JAD-151149] [PMID: 26967222]

[76] Cacabelos R. Donepezil in Alzheimer's disease: From conventional trials to pharmacogenetics. Neuropsychiatr Dis Treat 2007; 3(3): 303-33.
[PMID: 19300564]

[77] Seltzer B. Donepezil: an update. Expert Opin Pharmacother 2007; 8(7): 1011-23.
[http://dx.doi.org/10.1517/14656566.8.7.1011] [PMID: 17472546]

[78] Farlow MR. Clinical pharmacokinetics of galantamine. Clin Pharmacokinet 2003; 42(15): 1383-92.
[http://dx.doi.org/10.2165/00003088-200342150-00005] [PMID: 14674789]

[79] Seltzer B. Galantamine-ER for the treatment of mild-to-moderate Alzheimer's disease. Clin Interv

Aging 2010; 5: 1-6.
[PMID: 20169037]

[80]   Li DD, Zhang YH, Zhang W, Zhao P. Meta-analysis of randomized controlled trials on the efficacy and safety of donepezil, galantamine, rivastigmine, and memantine for the treatment of Alzheimer's disease. Front Neurosci 2019; 13: 472.
[http://dx.doi.org/10.3389/fnins.2019.00472] [PMID: 31156366]

[81]   Haake A, Nguyen K, Friedman L, Chakkamparambil B, Grossberg GT. An update on the utility and safety of cholinesterase inhibitors for the treatment of Alzheimer's disease. Expert Opin Drug Saf 2020; 19(2): 147-57.
[http://dx.doi.org/10.1080/14740338.2020.1721456] [PMID: 31976781]

[82]   Procter A. Abnormalities in non-cholinergic neurotransmitter systems in Alzheimer's disease Dementia. 2nd ed. Oxford: Edward Arnold 2000; pp. 433-42.

[83]   Rothman SM, Thurston JH, Hauhart RE. Delayed neurotoxicity of excitatory amino acids *In vitro* . Neuroscience 1987; 22(2): 471-80.
[http://dx.doi.org/10.1016/0306-4522(87)90347-2] [PMID: 3670595]

[84]   Marenco S, Weinberger DR. Therapeutic potential of positive AMPA receptor modulators in the treatment of neuropsychiatric disorders. CNS Drugs 2006; 20(3): 173-85.
[http://dx.doi.org/10.2165/00023210-200620030-00001] [PMID: 16529524]

[85]   Wang R, Reddy PH. Role of Glutamate and NMDA Receptors in Alzheimer's Disease. J Alzheimers Dis 2017; 57(4): 1041-8.
[http://dx.doi.org/10.3233/JAD-160763] [PMID: 27662322]

[86]   Parsons CG, Danysz W, Quack G. Memantine is a clinically well tolerated N-methyl-d-aspartate (NMDA) receptor antagonist—a review of preclinical data. Neuropharmacology 1999; 38(6): 735-67.
[http://dx.doi.org/10.1016/S0028-3908(99)00019-2] [PMID: 10465680]

[87]   Tariot PN, Federoff HJ. Current treatment for Alzheimer disease and future prospects. Alzheimer Dis Assoc Disord 2003; 17 (Suppl. 4): S105-13.
[http://dx.doi.org/10.1097/00002093-200307004-00005] [PMID: 14512816]

[88]   Rossom R, Adityanjee , Dysken M. Efficacy and tolerability of memantine in the treatment of dementia. Am J Geriatr Pharmacother 2004; 2(4): 303-12.
[http://dx.doi.org/10.1016/j.amjopharm.2004.12.006] [PMID: 15903287]

[89]   Calhoun A, King C, Khoury R, Grossberg GT. An evaluation of memantine ER + donepezil for the treatment of Alzheimer's disease. Expert Opin Pharmacother 2018; 19(15): 1711-7.
[http://dx.doi.org/10.1080/14656566.2018.1519022] [PMID: 30244611]

[90]   Pardo-Moreno T, González-Acedo A, Rivas-Domínguez A, *et al.* Therapeutic approach to Alzheimer's disease: Current treatments and new perspectives. Pharmaceutics 2022; 14(6): 1117.
[http://dx.doi.org/10.3390/pharmaceutics14061117] [PMID: 35745693]

[91]   Guo J, Wang Z, Liu R, Huang Y, Zhang N, Zhang R. Memantine, donepezil, or combination therapy—what is the best therapy for Alzheimer's disease? A network meta□analysis. Brain Behav 2020; 10(11): e01831.
[http://dx.doi.org/10.1002/brb3.1831] [PMID: 32914577]

[92]   Li G, Higdon R, Kukull WA, *et al.* Statin therapy and risk of dementia in the elderly. Neurology 2004; 63(9): 1624-8.
[http://dx.doi.org/10.1212/01.WNL.0000142963.90204.58] [PMID: 15534246]

[93]   Torrandell-Haro G, Branigan GL, Vitali F, Geifman N, Zissimopoulos JM, Brinton RD. Statin therapy and risk of Alzheimer's and age-related neurodegenerative diseases. Alzheimers Dement (N Y) 2020 Nov 25; 6(1): e12108.
[http://dx.doi.org/10.1002/trc2.12108] [PMID: 33283039]

[94]   Jick H, Zornberg GL, Jick SS, Seshadri S, Drachman DA. Statins and the risk of dementia. Lancet

2000; 356(9242): 1627-31.
[http://dx.doi.org/10.1016/S0140-6736(00)03155-X] [PMID: 11089820]

[95]   Waite L. Treatment for Alzheimer's disease: has anything changed? Aust Prescr 2015; 38(2): 60-3.
[http://dx.doi.org/10.18773/austprescr.2015.018] [PMID: 26648618]

[96]   Bui TT, Nguyen TH. Natural product for the treatment of Alzheimer's disease. J Basic Clin Physiol Pharmacol 2017; 28(5): 413-23.
[http://dx.doi.org/10.1515/jbcpp-2016-0147] [PMID: 28708573]

[97]   Iqubal A, Rahman SO, Ahmed M, *et al.* Current quest in natural bioactive compounds for Alzheimer's disease: Multi-targeted-designed-ligand based approach with preclinical and clinical based evidence. Curr Drug Targets 2021; 22(6): 685-720.
[http://dx.doi.org/10.2174/18735592MTEysMjQe4] [PMID: 33302832]

[98]   Xiao J, Shao R. Natural products for treatment of Alzheimer's disease and related diseases: understanding their mechanism of action. Curr Neuropharmacol 2013; 11(4): 337.
[http://dx.doi.org/10.2174/1570159X11311040001] [PMID: 24381527]

[99]   Venkatesan R, Ji E, Kim SY. Phytochemicals that regulate neurodegenerative disease by targeting neurotrophins: a comprehensive review. BioMed Research Intern 2015.

[100]   Singh A, Deshpande P, Gogia N. Exploring the efficacy of natural products in alleviating Alzheimer's disease. Neural Regen Res 2019; 14(8): 1321-9.
[http://dx.doi.org/10.4103/1673-5374.253509] [PMID: 30964049]

[101]   Liu Z, Zhou T, Ziegler AC, Dimitrion P, Zuo L. Oxidative stress in neurodegenerative diseases: from molecular mechanisms to clinical applications. Oxidative Med Cellular Longevity 2017.

[102]   Rani V, Deep G, Singh RK, Palle K, Yadav UCS. Oxidative stress and metabolic disorders: Pathogenesis and therapeutic strategies. Life Sci 2016; 148: 183-93.
[http://dx.doi.org/10.1016/j.lfs.2016.02.002] [PMID: 26851532]

[103]   Prasad KN, Hovland AR, Cole WC, *et al.* Multiple antioxidants in the prevention and treatment of Alzheimer disease: analysis of biologic rationale. Clin Neuropharmacol 2000; 23(1): 2-13.
[http://dx.doi.org/10.1097/00002826-200001000-00002] [PMID: 10682224]

[104]   von Bernhardi R, Eugenín-von Bernhardi L, Eugenín J. Microglial cell dysregulation in brain aging and neurodegeneration. Front Aging Neurosci 2015; 7: 124.
[http://dx.doi.org/10.3389/fnagi.2015.00124] [PMID: 26257642]

[105]   Streit WJ, Mrak RE, Griffin WST. Microglia and neuroinflammation: a pathological perspective. J Neuroinflammation 2004; 1(1): 14.
[http://dx.doi.org/10.1186/1742-2094-1-14] [PMID: 15285801]

[106]   Sandberg M, Patil J, D'Angelo B, Weber SG, Mallard C. NRF2-regulation in brain health and disease: Implication of cerebral inflammation. Neuropharmacology 2014; 79: 298-306.
[http://dx.doi.org/10.1016/j.neuropharm.2013.11.004] [PMID: 24262633]

[107]   Cooper EL, Ma MJ. Alzheimer Disease: Clues from traditional and complementary medicine. J Tradit Complement Med 2017; 7(4): 380-5.
[http://dx.doi.org/10.1016/j.jtcme.2016.12.003] [PMID: 29034183]

[108]   Olajide OA, Bhatia HS, De Oliveira AC, Wright CW, Fiebich BL. Inhibition of neuroinflammation in LPS-activated microglia by cryptolepine. Evidence-Based Complementary and Alternative Medicine. 2013; 2013.

[109]   Gregory J, Vengalasetti YV, Bredesen DE, Rao RV. Neuroprotective Herbs for the Management of Alzheimer's Disease. Biomolecules 2021; 11(4): 543.
[http://dx.doi.org/10.3390/biom11040543] [PMID: 33917843]

[110]   Mullan K, Williams MA, Cardwell CR, *et al.* Serum concentrations of vitamin E and carotenoids are altered in Alzheimer's disease: A case☐control study. Alzheimers Dement (N Y) 2017; 3(3): 432-9.

[http://dx.doi.org/10.1016/j.trci.2017.06.006] [PMID: 29067349]

[111] Yuan C, Chen H, Wang Y, Schneider JA, Willett WC, Morris MC. Dietary carotenoids related to risk of incident Alzheimer dementia (AD) and brain AD neuropathology: a community-based cohort of older adults. Am J Clin Nutr 2021; 113(1): 200-8.
[http://dx.doi.org/10.1093/ajcn/nqaa303] [PMID: 33184623]

[112] Cho KS, Shin M, Kim S, Lee SB. Recent advances in studies on the therapeutic potential of dietary carotenoids in neurodegenerative diseases. Oxidative medicine and cellular longevity. 2018; 2018.
[http://dx.doi.org/10.1155/2018/4120458]

[113] Rivera DS, Lindsay C, Codocedo JF, et al. Andrographolide recovers cognitive impairment in a natural model of Alzheimer's disease (Octodon degus). Neurobiol Aging 2016; 46: 204-20.
[http://dx.doi.org/10.1016/j.neurobiolaging.2016.06.021] [PMID: 27505720]

[114] Yang R, Liu S, Zhou J, Bu S, Zhang J. Andrographolide attenuates microglia-mediated Aβ neurotoxicity partially through inhibiting NF-κB and JNK MAPK signaling pathway. Immunopharmacol Immunotoxicol 2017; 39(5): 276-84.
[http://dx.doi.org/10.1080/08923973.2017.1344989] [PMID: 28669260]

[115] Zhu X, Perry G, Smith MA, Wang X. Abnormal mitochondrial dynamics in the pathogenesis of Alzheimer's disease. J Alzheimers Dis 2013; 33(0 1) (Suppl. 1): S253-62.
[PMID: 22531428]

[116] Du H, Yan SS. Mitochondrial permeability transition pore in Alzheimer's disease: Cyclophilin D and amyloid beta. Biochim Biophys Acta Mol Basis Dis 2010; 1802(1): 198-204.
[http://dx.doi.org/10.1016/j.bbadis.2009.07.005] [PMID: 19616093]

[117] Geng J, Liu W, Xiong Y, et al. Andrographolide sulfonate improves Alzheimer-associated phenotypes and mitochondrial dysfunction in APP/PS1 transgenic mice. Biomed Pharmacother 2018; 97: 1032-9.
[http://dx.doi.org/10.1016/j.biopha.2017.11.039] [PMID: 29136781]

[118] Das S, Mishra KP, Ganju L, Singh SB. Andrographolide - A promising therapeutic agent, negatively regulates glial cell derived neurodegeneration of prefrontal cortex, hippocampus and working memory impairment. J Neuroimmunol 2017; 313: 161-75.
[http://dx.doi.org/10.1016/j.jneuroim.2017.11.003] [PMID: 29146293]

[119] Rivera DS, Inestrosa NC, Bozinovic F. On cognitive ecology and the environmental factors that promote Alzheimer disease: lessons from Octodon degus (Rodentia: Octodontidae). Biol Res 2016; 49(1): 10.
[http://dx.doi.org/10.1186/s40659-016-0074-7] [PMID: 26897365]

[120] Serrano FG, Tapia-Rojas C, Carvajal FJ, Hancke J, Cerpa W, Inestrosa NC. Andrographolide reduces cognitive impairment in young and mature AβPPswe/PS-1 mice. Mol Neurodegener 2014; 9(1): 61.
[http://dx.doi.org/10.1186/1750-1326-9-61] [PMID: 25524173]

[121] Wang L, Cao F, Zhu L, et al. Andrographolide impairs alpha-naphthylisothiocyanate-induced cholestatic liver injury in vivo. J Nat Med 2019; 73(2): 388-96.
[http://dx.doi.org/10.1007/s11418-018-01275-3] [PMID: 30617707]

[122] Yang CH, Yen TL, Hsu CY, Thomas PA, Sheu JR, Jayakumar T. Multi-targeting andrographolide, a novel NF-κB inhibitor, as a potential therapeutic agent for stroke. Int J Mol Sci 2017; 18(8): 1638.
[http://dx.doi.org/10.3390/ijms18081638] [PMID: 28749412]

[123] Guo W, Liu W, Chen G, et al. Water-soluble andrographolide sulfonate exerts anti-sepsis action in mice through down-regulating p38 MAPK, STAT3 and NF-κB pathways. Int Immunopharmacol 2012; 14(4): 613-9.
[http://dx.doi.org/10.1016/j.intimp.2012.09.002] [PMID: 23036579]

[124] Shih RH, Wang CY, Yang CM. NF-kappaB signaling pathways in neurological inflammation: a mini review. Front Mol Neurosci 2015; 8: 77.
[http://dx.doi.org/10.3389/fnmol.2015.00077] [PMID: 26733801]

CHAPTER 9

The Importance of Andrographolide and its Analogs in Prostate Cancer

Kranthi Kumar Kotha[1,#], Siddhartha Lolla[2,#], Mopuri Deepa[3,†], Gopinath Papichettypalle[4,†], Ravishankar Ram Mani[5], Narahari N. Palei[6], Arghya Kusum Dhar[7], Priyanka Keshri[8], Alagusundaram Muthumanickam[8], Mohana Vamsi Nuli[9], Saijyothi Ausali[10,*] and Vinod K. Nelson[9,*]

[1] *Departement of. Pharmaceutics, College of Pharmaceutical Sciences, Dayananda Sagar University, Bengaluru, Karnataka 560078, India*

[2] *Department of Pharmacology, GITAM School of Pharmacy, Gandhi Institute of Technology and Management Deemed to be University, Hyderabad, Telangana, India*

[3] *Departement of Pharmaceutical Chemistry, Annamacharya College of Pharmacy, Razampet, Andhra Pradesh, India*

[4] *Department of Pharmaceutical Chemistry, GITAM School of Pharmacy, GITAM University Hyderabad Campus, Rudraram, Sangareddy, Telangana State, India*

[5] *Faculty of Pharmaceutical Sciences, UCSI University, Cheras, Kuala Lumpur 56000, Malaysia*

[6] *AMITY Institute of Pharmacy, AMITY University Lucknow Campus, Uttar Pradesh-226010, India*

[7] *School of Pharmacy, The Neotia University, Sarisha, West Bengal-743368, India*

[8] *Department of Pharmaceutics, School of Pharmacy, ITM University, Gwalior, Madhya Pradesh, India*

[9] *Centre for Global Health Research, Saveetha Medical College and Hospital, Saveetha Institute of Medical and Technical Sciences, Chennai 602105, Tamil Nadu, India*

[10] *MNR College of Pharmacy, MNR Higher Education and Research Academy Campus, MNR Nagar, Sangareddy-502294, India*

Abstract: One of the most common cancers in males is prostate cancer, which frequently appears later in life after 65 years. Prostate cancer is the second most frequent disease in men globally, according to the World Health Organization (WHO), with 1.3 million new cases identified in 2018. Although the composite molecular mechanisms that cause prostate cancer are still not fully understood, certain important

[*] **Corresponding authors Vinod K. Nelson and Saijyothi Ausali:** Centre for Global Health Research, Saveetha Medical College and Hospital, Saveetha Institute of Medical and Technical Sciences, Chennai 602105, Tamil Nadu, India;
MNR College of Pharmacy, MNR Higher Education and Research Academy campus, MNR Nagar, Sangareddy-502294, India; E-mails: vinod.kumar457@gmail.com; saijyothi.28.sj@gmail.com
[#] These authors share the first author of this work
[†] These authors share a second author in this work

S. Karuppusamy, Vinod K. Nelson & T. Pullaiah (Eds.)
All rights reserved-© 2024 Bentham Science Publishers

factors have been identified. These include mutations in the androgen receptor gene and the tumor suppressor gene known as prostate cancer gene 1 (PCA1) or "BRCA1", which are linked to prostate cancer. Furthermore, overproduction of prostate-specific antigen (PSA) and changes in the concentrations or functions of particular proteins, such as cyclin-dependent kinase 4 (CDK4), function as indicators of prostate cancer and aid in its progression. Age, family history, ethnicity, food, obesity, and exposure to specific chemicals and hormones are risk factors. Depending on the stage of the disease and the patient's general condition, the main treatment options for prostate cancer include surgery, radiation therapy, hormone therapy, chemotherapy, immunotherapy, and active surveillance. Examining several strategies, natural products—especially those derived from plants—have shown signs of having anti-cancer qualities and are being researched as possible treatments for prostate cancer. Among these, andrographolide—a diterpenoid lactone compound—has attracted attention. It is extracted from the leaves of the *Andrographis paniculata* plant, traditionally used in Chinese and Ayurvedic medicine. Andrographolide and its analogs are being studied for their potential to treat a variety of malignancies, including prostate cancer, due to their well-known pharmacological actions, which include anti-inflammatory, anticancer, antiviral, and antioxidant qualities. Studies show that they have antiproliferative, pro-apoptotic, and antimetastatic properties in animal models and prostate cancer cell lines, suggesting they may be a valuable treatment for prostate cancer.

Keywords: Andrographolide, analogs, Antioxidants, Anti-cancer activity, Natural products, Prostate cancer.

INTRODUCTION

In 2018, prostate cancer (PC) was placed as the second most widespread cancer in men, after lung cancer. Approximately 1,276,106 new cases were reported every year, out of which, 358,989 deaths were noted, representing 3.8% of all cancer-related deaths in males [1]. Globally, the mean age at diagnosis for prostate cancer is 66, and both the death and prevalence rates of the disease show an age-related relationship [2]. Comparing African American men to their White counterparts, the prevalence of PC was 1.58%, and the fatality rate was nearly twice as high [1]. This discrepancy suggests that social, environmental, and genetic influences vary. By 2040, 2.2 million PC instances are predicted, and variations in death rates are projected [3].

Prostate cancer develops slowly in the early stages and advances silently. Its asymptomatic nature makes the treatment complex and unpretentious. Its symptoms include enlargement of the prostatic gland, increased frequency of urination, and nocturnal urination. As the disease progresses to the bone metastatic stage, urine incontinence and back pain are experienced by the patient. Prostate-specific antigen (PSA > four ng/mL), a glycoprotein that is generally expressed by prostate tissue, is often expressed at increased levels that aid in the diagnosis of prostate cancer [4]. Tissue biopsy remains the primary method for confirming suspected cancer, even though individuals without cancer may exhibit elevated PSA levels. Unlike many other cancers, the cause of prostate cancer has been broadly researched and remains unclear. Renowned risk factors for PC include higher age, ethnicity, genetic variables, and a family history of cancer, and it is the primary cancer diagnosed in aged men [5]. Increasingly, older men are indeed being screened for prostate cancer as men live longer lives, and PSA screening has become more common. Prevalence rates of PC reveal notable discrepancies across different locations and populations. Globally, 1.2 million new PC cases were reported in 2018, constituting 7.1% of all malignancies among the male population [6]. The occurrence of PC considerably differs among countries. Oceania recorded the maximum age-standardized rate (ASR) at 79.1 per 100,000 persons, followed by North America (73.7) and Europe (62.1) [6]. On the contrary, the prevalence rates in Asia and Africa are relatively lower than those mentioned above, *i.e.*, 26.6 and 11.5, respectively [6]. While there are noteworthy racial differences in the occurrence of PC, in the USA, White people have the second-lowest incidence, followed by Alaska Natives and Asian or Pacific Islander people [7, 8]. The frequency and fatality rates for PC are elevated among males of Afro-American descent [7]. This indicates that Afro-American men might hold definite genetic factors that raise their probability of developing prostate cancer mutations. Moreover, these mutations appear to be a more destructive form of cancer. The more prevalent 8q24 variants are known for enhancing the risk of PC among Afro-American men [9]. According to specific research, Afro-Americans cover most gene mutations that govern cell death, including BCL2, or inhibit malignancies, such as EphB2 [1, 10]. Afro-American inheritance is another factor related to hereditary and biological abnormalities, while insufficient surveillance and belated presentation cannot be ruled out. However, a 2007 study by Oliver found that Afro-Americans are notably less prone than Caucasian men to early diagnosis of PC [15]. Additionally, there is a noticeable disparity in prostate cancer mortality rates among the regions. In 2018, Central America reported the maximum death rate at 10.7 per 100,000, with Western Europe and Australia/New Zealand closely following at 10.2 [6]. In Asia, the mortality rates are diverse with regions: South-Central at 3.3, Eastern at 4.7, and South-Eastern Asia at approximately 5.4. Meanwhile, Northern Africa had the lowest mortality rate (5.8) compared to other areas. Asia contributed to 33.0% (118,427) of all prostate cancer fatalities; at the same time, Europe contributed 29.9% (107,315) [11].

About 20% of men diagnosed with PC have a previous family history indicative of the possibility of a potential connection to inherited genes, in addition to exposure to environmental toxins and universal lifestyle choices [1]. Research specifies that the hereditary genetic background contributes to 5% of the risk of developing PC. The X chromosome, housing the androgen receptor (AR) gene, is concerned with this process. Minute deletions in the AR gene are linked through sporadic and genetic forms of prostate cancer and point towards the role of the X chromosome in the transmission of PC [12]. Diet (overconsumption of fat and red meat, less use of fruit and vegetables, vitamin supplements, and coffee), excess weight, consumption of alcohol, lack of physical activity, inflammation, high blood sugar, infectious diseases, and environmental exposure to toxicants or ionizing radiation are all risk factors for prostate cancer. Research findings on immigrants migrating from low-risk regions in developing nations to high-risk areas in developed countries revealed how the transition to a "Westernized" lifestyle increased prostate cancer incidence, implying that dietary patterns play a considerable role in the growth of PC. Several studies have shown that some foods are even protective while others are linked to greater risk. The consumption of meat, fat, and dairy items per person is positively correlated with prostate mortality in numerous ecological studies. High fat intake is linked to a significant rise in the risk of PC, according to recent data on persons under 60 [13]. Heavy alcohol consumption has been correlated to various human cancers, including PC. The relative risks connected with consuming one to four drinks of alcohol per day range from 1.05 to 1.21, stressing the potential impact on prostate health [14]. For many human malignancies, both direct and indirect cigarette smoke exposure is related and leads to carcinogenesis. The link between smoking and increased risk of prostate cancer may speed up its development. Contact with various environmental variables like insecticides and herbicides enhances the chance of developing cancer and affects the gradual approach of prostate tumorigenesis. According to studies, herbicides like Agent Orange (AO) [138] and insecticides like Chlordecone (also known as Kepone) were involved [16]. Bisphenol A (BPA) is a significant chemical present in packed foods, which causes the advancement of PC [17]. Despite the high occurrence of PC, most cases are diagnosed when the cancer is confined to the prostate gland alone. In the USA, men who are diagnosed with PC have a survival rate of about five years in 98% of cases [18]. Data from the Eurocare project (EUROCARE-5) on patients diagnosed with PC between 2003 and 2007 found a 5-year survival rate of 83% [19]. Euro care project data (EUROCARE-5) for persons diagnosed with PC between 2003 and 2007 discovered a 5-year survival rate of 83% [19]. Furthermore, survival rates have increased across Europe, with the Eastern European nations exhibiting the most significant improvements.

The general principle for most cancers is diagnosing and treating early. Early treatment and probable side effects can be avoided by carefully practicing active scrutiny because many prostate cancers have a gradual and usually slothful course (classified as "low-risk" tumors). Despite progress in the perception of the etiopathogenesis of PC and the significant lifelong risk that men face, there is still a requirement for an effective chemotherapeutic drug that can be provided safely to enhance men's lives.

The "androgen theory", supported by a sizable body of historical and contemporary evidence, holds that androgens have a function in the pathogenesis and development of PC. Huggins and Hodges stated that androgens were involved in the growth and development of PC in 1941 after studying the advantages of castration in PC patients [20]. *In vitro* studies have revealed that well-differentiated PC cell lines react to androgen activation and induce apoptosis in response to androgen elimination. Similarly, *in vivo,* androgen hormones promote carcinogenesis and xenografted development in animal models, and when androgens are removed, tumors decrease. For more than 70 years, the basis of clinical treatment for metastatic PC has been the inhibition of AR signaling with Androgen Deprivation Therapy (ADT). ADT, now used, comprises pharmacological or surgical castration employing agonists or antagonists of the luteinizing-releasing hormone together with or without anti-androgen medications [21]. The formation of mCRPC makes cancer cells resistant, even though ADT delivers nearly guaranteed remission lasting 1-2 years in most patients (metastatic castration-resistant PC). Docetaxel, an anti-cancer agent that acts on microtubules, was permitted to be used in patients with metastatic colorectal cancer in 2004. Nevertheless, it only provided a minor median extension of 2.5 months until acquired resistance to the drug developed.

Finasteride and dutasteride, which are 5-α reductase inhibitors, convert testosterone hormone into active dihydrotestosterone, a prevailing and powerful androgen derivative of the prostate gland implicated in embryogenesis, growth, and along with the possibility of progression or hostility of PC [22]. Statin drugs block lipid synthesis, notably cholesterol. Despite inconsistent results, they are also linked to better outcomes following radical prostatectomy and radiation therapy. Toremifene is a selective estrogen receptor modulator [23]. A phase II trial demonstrated a negligible hazard; however, there was no discernible reduction in a phase III trial [28]. An immunotherapeutic agent, Sipuleucel-T [24], and two androgen signaling inhibitors, including Abiraterone and Enzalutamide [26], another chemotherapeutic agent, Cabazitaxel [25], and an alpha-emitting bone-seeking radioisotope [27] were the other five medications approved by FDA for the treatment of CRPC.

Although there was advancement in the treatment options and strategies, there is still a persistent increase in prostate cancer-related deaths all over the world. Apart from the effectiveness of the treatment, the side effects they pose have been an enormous burden to deal with even after the completion of the treatment regimen. Apart from several general physical side effects observed in the case of localized treatment with hormonal and surgery or systemic therapy with chemotherapy, there are side effects, including loss of libido, erectile dysfunction, less semen/dry orgasm, and a smaller penis. There are few observed sexual side effects with prostate cancer treatment, which are sometimes reversible and sometimes not. Apart from these, emotional and social side effects also surface, such as anxiety, sorrow, and irritation. Moreover, the current treatment is not affordable to many people and is a financial concern. Owing to all these existing culprits in the available treatment, researchers are continuously searching to design new drugs or discover naturally derived substances that can be effective, safe, and affordable.

Among these, natural product discovery has been widely done owing to the shortage of successful therapies with negligible adverse effects. Plant and microbial-derived compounds may be less hazardous and more practical than allopathic anti-cancer drugs. Several anticancer drugs have been originated from natural sources. Alternative medicinal systems, including Ayurveda, Unani, and Traditional Chinese Medicine, where natural products are used as therapeutic agents, are promised anti-cancer agents. Approximately 2.1 million pharmacologically active agents having drug-like properties have been discovered [29]. In the drug development process, some natural compounds have emerged as therapeutic agents to treat various cancers, like vinblastine, vincristine, vindesine, Epipodophyllotoxins, taxanes (paclitaxel and docetaxel), and camptothecin analogs. Recent experimental, clinical, and epidemiological studies show that certain nutritionally benefit compounds, including lycopene, sulforaphane, indole-3-carbinol, epigallocatechin gallate, curcumin, piperine, quercetin, resveratrol, play an essential role in PC prevention and progression. Thus, these compounds have gained much attention in developing new drug molecules to combat PC [30]. Similarly, several secondary metabolites and chemical constituents have been isolated and explored for their beneficial effect on prostate cancer.

Andrographolide (AGP), a diterpene lactone molecule derived from *Andrographis paniculata*, has been widely utilized in clinical settings for its anti-inflammatory and antibacterial properties, cardiovascular protection, and immunological modulation. According to recent research, AGP is a potent anti-cancer drug that promotes cancer cell death [31]. AGP exerted its anti-cancer effect on breast cancer cells through an apoptosis-inducing mechanism [32]. AGP increased the radio sensitivity of oesophageal cancer cells *in vitro*, resulting in severe apoptosis [33]. Similarly, AGP was discovered to repeal the resistance phenotype of cancer cells to anti-cancer medications, increasing treatment efficacy [34]. Previous research has suggested that AGP suppresses prostate cancer through cell cycle modulation. It is worth noting that when taken with anticancer medications or biological treatments, AGP can significantly limit tumor genesis and progression.

Furthermore, AGP typically improves the vulnerability of cancer cells to apoptosis [35]. This chapter briefly discusses prostate cancer, its risk factors, current treatments, and drug targets, along with the critical role of AGP and its analog in treating cancer.

Risk Factors of Prostate Cancer

PC usually occurs in a population of more than 65 years old. Approximately one person is diagnosed in six members. The following are the potential risk factors of PC.

Age

Older men experience a lower survival rate and are likely to develop high-risk prostate cancer, so age is an influential factor in selecting the type of treatment [36]. However, age of 40 years in black men is a potential risk factor than in white men without a family history [37].

Ethnicity

Recent research suggests that ethnicity is a crucial prostate cancer risk factor. The prevalence and death rate of PC is higher in Indonesian and South American males than in white men. Asian males often have the lowest rates of prostate cancer, which are correlated not only with genetic vulnerability but also with dietary, lifestyle, and environmental variables [38]. According to National Cancer Institute data, African American males have much higher rates of Prostate cancer (54.2/100,000 compared to 24.7/100,000), superior to other ethnic groups. Chromosome 8q24 mutations are more ubiquitous in Afro-American men and are associated with PC risk. Furthermore, Afro-Americans have higher rates of polymorphisms in EphB2 and BCL2 genes [39].

Family History

Family history is a well-known risk factor for PC among males [40]. Five specific single-nucleotide polymorphisms enclose a considerable relationship with the occurrence and mortality of PC predominantly when combined with a family history of the disease. A study observed a 2.3-fold higher incidence of PC among individuals with a father or brother affected by the disease under 60 years old (95% confidence interval (CI) =1.76-3.12). PC risk may carry a hereditary factor, with genes from seven distinct loci implicated. Nevertheless, the role of these genes in PC development remains uncertain and may contribute less than 5-10% of the overall risk [41].

Insulin-Like Growth Factors

Insulin-like growth factors inhibit apoptosis, promote cell division, and play an imperative role in PC biology, exerting mitogenic and anti-apoptotic effects [42]. Several studies have established a link between serum levels of IGF-1 and the risk of PC. Mainly, the European population exhibits high circulating IGF-1, a factor optimistically connected with a heightened incidence of PC [43].

Sexually Transmitted Disease

Sexually transmitted diseases and their relation were well described. McNicol and Dodd revealed the presence of human papillomavirus types 16 and 18 in healthy and malignant human prostate cells [44]. This study was further supported by Southern blot and polymerase chain reaction analysis to detect high-risk HPVs in prostate cancer tissues. Thirteen published studies focused on investigating HPVs in PC, revealing a prevalence ranging from 4.2% to 53% [44].

Obesity

The advancement and aggression of PC are linked to obesity and body mass index (BMI). Obesity increases insulin resistance and reduces glucose uptake, especially when combined with physical inactivity. Insulin encourages the growth and proliferation of healthy cells and accelerates the development of prostate cancer [45, 46]. Further, a rise in fat, ROS levels, and oxidative stress causes the cells to undergo DNA damage and peroxidation [47]. Increased ROS, leukotrienes, and prostaglandins from fat metabolism alter basal metabolism, insulin growth factor, and tumor proliferation to promote prostate carcinogenesis [13].

Smoking

Tobacco and cigarette smoke emits many toxicants, many of which are cancer-causing agents [48]. To exercise their carcinogenic impact, however, cigarette smoke components like polycyclic aromatic hydrocarbons have to activate the metabolism, evade detoxifying procedures, and then attach to DNA. Thus, the impact of smoking on PC may be altered by functional polymorphisms in genes implicated in polycyclic aromatic hydrocarbon metabolism and detoxification [49]. Men who smoke were shown to have higher amounts of the hormones androsterone and testosterone in their blood than non-smokers, which may raise their risk of developing PC or speed up the progression of the disease [50].

Alcohol Consumption

One of the noteworthy risk factors for cancer in humans is alcohol intake, and it is the primary variable that should be avoided. Alcohol intake is typically measured in drinks per day, and its use, hefty consumption, may increase the risk of certain malignancies, like PC [51]. There is data on the effect of alcohol on polymorphisms of genes coding for DNA repair, folate metabolism, and ethanol metabolism enzymes (alcohol dehydrogenase) [10, 52]. However, some cohort researchers have found a tenuous link between alcohol consumption and mortality of PC, while other investigations have found no link at all [53].

Vasectomy

Approximately 500,000 vasectomy surgeries are performed annually in the USA, making it a popular method of male contraception. A few studies have correlated it to a higher risk of PC [54]. There is no established biological mechanism that could account for the link between vasectomy and PC. Data were constrained in studies showing low relative risks due to methodological issues and possible prejudice, such as detection and misclassification bias [55].

Diet

Rising testosterone levels in PC and a more fatty diet have frequently been related to a higher risk of PC [56]. Similarly, consumption of meat and cancer incidence and mortality have a link to carcinogenesis [57]. According to Rohman *et al.* [40], males who consume more processed meat every week than one serving have a higher chance of developing PC. Thus, American black men with an excessive red meat diet had a high risk of PC [58]. Recent studies reveal that high calcium content and milk and dairy consumption raise the level of saturated fats, leading to more significant PC risks [59]. The involvement of calcium in the progression of PC is biologically plausible. Intracellular calcium pools have been demonstrated to regulate PC cell proliferation and apoptotic susceptibility. Therefore, trivial changes in calcium homeostasis may cause PC cells to proliferate, differentiate, and undergo apoptosis more frequently [60].

Drugs Targets in Prostate Cancer

Several targets have been connected with PC; a few critical targets are briefed below.

Targets Associated with Androgen Receptor Axis

The androgen receptor (AR) is recognized as a ligand-dependent transcription factor in the nuclear receptor family. This receptor is essential for the growth and expansion of PC [61]. AR has four dominos and, upon interaction with its ligand, translocates to the nucleus to allow contacts between motifs in the DNA binding domine and ligand binding domine. The dimerization of receptors differentiates response elements on cognate DNA in both intra- and intergenic regulatory regions, proximal or distal to the androgen target gene [62]. Hence, this receptor plays a fundamental part in the proliferation of PCs, and targeting AR is essential in PC management. Currently, androgen deprivation therapy, relating to pharmaceutical castration, is considered the most successful approach [63, 64]. An additional mechanism contributing to androgen-independent proliferation in PC is ligand perplexity, which originates from mutations in the AR gene leading to amino acid modification in the LBD, causing a lack of ligand specificity and selectivity [65].

F876L, T877A, L701H, and W741L have altered fragments of the androgen receptors that combine with other hormones like sex hormones and corticoids to trigger the AR signaling mechanism and promote cancer development [66]. AR stimulation through ligand-independent processes is the third pathway of androgen-independent PC formation [67]. Indeed, ligands activating tyrosine kinase receptors like epidermal growth factor and IGF-1 help activate the AR *via* the PI3K/Akt/mTOR mechanism [68, 69]. Finally, recent reports show that multiple AR pre-mRNAs are absent of LBD, leading to activation of the AR-terminal and allowing castration-resistant proliferation [70]. Targeting these signaling cascades and mutations responsible for modulation of the AR axis has been shown to inhibit PC.

Targets Associated with Proliferation

When activated, the receptor tyrosine kinase EGFR is connected to increased cell survival and proliferation, which illustrates why EGFR is typically abundantly expressed in epithelial malignancies such as PC. It stimulates many downstream signaling pathways upon binding with its specialized ligands, such as EGF and TGFa, including PI3K/Akt/mTOR, MAPK, Hedgehog (Hb) signaling, and NF-kB, each of which has been a therapeutic target [71]. Targeting EGFR and its related downstream kinase activities have been shown to significantly suppress prostate cancer proliferation.

The insulin growth factor-1 alignment is a signal transduction complex related to several tumorigenic processes, including cancer development, metabolism, and endurance. It entails the association of the IGF-1 and IGF-2 with their concerned receptor sites and its activation results in the activation of down regulatory signals like PI3K/AKT and MAPK [72]. Ironically, the IGF axis is an accepted target in PC treatment.

As a result, it is validated that the creation of new PI3K inhibitors is capable of inhibiting castration-resistant PC development and survival [74]. NF-B promotes tumor invasion and chemoresistance during PC development. NF-B activation is linked with AR loss and castration resistance, producing carcinogenesis and therapeutic resistance in PC [73].

The Wnt pathway is also important in the development of castration-resistant PC, according to genome sequencing and gene expression investigations [75, 76]. Wnt signaling has also been a potential target in inhibiting cancer growth and resistance. Several apoptosis-related targets have also been identified in prostate cancer. Many medications are designed to induce apoptosis by targeting and engaging cell membrane DR, changing the Bad/BCL-2 ratio, escalating p21 levels, and activating caspases and PARP breakage [77 - 82].

Targets Associated with Cancer Cell Metabolism

Tumor cell metabolism is often characterized by more flow of glucose *via* glycolysis and HMP shunt, making it a valuable therapeutic target. Treatments that disrupt these processes and/or transfer fermentation of lactic acid to oxidative phosphorylation in mitochondria have shown potential in lowering tumor development [83]. As previously stated, cancer cells require increased glucose absorption to meet their elevated requirement for the growth and proliferation of cells. It is accomplished by an enhanced diffusion process mediated by glucose transporters (GLUTs). These transporters are targeted and modulated to alter glucose uptake and inhibit metabolism in cancer cells.

Many investigations have shown that previous non-invasive PC is distinguished with augmented lipid synthesis apart from extracellular/circulating lipid levels [84, 85]. Increased *de novo* lipogenesis has been linked to PC cells' demand for more energy, creation of membranes, escape from normal death of cells, and regulation of several intra-cellular proliferative mechanisms [86, 87]. As a result, the specific lipid metabolic properties of PCa constitute an ideal target for cancer therapy.

Targets Associated with Cancer Metastasis

Transfer of malignant cells (metastasis) from the main tumor to other bodily tissues and organs is an important phase during PC. Shifting from epithelial-t--mesenchymal is the essential feature of metastasis and involves an important transition in the expression of adhesion molecules that regulate the interaction of tumor cells through the extra-cellular matrix and their surroundings. Many signaling cascades, including as PI3K/Akt and Wnt-catenin, are known to perpetuate EMT, culminating in metastasis [88 - 90]. Further, MMP-2 and MMP-9 have been linked to tumor invasiveness, including PCa among all matrix metalloproteinases (MMPs) involved in ECM destruction [91 - 93]. These levels were reduced following treatment with several nutraceuticals, and this often coincides with MAPK inactivation [81, 94, 95]. The normal epithelial CD44 standard (CD445) is eliminated in tumors, but the pro-invasive splice alternative isoform CD447-10 is abundantly expressed [96]. CD44 is also utilized as a target by various drugs for the treatment of prostate cancer.

Targeting Angiogenesis

A significant cancer-derived angiogenic factor is vascular endothelial growth factor expressed as VEGFR-1 and VEGFR-2, related to tyrosine kinase. VEGFR-2 is more significant in driving the proliferation of endothelial cells, migration, and formation of the tube by engaging a variety of downstream signals, including PI3K/Akt and MAPKs [97]. Hypoxia and transforming growth factor-Beta are key targets implicated in the rise in VEGF release [98]. Similarly, extracellular calcium-binding glycoprotein TSP-1 is a 450 kDa that also functions as a potent endogenous anti-angiogenic target [99].

Targeting Cancer Stem Cells

Prostate cancer stem cells (PCSCs) are tiny fractions similar to stem-like cells that can self-renew and differentiate, along with tutor-initiating and spreading capabilities. Markers present on the surface of the cell, including CD133, CD44, and a261 integrin, are routinely utilized to perceive and enhance PCSCs. PCSCs are now being studied extensively for anti-cancer drug development because of their resistance to traditional treatments, contribution to metastasis or relapse, and development of castration-resistant PC [100].

Apart from these targets, several continuing research studies on prostate cancer have been elucidating various other novel proteins and pathways as targets that can be exploited by developing drugs against them to eradicate cancer in an effective way [101].

Furthermore, epigenetic changes lead to continuing, inheritable modifications in gene expression without affecting genetic sequences or the function of a particular gene. PC demonstrates an 'epigenetic catastrophe', where the modifications occurring in the early stages of tumor initiation continue all through malignancy progression. Given its slow onset and gradual advancement, prostate cancer becomes an ideal candidate for chemoprevention through the use of epigenetic modulators. A range of studies exploring the potential of several DNA methylase inhibitors and histone deacetylase inhibitors as treatments for PC. These drugs include Vidaza, Decitabine Panabinostat, Vorinostat, and Romidepsin (HDAC class I inhibitor) [102].

Current Treatment Strategies and Side Effects of Prostate Cancer

Local Treatments

<u>*Surgery*</u>

• Radical prostatectomy is a process in which the entire prostate gland and seminal vesicles are surgically removed; the excision of pelvic lymph nodes is another option. However, this may affect the sexual function of the patient. Another negative impact of radical prostatectomy on testosterone levels is incontinence.

• Robotic or laparoscopic prostatectomy is another procedure adopted to reduce invasiveness than a radical prostatectomy and may result in a shorter recovery period. A camera and tools are placed into the patient's belly through tiny keyhole incisions. The robotic devices are then directed by the surgeon to extract the prostate. The advantages of this procedure including less bleeding and discomfort than open prostatectomy.

<u>*Radiation therapy*</u>

Radiation treatment using an external beam is the most common kind of therapy in PC. Treating a person with a higher daily dose of radiotherapy over a shorter amount of time rather than lesser doses over a greater amount of time is referred to as accelerated radiation therapy. Moderate hypofraction radiation treatment regimens typically consist of 20 to 28 sessions. Hypofractionated radiation therapy may benefit individuals diagnosed with low-risk prostate cancer who might need or favor intervention overactive monitoring, along with individuals with medium or elevated-risk prostate cancer who are getting external-beam irradiation to the prostate and presumably the pelvic lymph nodes. This treatment can lead to some side effects that include an increased desire to urinate, sexual function issues, bowel function issues like diarrhea, rectal discomfort, rectal bleeding, and weariness during treatment.

<u>*Hormonal Therapy*</u>

Hormonal therapy is a crucial and efficient treatment option for PC since reducing levels of androgen hormones can help limit the disease's development. Testosterone is the most prevalent androgen involved in PC, and pharmacologically active antagonists of testosterone are employed in the management of PC. Hormonal therapy is employed in PC in several circumstances, including localized, locally advanced, metastatic prostate cancer, as well as to raise PSA levels after regionalized prostate surgical treatment and/or radiation therapy. For the treatment of advanced-stage PC, the FDA has approved the monthly injection of degarelix (Firmagon). This medication's potential to trigger a serious allergic reaction is one of its negative effects.

Androgen receptor inhibitors are another prominent choice in PC. These drugs prevent testosterone from functioning. Older AR inhibitors are in the form of pills and include bicalutamide, flutamide, and nilutamide. Apalutamide, darolutamide, and enzalutamide are more recent AR inhibitors. Androgen Synthesis inhibitors are also employed in the treatment of PC. Androgen synthesis inhibitors hinder cells from generating testosterone by blocking an enzyme called CYP17. Ketoconazole and Abiraterone are androgen synthesis blockers that are no longer often used due to several medication interactions. Hormonal treatment has several negative effects, including erectile dysfunction (ED), sexual arousal loss, fatigue, gynecomastia, and hot flashes. Further other effects include depression, loss of memory, cognitive deficits, heart disease, weight increase, and osteopenia.

Chemotherapy

Chemotherapy is a commonly used treatment option to eradicate the majority of malignancies. This might help both advanced or castration-resistant prostate cancer and recently diagnosed or castration-sensitive metastatic prostate cancer. A chemotherapeutic regimen, or schedule, generally consists of a set number of cycles spread out over a set time period.

In most cases, conventional chemotherapy begins with docetaxel and prednisone. This combination helps newly diagnosed patients or castration-sensitive metastatic prostate cancer extend life and prevent the illness from developing and spreading. Cabazitaxel is another approved drug for the management of metastatic castration-resistant PC act by blocking microtubules.

Medicinal Plants and Phytocompounds used in PC Treatment

Microbial and plant-derived compounds may be less hazardous and more useful than traditional anti-cancer drugs. As a result, several of these agents are in clinical trials; however, they have certain limitations, such as low bioavailability [103, 104]. The available natural anticancer agents include podophyllotoxins, vinca alkaloids, and camptothecins [105]. These compounds reveal multiple pharmacological activities, like anti-inflammatory [106] and anticancer [107, 108] properties. Terpenes and terpenoids are another category of phytocompounds that provide promising new paths for the identification of novel medication candidates in the arena of cancer treatment. Terpenoids cause apoptosis in prostate cancer cell lines or xenografts, which leads to tumor cell proliferation and growth inhibition. Several mechanisms are involved in the induction of apoptosis by various terpenoids, such as inhibiting the ubiquitin-proteasome and NF-B pathways, which is related to an increase in proapoptotic protein Bax and a reduction in anti-apoptotic protein Bcl-2, resulting in cytochrome c release, caspase activation, and apoptotic cell death [82]. Recent research has shown that δ-tocotrienol, present in rice bran and palm oil [109], may induce both apoptosis and paraptosis of various cancer cell lines [63]. Another compound, apigenin, inhibits PCSC development by increasing p21 and p27 protein levels in a dose-dependent manner. Furthermore, apigenin administration reduces the expression of the pluripotency marker Oct3/4 protein *via* the PI3K/Akt/NF-B pathway [110 - 112]. Quercetin is a penta-hydroxylated flavonol that possesses anti-cancer and chemopreventive properties in LNCaP cell lines. Quercetin complex with androgen receptor at specific protein 1 and c-Jun inhibits AR activity and also reduces expression of androgen-associated genes like ornithine decarboxylase and NKX3.1 [113, 114]. Fisetin, a fruit flavone confirmed in PC, selectively binds to the AR LBD and suppresses tumor development *in vivo* [115]. Curcumin is a polyphenol derived from *Curcuma longa,* a potential anticancer agent that reduces the expression of AR and AR-related cofactors like activator protein-1 (AP-1), NF-kB, CREB-binding protein (CBP), and NKX3.1 in PC cell lines and xenograft models [116, 117].

The other biologically active phytocompounds, including luteolin, quercetin, genistein, and resveratrol, reduce EGFR levels and restrict their inherent tyrosine kinase activity along with ligand-induced activation in various PC cell models and animal models. Silibinin is another anti-cancer molecule acting on the IGF axis that aborts cancer development, survival, and metabolism in cancer cell lines [118, 119].

NF-κB promotes tumor invasion and chemoresistance during PC development. Certain compounds like genistein, sulforaphane, ursolic acid, tocotrienol, and celastrol down-regulate NF-κB in the PC cell line to elicit anticancer effects [120 - 122]. Wnt inhibitors are other promising compounds that reduce PC development in pre-clinical investigations. Few drug molecules are in phase I studies but have not yet been given to PC patients [76, 75]. Interestingly, quercetin, curcumin, genistein, and silibinin treatment of PC cells resulted in growth reduction *via* Wnt cascade modification [123].

Some phytochemical compounds are also involved in the abruption of tumor cell metabolism, causing cessation of tumor growth. Transporters involved in glucose transport, *i.e.,* enzymes occupied in glucose and lipid metabolism in cancer cells, have also been targets of several natural compounds like apigenin, phloretin, sulforaphane (inhibit glucose metabolism and transport), and certain other compounds like quercetin, luteolin, sulforaphane and kaempferol involved in lipid metabolism [89, 120, 124]. Apart from these, angiogenesis and cancer stem cells have also been targeted by natural products in prostate cancer setups and have been shown to exhibit excellent potency compared to existing treatments [91, 120].

Andrographolide and its Analog's Role in Prostate Cancer

Andrographolide (AGP) is the main biologically active secondary metabolite of *Andrographis paniculata*. It is a bicyclic diterpenoid lactone with significant anticancer effects, including in prostate cancer, as demonstrated by earlier research, and its efficacy was attributed to a variety of pathways. Through the modulation of pro-inflammatory cytokines like IL-6 and chemokines like CXCL11, CXCR3, and CXCR7, as well as particular cell cycle regulators like cyclin-dependent kinases, andrographolide has been shown to hinder tumor formation in prostate cancer cells [125 - 127].

Interleukin -6 functions as a growth factor in androgen-dependent LNCaP, PC-3, and DU145 cells [129]. These cells were used to elucidate the selectivity of andrographolide on the way to block IL-6. LNCaP cells reveal an absence of IL-6 but express its receptor, whereas DU145 and PC-3 show a constitutive IL-6 autocrine loop. In the earlier situation, AGP demonstrated the capacity to inhibit the paracrine IL-6-stimulated mechanism, which includes JAK/STAT, MAPK/Erk phosphorylation, and PI3K/AKT Akt phosphorylation pathways. The androgen dependence of the cancer cells, status of p53, and prostate-specific antigen (PSA) are attributed to the sensitivity of prostate cancer cells towards AGP [127]. Likewise, AGP exhibits higher cytotoxic selectivity for PC-3 cells (GI50 = 1.5 mM), which are independent of androgen and express PSA, yet lack p53. AGP treatment to mice xenografted with DU145 cells significantly inhibited tumor development while having no visible adverse consequences. Initiating apoptosis was signified as another mechanistic approach of AGP to act against tumor suppression. 10mM of AGP stimulated apoptosis and could inhibit prostate cancer cell growth [125]. Apoptosis by AGP was brought about by modulating the PARP, caspases, and Bcl-2 family members involved in the intrinsic pathway [130]. When treated with 10 mM AGP, about 86% of PC-3 cells were identified to be in the early and late phases of apoptosis 9 [35]. Similarly, another study supported this apoptosis-inducing property and discovered that andrographolide induces an apoptotic mechanism *via* the activation of the caspase mechanism and boosting the expression of Bax and Bid belonging to the pro-apoptotic Bcl-2 family [127]. Additionally, AGP inhibited the G-2/M phase of the cell cycle by down-regulating the cyclin-dependent kinase (CDK) 1 expression. Andrographolide, in addition, promotes p53 and free radical-dependent TRAIL-mediated apoptotic cell death in PC-3 cells by increasing the DR4 and DR5 receptor expression along with activating the caspase-8/caspase-3 pathway [35]. In another report, C4-2b cells' growth and survival were inhibited by AGP treatment [126]. AGP has been demonstrated to influence and inhibit cell cycle progression by altering the regulators of the cell cycle, such as cyclin B1, cyclin A2, and cyclin E2, as well as CXCR3 or CXCR7 chemokine receptors. After AGP treatment, cyclin A2 levels rose in all prostate cancer cell lines, and cytokine B1 levels were augmented in LNCaP and PC3, albeit reduced in C4-2b, and remained unchanged in DU-145 cells. There was a reduction only in cyclin E2 levels in PC3 and DU-145 cells. AGP affected PC cell survival in a dosage-dependent way with no effect on primary epithelial cells of the prostate. It also changed the phosphorylation of Rb, H3, Weel, and CDC2 in all prostate cancer cells [126]. Additionally, in prostate cancer cells, receptor-ligand axes (C-X-C motif of CXCL11-CXCR3/7) were also diminished by AGP treatment, which resulted in the downregulation of cell viability and stalled migration of cells. Conversely, andrographolide exhibits a potent anti-angiogenic activity [131, 132]. Lately, few mechanistic studies revealed that AGP could exhibit metabolic changes, alter mitochondrial bioenergetics, and produce ROS in the mitochondria of PC cells. The genes associated with carbohydrate metabolism in the PC cell lines were found to be altered with AGP treatment [133]. Additionally, treatment resulted in the inhibition of mitochondrial activity in PC3 and 22Rv1 prostate cancer cell lines, causing a metabolic phenotype that resulted in cancer cell death. AGP treatment displayed a transformed ATP production ratio between glycolysis-ATP production and mitochondrial-AP in prostate cancer cell lines like PC3 and 22RV1. In 22Rv1 cells treated with AGP, mitochondrial membrane potential analysis reveals membrane depolarization. Furthermore, mitochondrial ROS generation was increased 1.4-fold in 22Rv1 cells when treated with AGP for 24 hours [133, 134].

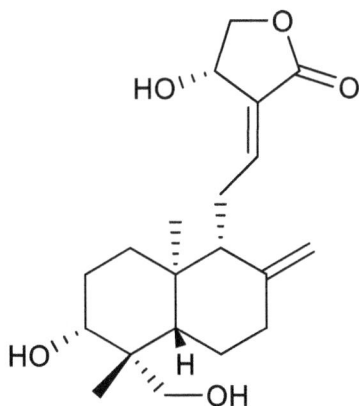

[1] Andrographolide

Owing to all these significant antitumor properties exhibited by AGP, few researchers designed synthetic and semi-synthetic derivatives of AGP to investigate anticancer potential against PC, and few compounds were reported. To enhance AGP's antitumor effectiveness, a derivative known as 3, 19-(3-chlor--4-fluorobenzylidene) andrographolide (SRJ23) (Structure 2) was synthesized and shown to preferentially inhibit the development of PC cells [135]. When compared to the parent chemical AGP (GI50 = 19.95 mM), SRJ23 (GI50 = 0.4 mM) triggered cell cycle arrest in the G2/M phase, which coincided with a decline in CDKI expression and apoptosis of PC-3 cells through the activation of the mitochondrial caspase-cascade signal pathway [128].

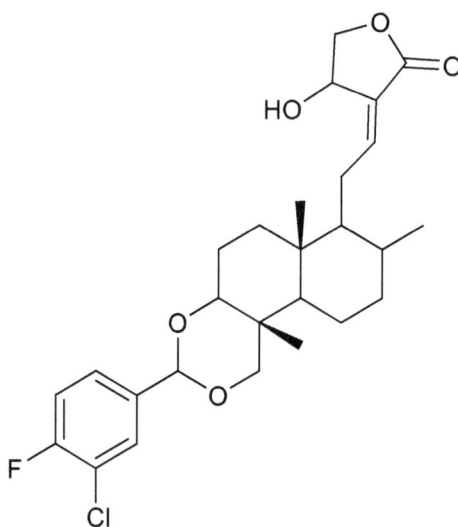

[2] SRJ23

Another study designed 38 analogs of andrographolide *via* the modification of C-12 and 14-OH positions with the introduction of novel hetero aromatic or aromatic thioether into the structure. All the analogs designed exhibited superior activity when compared to AGP. Among these compounds, seven compounds 3, 4, 5, 6, 7, 8, and 9 (isopropylideneandrographolide analogs) displayed substantial anticancer activity towards PC cell line PC3 along with breast cancer cell lines (MCF-7 and MDA-MB-231). They also elucidated that heteroaromatic thioether containing C-12 andrographolide derivatives possessed comparatively more anti-prostate cancer activity than the compounds with aromatic thioether modification. Further, the study also reported that the length of the linker and the substitution sequence on the aromatic ring had no effect on the activity of the C-14 analogs [136].

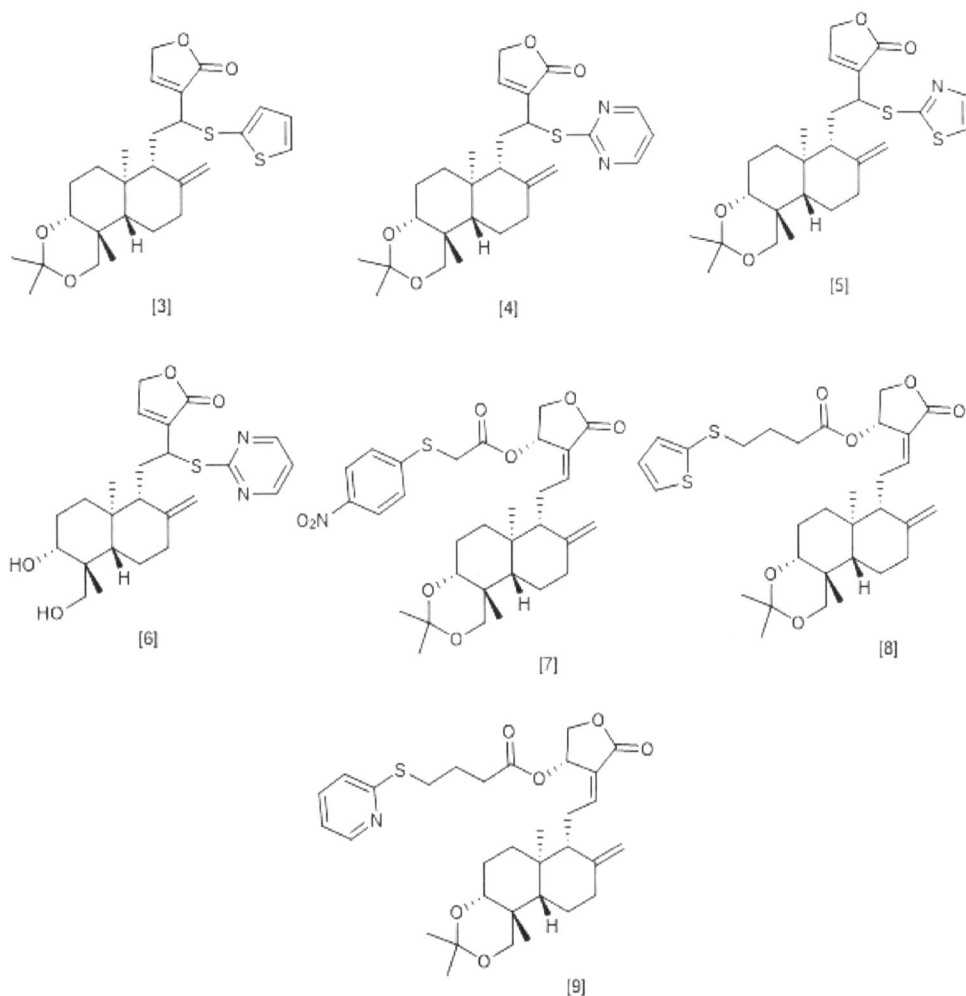

[3]   [4]   [5]

[6]   [7]   [8]

[9]

Another andrographolide derivative, 19-tert-butyldiphenylsilyl-8,7-epoxy andrographolide (3A.1) (Structure 10), was reported to possess anticancer activity against several cancers. The compound was examined for its mechanistic approach in inhibiting aggressive metastatic castration-resistant PC, alone and in combination with docetaxel (DTX) or cabazitaxel (CBZ). 3A.1 alone displayed a time and concentration-dependent inhibition of mCRPC. However, when given in combination with taxanes DTX and CBZ, it resulted in a reduced required dose of both taxanes. Further, it was elucidated that the treatment of 3A.1 stimulated apoptosis, augmented heat shock proteins (Hsp70, Hsp40, Hsp27, and Hsp90), and diminished MAT2A, which was evidenced to be associated with invasion and cell migration. Further, the compound was also shown to alter the differentially exhibited genes associated with cell migration, cancer progression pathways, DNA damage, hypoxia, and autophagy (MMP1, MMP9, HIF-1α, Bag-3, H2AX, HMOX1, PSRC1). All these results suggested that compound 3A. 1 was shown to synergistically enhance the anticancer potency of taxanes against aggressive cancer [137].

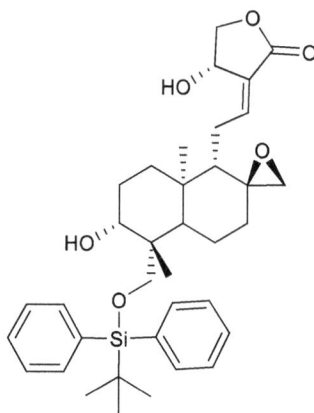

[10] 3A.1

CONCLUSION

Prostate cancer is frequently observed as a malignancy among males, and it most commonly affects older men. Prostate cancer's molecular pathways are complicated and not fully understood. However, certain crucial actors have been found, including genetic abnormalities linked to prostate cancer in the tumor suppressor gene known as prostate cancer gene 1 (PCA1) or "BRCA1", as well as alterations in the androgen receptor gene. Changes in the levels or activity of some proteins, such as cyclin-dependent kinase 4 (CDK4), as well as an increase in the synthesis of the protein PSA (prostate-specific antigen), which may be used as a diagnostic for prostate cancer, all play a part in prostate cancer. Investigations are being done on natural compounds as potential therapeutics for prostate cancer since they have been shown to have potential anti-cancer properties. This type of phytocompound is andrographolide and its derivatives, a diterpenoid lactone chemical used for centuries in alternative medicine. It is found in the leaves of the *Andrographis paniculata* plant. Numerous studies have examined andrographolide and its analogs as potential compounds to treat cancer and a variety of malignancies, including prostate cancer. It has been shown that andrographolide and its structural analogs have anti-proliferative, pro-apoptotic, and anti-metastatic effects on prostate cancer cell lines and animal models, underscoring its applicability as a potential alternative therapy for prostate cancer.

REFERENCES

[1]   Rawla P. Epidemiology of Prostate Cancer. World J Oncol 2019; 10(2): 63-89.
[http://dx.doi.org/10.14740/wjon1191] [PMID: 31068988]

[2]   Daniyal M, Siddiqui ZA, Akram M, Asif HM, Sultana S, Khan A. Epidemiology, etiology, diagnosis and treatment of prostate cancer. Asian Pac J Cancer Prev 2014; 15(22): 9575-8.
[http://dx.doi.org/10.7314/APJCP.2014.15.22.9575] [PMID: 25520069]

[3]   Pandit AA, Gressler LE, Halpern MT, Kamel M, Payakachat N, Li C. Racial/Ethnic Disparities in Patient Care Experiences among Prostate Cancer Survivors: A SEER-CAHPS Study. Curr Oncol 2022; 29(11): 8357-73.
[http://dx.doi.org/10.3390/curroncol29110659] [PMID: 36354719]

[4]   Balk SP, Ko YJ, Bubley GJ. Biology of prostate-specific antigen. J Clin Oncol 2003; 21(2): 383-91.
[http://dx.doi.org/10.1200/JCO.2003.02.083] [PMID: 12525533]

[5]   Heinzer H, Steuber T. Prostate cancer in the elderly. Urol Oncol 2009; 27(6): 668-72.
[http://dx.doi.org/10.1016/j.urolonc.2009.07.015] [PMID: 19879477]

[6]   Bray F, Ferlay J, Soerjomataram I, Siegel RL, Torre LA, Jemal A. Global cancer statistics 2018: GLOBOCAN estimates of incidence and mortality worldwide for 36 cancers in 185 countries. CA Cancer J Clin 2018; 68(6): 394-424.
[http://dx.doi.org/10.3322/caac.21492] [PMID: 30207593]

[7]   Giaquinto AN, Miller KD, Tossas KY, Winn RA, Jemal A, Siegel RL. Cancer statistics for African American/Black People 2022. CA Cancer J Clin 2022; 72(3): 202-29.
[http://dx.doi.org/10.3322/caac.21718] [PMID: 35143040]

[8]   Johnson JA, Moser RP, Ellison GL, Martin DN. Associations of prostate-specific antigen (PSA) testing in the US population: Results from a national cross-sectional survey. J Community Health 2021; 46(2): 389-98.
[http://dx.doi.org/10.1007/s10900-020-00923-8] [PMID: 33064229]

[9]   Haiman CA, Patterson N, Freedman ML, et al. Multiple regions within 8q24 independently affect risk for prostate cancer. Nat Genet 2007; 39(5): 638-44.
[http://dx.doi.org/10.1038/ng2015] [PMID: 17401364]

[10]   Perdana NR, Mochtar CA, Umbas R, Hamid AR. The risk factors of prostate cancer and its prevention: A literature review. Acta Med Indones 2016; 48(3): 228-38.
[PMID: 27840359]

[11]   Culp MB, Soerjomataram I, Efstathiou JA, Bray F, Jemal A. Recent global patterns in prostate cancer incidence and mortality rates. Eur Urol 2020; 77(1): 38-52.
[http://dx.doi.org/10.1016/j.eururo.2019.08.005] [PMID: 31493960]

[12]   Quigley CA, Bellis AD, Marschke KB, El-Awady MK, Wilson EM, French FS. Androgen receptor defects: historical, clinical, and molecular perspectives. Endocr Rev 1995; 16(3): 271-321.
[http://dx.doi.org/10.1210/edrv-16-3-271] [PMID: 7671849]

[13]   Lophatananon A, Archer J, Easton D, et al. Dietary fat and early-onset prostate cancer risk. Br J Nutr 2010; 103(9): 1375-80.
[http://dx.doi.org/10.1017/S0007114509993291] [PMID: 20082736]

[14]   Platz EA, Leitzmann MF, Rimm EB, Willett WC, Giovannucci E. Alcohol intake, drinking patterns, and risk of prostate cancer in a large prospective cohort study. Am J Epidemiol 2004; 159(5): 444-53.
[http://dx.doi.org/10.1093/aje/kwh062] [PMID: 14977640]

[15]   Reddy A, Roberts R, Shenoy D, Packianathan S, Giri S, Vijayakumar S. Prostate cancer screening guidelines for African American veterans: A new perspective. J Natl Med Assoc 2020; 112(5): 448-53.
[http://dx.doi.org/10.1016/j.jnma.2018.10.010] [PMID: 30409717]

[16]   Multigner L, Ndong JR, Giusti A, et al. Chlordecone exposure and risk of prostate cancer. J Clin

Oncol 2010; 28(21): 3457-62.
[http://dx.doi.org/10.1200/JCO.2009.27.2153] [PMID: 20566993]

[17] Di Donato M, Cernera G, Giovannelli P, *et al.* Recent advances on bisphenol-A and endocrine disruptor effects on human prostate cancer. Mol Cell Endocrinol 2017; 457: 35-42.
[http://dx.doi.org/10.1016/j.mce.2017.02.045] [PMID: 28257827]

[18] Siegel DA, O'Neil ME, Richards TB, Dowling NF, Weir HK. Prostate Cancer Incidence and Survival, by Stage and Race/Ethnicity — United States, 2001–2017. MMWR Morb Mortal Wkly Rep 2020; 69(41): 1473-80.
[http://dx.doi.org/10.15585/mmwr.mm6941a1] [PMID: 33056955]

[19] Marhold M, Kramer G, Krainer M, Le Magnen C. The prostate cancer landscape in Europe: Current challenges, future opportunities. Cancer Lett 2022; 526: 304-10.
[http://dx.doi.org/10.1016/j.canlet.2021.11.033] [PMID: 34863887]

[20] Huggins C, Scott WW. Bilateral adrenalectomy in prostatic cancer: Clinical features and urinary excretion of 17-ketosteroids and estrogen. Ann Surg 1945; 122(6): 1031-41.
[http://dx.doi.org/10.1097/00000658-194512260-00012] [PMID: 17858696]

[21] Schröder F, Crawford ED, Axcrona K, Payne H, Keane TE. Androgen deprivation therapy: past, present and future. BJU Int 2012; 109(s6) (Suppl. 6): 1-12.
[http://dx.doi.org/10.1111/j.1464-410X.2012.11215.x] [PMID: 22672120]

[22] Hirshburg JM, Kelsey PA, Therrien CA, Gavino AC, Reichenberg JS. Adverse effects and safety of 5-alpha reductase inhibitors (finasteride, dutasteride): A systematic review. J Clin Aesthet Dermatol 2016; 9(7): 56-62.
[PMID: 27672412]

[23] Patel MI, Subbaramaiah K, Du B, *et al.* Celecoxib inhibits prostate cancer growth: evidence of a cyclooxygenase-2-independent mechanism. Clin Cancer Res 2005; 11(5): 1999-2007.
[http://dx.doi.org/10.1158/1078-0432.CCR-04-1877] [PMID: 15756026]

[24] Kantoff PW, Higano CS, Shore ND, *et al.* Sipuleucel-T immunotherapy for castration-resistant prostate cancer. N Engl J Med 2010; 363(5): 411-22.
[http://dx.doi.org/10.1056/NEJMoa1001294] [PMID: 20818862]

[25] Paller CJ, Antonarakis ES. Cabazitaxel: a novel second-line treatment for metastatic castration-resistant prostate cancer. Drug Des Devel Ther 2011; 5: 117-24.
[PMID: 21448449]

[26] de Wit R, de Bono J, Sternberg CN, *et al.* CARD Investigators. Cabazitaxel *versus* abiraterone or enzalutamide in metastatic prostate cancer. N Engl J Med 2019; 381(26): 2506-18.
[http://dx.doi.org/10.1056/NEJMoa1911206] [PMID: 31566937]

[27] Du Y, Dizdarevic S. Molecular radiotheragnostics in prostate cancer. Clin Med (Lond) 2017; 17(5): 458-61.
[http://dx.doi.org/10.7861/clinmedicine.17-5-458] [PMID: 28974599]

[28] Rittmaster RS, Fleshner NE, Thompson IM. Pharmacological approaches to reducing the risk of prostate cancer. Eur Urol 2009; 55(5): 1064-74.
[http://dx.doi.org/10.1016/j.eururo.2009.01.037] [PMID: 19200641]

[29] Shanmugam MK, Lee JH, Chai EZP, *et al.* Cancer prevention and therapy through the modulation of transcription factors by bioactive natural compounds. Semin Cancer Biol 2016; 40-41: 35-47.
[http://dx.doi.org/10.1016/j.semcancer.2016.03.005] [PMID: 27038646]

[30] Mokbel K, Wazir U, Mokbel K. Chemoprevention of prostate cancer by natural agents: Evidence from molecular and epidemiological studies. Anticancer Res 2019; 39(10): 5231-59.
[http://dx.doi.org/10.21873/anticanres.13720] [PMID: 31570421]

[31] Mishra SK, Tripathi S, Shukla A, Oh SH, Kim HM. Andrographolide and analogs in cancer prevention. Front Biosci (Elite Ed) 2015; 7(2): 255-66.

[PMID: 25553378]

[32]   Banerjee M, Chattopadhyay S, Choudhuri T, *et al.* Cytotoxicity and cell cycle arrest induced by andrographolide lead to programmed cell death of MDA-MB-231 breast cancer cell line. J Biomed Sci 2016; 23(1): 40.
[http://dx.doi.org/10.1186/s12929-016-0257-0] [PMID: 27084510]

[33]   Wang ZM, Kang YH, Yang X, *et al.* Andrographolide radiosensitizes human esophageal cancer cell line ECA109 to radiation *in vitro*. Dis Esophagus 2016; 29(1): 54-61.
[http://dx.doi.org/10.1111/dote.12255] [PMID: 25059546]

[34]   Zhou J, Ong CN, Hur GM, Shen HM. Inhibition of the JAK-STAT3 pathway by andrographolide enhances chemosensitivity of cancer cells to doxorubicin. Biochem Pharmacol 2010; 79(9): 1242-50.
[http://dx.doi.org/10.1016/j.bcp.2009.12.014] [PMID: 20026083]

[35]   Zhang X-S, Wei R-J, He DL. Andrographolide sensitizes prostate cancer cells to TRAIL-induced apoptosis. Asian J Androl 2018; 20(2): 200-4.
[http://dx.doi.org/10.4103/aja.aja_30_17] [PMID: 28869219]

[36]   Howlader N, Noone AM, Krapcho M, *et al.* SEER cancer statistics review, 1975-2009 (vintage 2009 populations), National Cancer Institute. Bethesda, MD.

[37]   Vickers AJ, Cronin AM, Björk T, *et al.* Prostate specific antigen concentration at age 60 and death or metastasis from prostate cancer: case-control study. BMJ 2010; 341(sep14 1): c4521.
[http://dx.doi.org/10.1136/bmj.c4521] [PMID: 20843935]

[38]   Wu I, Modlin CS. Disparities in prostate cancer in African American men: What primary care physicians can do. Cleve Clin J Med 2012; 79(5): 313-20.
[http://dx.doi.org/10.3949/ccjm.79a.11001] [PMID: 22550073]

[39]   Powell IJ, Bollig-Fischer A. Minireview: the molecular and genomic basis for prostate cancer health disparities. Mol Endocrinol 2013; 27(6): 879-91.
[http://dx.doi.org/10.1210/me.2013-1039] [PMID: 23608645]

[40]   Kwabi-Addo B, Wang S, Chung W, *et al.* Identification of differentially methylated genes in normal prostate tissues from African American and Caucasian men. Clin Cancer Res 2010; 16(14): 3539-47.
[http://dx.doi.org/10.1158/1078-0432.CCR-09-3342] [PMID: 20606036]

[41]   Sridhar G, Masho SW, Adera T, Ramakrishnan V, Roberts JD. Association between family history of cancers and risk of prostate cancer. J Men's Health 2010; 7(1): 45-54.
[http://dx.doi.org/10.1016/j.jomh.2009.10.006]

[42]   Gennigens C, Menetrier-Caux C, Droz JP. Insulin-Like Growth Factor (IGF) family and prostate cancer. Crit Rev Oncol Hematol 2006; 58(2): 124-45.
[http://dx.doi.org/10.1016/j.critrevonc.2005.10.003] [PMID: 16387509]

[43]   Ryan CJ, Haqq CM, Simko J, *et al.* Expression of insulin-like growth factor-1 receptor in local and metastatic prostate cancer. Urol Oncol 2007; 25(2): 134-40.
[http://dx.doi.org/10.1016/j.urolonc.2006.07.019] [PMID: 17349528]

[44]   Al Moustafa AE. Involvement of human papillomavirus infections in prostate cancer progression. Med Hypotheses 2008; 71(2): 209-11.
[http://dx.doi.org/10.1016/j.mehy.2008.03.036] [PMID: 18468811]

[45]   Kaaks R, Stattin P. Obesity, endogenous hormone metabolism, and prostate cancer risk: a conundrum of "highs" and "lows". Cancer Prev Res (Phila) 2010; 3(3): 259-62.
[http://dx.doi.org/10.1158/1940-6207.CAPR-10-0014] [PMID: 20179295]

[46]   McBride RB. Obesity and aggressive prostate cancer bias and biomarkers. Columbia University 2012.

[47]   Bartsch H, Nair J. Oxidative stress and lipid peroxidation-derived DNA-lesions in inflammation driven carcinogenesis. Cancer Detect Prev 2004; 28(6): 385-91.
[http://dx.doi.org/10.1016/j.cdp.2004.07.004] [PMID: 15582261]

[48] Huncharek M, Haddock KS, Reid R, Kupelnick B. Smoking as a risk factor for prostate cancer: a meta-analysis of 24 prospective cohort studies. Am J Public Health 2010; 100(4): 693-701.
[http://dx.doi.org/10.2105/AJPH.2008.150508] [PMID: 19608952]

[49] Li J, Thompson T, Joseph DA, Master VA. Association between smoking status, and free, total and percent free prostate specific antigen. J Urol 2012; 187(4): 1228-33.
[http://dx.doi.org/10.1016/j.juro.2011.11.086] [PMID: 22335864]

[50] Gutt R, Tonlaar N, Kunnavakkam R, Karrison T, Weichselbaum RR, Liauw SL. Statin use and risk of prostate cancer recurrence in men treated with radiation therapy. J Clin Oncol 2010; 28(16): 2653-9.
[http://dx.doi.org/10.1200/JCO.2009.27.3003] [PMID: 20421534]

[51] Rizos Ch, Papassava M, Golias Ch, Charalabopoulos K. Alcohol consumption and prostate cancer: a mini review. Exp Oncol 2010; 32(2): 66-70.
[PMID: 20693964]

[52] Rohrmann S, Linseisen J, Key TJ, et al. Alcohol consumption and the risk for prostate cancer in the European Prospective Investigation into Cancer and Nutrition. Cancer Epidemiol Biomarkers Prev 2008; 17(5): 1282-7.
[http://dx.doi.org/10.1158/1055-9965.EPI-07-2888] [PMID: 18483352]

[53] Davenport MT, Zhang CA, Leppert JT, Brooks JD, Eisenberg ML. Vasectomy and the risk of prostate cancer in a prospective US Cohort: Data from the NIH☐AARP Diet and Health Study. Andrology 2019; 7(2): 178-83.
[http://dx.doi.org/10.1111/andr.12570] [PMID: 30714352]

[54] Holt SK, Salinas CA, Stanford JL. Vasectomy and the risk of prostate cancer. J Urol 2008; 180(6): 2565-8.
[http://dx.doi.org/10.1016/j.juro.2008.08.042] [PMID: 18930503]

[55] Schwingl PJ, Meirik O, Kapp N, Farley TMM, Multicenter HRP. Prostate cancer and vasectomy: a hospital-based case–control study in China, Nepal and the Republic of Korea. Contraception 2009; 79(5): 363-8.
[http://dx.doi.org/10.1016/j.contraception.2008.11.015] [PMID: 19341848]

[56] Venkateswaran V, Klotz LH. Diet and prostate cancer: mechanisms of action and implications for chemoprevention. Nat Rev Urol 2010; 7(8): 442-53.
[http://dx.doi.org/10.1038/nrurol.2010.102] [PMID: 20647991]

[57] Gibson TM, Ferrucci LM, Tangrea JA, Schatzkin A. Epidemiological and clinical studies of nutrition. Semin Oncol 2010; 37(3): 282-96.
[http://dx.doi.org/10.1053/j.seminoncol.2010.05.011] [PMID: 20709210]

[58] Aronson WJ, Barnard RJ, Freedland SJ, et al. Growth inhibitory effect of low fat diet on prostate cancer cells: results of a prospective, randomized dietary intervention trial in men with prostate cancer. J Urol 2010; 183(1): 345-50.
[http://dx.doi.org/10.1016/j.juro.2009.08.104] [PMID: 19914662]

[59] Schultz C, Meier M, Schmid HP. Nutrition, dietary supplements and adenocarcinoma of the prostate. Maturitas 2011; 70(4): 339-42.
[http://dx.doi.org/10.1016/j.maturitas.2011.08.007] [PMID: 22001108]

[60] Hori S, Butler E, McLoughlin J. Prostate cancer and diet: food for thought? BJU Int 2011; 107(9): 1348-59.
[http://dx.doi.org/10.1111/j.1464-410X.2010.09897.x] [PMID: 21518228]

[61] Dai C, Heemers H, Sharifi N. Androgen signaling in prostate cancer. Cold Spring Harb Perspect Med 2017; 7(9): a030452.
[http://dx.doi.org/10.1101/cshperspect.a030452] [PMID: 28389515]

[62] Nadal M, Prekovic S, Gallastegui N, et al. Structure of the homodimeric androgen receptor ligand-binding domain. Nat Commun 2017; 8(1): 14388.

[http://dx.doi.org/10.1038/ncomms14388] [PMID: 28165461]

[63]   Fontana F, Raimondi M, Marzagalli M, Di Domizio A, Limonta P. Natural compounds in prostate cancer prevention and treatment: Mechanisms of action and molecular targets. Cells 2020; 9(2): 460.
[http://dx.doi.org/10.3390/cells9020460] [PMID: 32085497]

[64]   Teo MY, Rathkopf DE, Kantoff P. Treatment of advanced prostate cancer. Annu Rev Med 2019; 70(1): 479-99.
[http://dx.doi.org/10.1146/annurev-med-051517-011947] [PMID: 30691365]

[65]   Koivisto P, Kononen J, Palmberg C, *et al.* Androgen receptor gene amplification: a possible molecular mechanism for androgen deprivation therapy failure in prostate cancer. Cancer Res 1997; 57(2): 314-9.
[PMID: 9000575]

[66]   Buchanan G, Greenberg NM, Scher HI, Harris JM, Marshall VR, Tilley WD. Collocation of androgen receptor gene mutations in prostate cancer. Clin Cancer Res 2001; 7(5): 1273-81.
[PMID: 11350894]

[67]   Jenster G. Ligand-independent activation of the androgen receptor in prostate cancer by growth factors and cytokines. J Pathol 2000; 191(3): 227-8.
[http://dx.doi.org/10.1002/1096-9896(200007)191:3<227::AID-PATH636>3.0.CO;2-3]   [PMID: 10878541]

[68]   Green SM, Mostaghel EA, Nelson PS. Androgen action and metabolism in prostate cancer. Mol Cell Endocrinol 2012; 360(1-2): 3-13.
[http://dx.doi.org/10.1016/j.mce.2011.09.046] [PMID: 22453214]

[69]   Liu Y, Karaca M, Zhang Z, Gioeli D, Earp HS, Whang YE. Dasatinib inhibits site-specific tyrosine phosphorylation of androgen receptor by Ack1 and Src kinases. Oncogene 2010; 29(22): 3208-16.
[http://dx.doi.org/10.1038/onc.2010.103] [PMID: 20383201]

[70]   Sharifi N. Mechanisms of androgen receptor activation in castration-resistant prostate cancer. Endocrinology 2013; 154(11): 4010-7.
[http://dx.doi.org/10.1210/en.2013-1466] [PMID: 24002034]

[71]   Normanno N, De Luca A, Bianco C, *et al.* Epidermal growth factor receptor (EGFR) signaling in cancer. Gene 2006; 366(1): 2-16.
[http://dx.doi.org/10.1016/j.gene.2005.10.018] [PMID: 16377102]

[72]   Heidegger I, Kern J, Ofer P, Klocker H, Massoner P. Oncogenic functions of IGF1R and INSR in prostate cancer include enhanced tumor growth, cell migration and angiogenesis. Oncotarget 2014; 5(9): 2723-35.
[http://dx.doi.org/10.18632/oncotarget.1884] [PMID: 24809298]

[73]   Verzella D, Fischietti M, Capece D, *et al.* Targeting the NF-κB pathway in prostate cancer: a promising therapeutic approach? Curr Drug Targets 2016; 17(3): 311-20.
[http://dx.doi.org/10.2174/1389450116666150907100715] [PMID: 26343112]

[74]   Hsieh AC, Edlind MP. PI3K-AKT-mTOR signaling in prostate cancer progression and androgen deprivation therapy resistance. Asian J Androl 2014; 16(3): 378-86.
[http://dx.doi.org/10.4103/1008-682X.122876] [PMID: 24759575]

[75]   Yardy GW, Brewster SF. Wnt signalling and prostate cancer. Prostate Cancer Prostatic Dis 2005; 8(2): 119-26.
[http://dx.doi.org/10.1038/sj.pcan.4500794] [PMID: 15809669]

[76]   Murillo-Garzón V, Kypta R. WNT signalling in prostate cancer. Nat Rev Urol 2017; 14(11): 683-96.
[http://dx.doi.org/10.1038/nrurol.2017.144] [PMID: 28895566]

[77]   Ben-Eltriki M, Deb S, Adomat H, Tomlinson Guns ES. Calcitriol and 20(S)-protopanaxadiol synergistically inhibit growth and induce apoptosis in human prostate cancer cells. J Steroid Biochem Mol Biol 2016; 158: 207-19.

[http://dx.doi.org/10.1016/j.jsbmb.2015.12.002] [PMID: 26709138]

[78]   Lee DH, Szczepanski M, Lee YJ. Role of Bax in quercetin-induced apoptosis in human prostate cancer cells. Biochem Pharmacol 2008; 75(12): 2345-55.
[http://dx.doi.org/10.1016/j.bcp.2008.03.013] [PMID: 18455702]

[79]   Senthilkumar K, Elumalai P, Arunkumar R, *et al.* Quercetin regulates insulin like growth factor signaling and induces intrinsic and extrinsic pathway mediated apoptosis in androgen independent prostate cancer cells (PC-3). Mol Cell Biochem 2010; 344(1-2): 173-84.
[http://dx.doi.org/10.1007/s11010-010-0540-4] [PMID: 20658310]

[80]   Shankar S, Srivastava R. Involvement of Bcl-2 family members, phosphatidylinositol 3'-kinase/AKT and mitochondrial p53 in curcumin (diferulolylmethane)-induced apoptosis in prostate cancer. Int J Oncol 2007; 30(4): 905-18.
[http://dx.doi.org/10.3892/ijo.30.4.905] [PMID: 17332930]

[81]   Vijayababu MR, Kanagaraj P, Arunkumar A, Ilangovan R, Dharmarajan A, Arunakaran J. Quercetin induces p53-independent apoptosis in human prostate cancer cells by modulating Bcl-2-related proteins: a possible mediation by IGFBP-3. Oncol Res 2006; 16(2): 67-74.
[http://dx.doi.org/10.3727/000000006783981224] [PMID: 16898267]

[82]   Yang H, Ping Dou Q. Targeting apoptosis pathway with natural terpenoids: implications for treatment of breast and prostate cancer. Curr Drug Targets 2010; 11(6): 733-44.
[http://dx.doi.org/10.2174/138945010791170842] [PMID: 20298150]

[83]   Kalyanaraman B. Teaching the basics of cancer metabolism: Developing antitumor strategies by exploiting the differences between normal and cancer cell metabolism. Redox Biol 2017; 12: 833-42.
[http://dx.doi.org/10.1016/j.redox.2017.04.018] [PMID: 28448945]

[84]   Suburu J, Chen YQ. Lipids and prostate cancer. Prostaglandins Other Lipid Mediat 2012; 98(1-2): 1-10.
[http://dx.doi.org/10.1016/j.prostaglandins.2012.03.003] [PMID: 22503963]

[85]   Zadra G, Photopoulos C, Loda M. The fat side of prostate cancer. Biochim Biophys Acta Mol Cell Biol Lipids 2013; 1831(10): 1518-32.
[http://dx.doi.org/10.1016/j.bbalip.2013.03.010] [PMID: 23562839]

[86]   Rysman E, Brusselmans K, Scheys K, *et al.* De *novo* lipogenesis protects cancer cells from free radicals and chemotherapeutics by promoting membrane lipid saturation. Cancer Res 2010; 70(20): 8117-26.
[http://dx.doi.org/10.1158/0008-5472.CAN-09-3871] [PMID: 20876798]

[87]   Leon CG, Locke JA, Adomat HH, *et al.* Alterations in cholesterol regulation contribute to the production of intratumoral androgens during progression to castration☐resistant prostate cancer in a mouse xenograft model. Prostate 2010; 70(4): 390-400.
[http://dx.doi.org/10.1002/pros.21072] [PMID: 19866465]

[88]   Bhat FA, Sharmila G, Balakrishnan S, *et al.* Quercetin reverses EGF-induced epithelial to mesenchymal transition and invasiveness in prostate cancer (PC-3) cell line *via* EGFR/PI3K/Akt pathway. J Nutr Biochem 2014; 25(11): 1132-9.
[http://dx.doi.org/10.1016/j.jnutbio.2014.06.008] [PMID: 25150162]

[89]   Liu CH, Tang WC, Sia P, *et al.* Berberine inhibits the metastatic ability of prostate cancer cells by suppressing epithelial-to-mesenchymal transition (EMT)-associated genes with predictive and prognostic relevance. Int J Med Sci 2015; 12(1): 63-71.
[http://dx.doi.org/10.7150/ijms.9982] [PMID: 25552920]

[90]   Peng X, Zhou Y, Tian H, *et al.* Sulforaphane inhibits invasion by phosphorylating ERK1/2 to regulate E-cadherin and CD44v6 in human prostate cancer DU145 cells. Oncol Rep 2015; 34(3): 1565-72.
[http://dx.doi.org/10.3892/or.2015.4098] [PMID: 26134113]

[91]   Chien MH, Lin YW, Wen YC, *et al.* Targeting the SPOCK1-snail/slug axis-mediated epithelial-t-

-mesenchymal transition by apigenin contributes to repression of prostate cancer metastasis. J Exp Clin Cancer Res 2019; 38(1): 246.
[http://dx.doi.org/10.1186/s13046-019-1247-3] [PMID: 31182131]

[92] Khan MI, Adhami VM, Lall RK, *et al.* YB-1 expression promotes epithelial-to-mesenchymal transition in prostate cancer that is inhibited by a small molecule fisetin. Oncotarget 2014; 5(9): 2462-74.
[http://dx.doi.org/10.18632/oncotarget.1790] [PMID: 24770864]

[93] Senthilkumar K, Arunkumar R, Elumalai P, *et al.* Quercetin inhibits invasion, migration and signalling molecules involved in cell survival and proliferation of prostate cancer cell line (PC☐3). Cell Biochem Funct 2011; 29(2): 87-95.
[http://dx.doi.org/10.1002/cbf.1725] [PMID: 21308698]

[94] Chien CS, Shen KH, Huang JS, Ko SC, Shih YW. Antimetastatic potential of fisetin involves inactivation of the PI3K/Akt and JNK signaling pathways with downregulation of MMP-2/9 expressions in prostate cancer PC-3 cells. Mol Cell Biochem 2010; 333(1-2): 169-80.
[http://dx.doi.org/10.1007/s11010-009-0217-z] [PMID: 19633975]

[95] Yang J, Wang C, Zhang Z, *et al. Retracted:* Curcumin inhibits the survival and metastasis of prostate cancer cells *via* the Notch☐1 signaling pathway. Acta Pathol Microbiol Scand Suppl 2017; 125(2): 134-40.
[http://dx.doi.org/10.1111/apm.12650] [PMID: 28120490]

[96] Chen C, Zhao S, Karnad A, Freeman JW. The biology and role of CD44 in cancer progression: therapeutic implications. J Hematol Oncol 2018; 11(1): 64.
[http://dx.doi.org/10.1186/s13045-018-0605-5] [PMID: 29747682]

[97] Simons M, Gordon E, Claesson-Welsh L. Mechanisms and regulation of endothelial VEGF receptor signalling. Nat Rev Mol Cell Biol 2016; 17(10): 611-25.
[http://dx.doi.org/10.1038/nrm.2016.87] [PMID: 27461391]

[98] Krock BL, Skuli N, Simon MC. Hypoxia-induced angiogenesis: good and evil. Genes Cancer 2011; 2(12): 1117-33.
[http://dx.doi.org/10.1177/1947601911423654] [PMID: 22866203]

[99] Shi X, Deepak V, Wang L, *et al.* Thrombospondin-1 is a putative target gene of Runx2 and Runx3. Int J Mol Sci 2013; 14(7): 14321-32.
[http://dx.doi.org/10.3390/ijms140714321] [PMID: 23846726]

[100] Skvortsov S, Skvortsova II, Tang DG, Dubrovska A. Concise Review: Prostate Cancer Stem Cells: Current Understanding. Stem Cells 2018; 36(10): 1457-74.
[http://dx.doi.org/10.1002/stem.2859] [PMID: 29845679]

[101] Vainio P, Mpindi JP, Kohonen P, *et al.* High-throughput transcriptomic and RNAi analysis identifies AIM1, ERGIC1, TMED3 and TPX2 as potential drug targets in prostate cancer. PLoS One 2012; 7(6): e39801.
[http://dx.doi.org/10.1371/journal.pone.0039801] [PMID: 22761906]

[102] Perry AS, Watson RWG, Lawler M, Hollywood D. The epigenome as a therapeutic target in prostate cancer. Nat Rev Urol 2010; 7(12): 668-80.
[http://dx.doi.org/10.1038/nrurol.2010.185] [PMID: 21060342]

[103] De Luca V, Salim V, Atsumi SM, Yu F. Mining the biodiversity of plants: a revolution in the making. Science 2012; 336(6089): 1658-61.
[http://dx.doi.org/10.1126/science.1217410] [PMID: 22745417]

[104] Wurtzel ET, Kutchan TM. Plant metabolism, the diverse chemistry set of the future. Science 2016; 353(6305): 1232-6.
[http://dx.doi.org/10.1126/science.aad2062] [PMID: 27634523]

[105] Gershenzon J, Dudareva N. The function of terpene natural products in the natural world. Nat Chem

Biol 2007; 3(7): 408-14.
[http://dx.doi.org/10.1038/nchembio.2007.5] [PMID: 17576428]

[106] Andrade LN, de Sousa DP. Sesquiterpenes from Essential Oils and Anti-Inflammatory Activity. Nat Prod Commun 2015; 10(10): 1767-74.
[PMID: 26669122]

[107] De Cássia da Silveira e Sá R, Andrade L, De Sousa D. A review on anti-inflammatory activity of monoterpenes. Molecules 2013; 18(1): 1227-54.
[http://dx.doi.org/10.3390/molecules18011227] [PMID: 23334570]

[108] Sobral MV, Xavier AL, Lima TC, de Sousa DP. Antitumor activity of monoterpenes found in essential oils. ScientificWorldJournal 2014; 2014: 1-35.
[http://dx.doi.org/10.1155/2014/953451] [PMID: 25401162]

[109] Montagnani Marelli M, Marzagalli M, Fontana F, Raimondi M, Moretti RM, Limonta P. Anticancer properties of tocotrienols: A review of cellular mechanisms and molecular targets. J Cell Physiol 2019; 234(2): 1147-64.
[http://dx.doi.org/10.1002/jcp.27075] [PMID: 30066964]

[110] Erdogan S, Turkekul K, Dibirdik I, Doganlar ZB, Doganlar O, Bilir A. Midkine silencing enhances the anti–prostate cancer stem cell activity of the flavone apigenin: cooperation on signaling pathways regulated by ERK, p38, PTEN, PARP, and NF-κB. Invest New Drugs 2020; 38(2): 246-63.
[http://dx.doi.org/10.1007/s10637-019-00774-8] [PMID: 30993586]

[111] Erdogan S, Turkekul K, Serttas R, Erdogan Z. The natural flavonoid apigenin sensitizes human CD44 $^+$ prostate cancer stem cells to cisplatin therapy. Biomed Pharmacother 2017; 88: 210-7.
[http://dx.doi.org/10.1016/j.biopha.2017.01.056] [PMID: 28107698]

[112] Rauf A, Imran M, Khan IA, *et al.* Anticancer potential of quercetin: A comprehensive review. Phytother Res 2018; 32(11): 2109-30.
[http://dx.doi.org/10.1002/ptr.6155] [PMID: 30039547]

[113] Yuan H, Pan Y, Young CYF. Overexpression of c-Jun induced by quercetin and resverol inhibits the expression and function of the androgen receptor in human prostate cancer cells. Cancer Lett 2004; 213(2): 155-63.
[http://dx.doi.org/10.1016/j.canlet.2004.04.003] [PMID: 15327830]

[114] Yuan H, Young CYF, Tian Y, Liu Z, Zhang M, Lou H. Suppression of the androgen receptor function by quercetin through protein–protein interactions of Sp1, c-Jun, and the androgen receptor in human prostate cancer cells. Mol Cell Biochem 2010; 339(1-2): 253-62.
[http://dx.doi.org/10.1007/s11010-010-0388-7] [PMID: 20148354]

[115] Lall RK, Adhami VM, Mukhtar H. Dietary flavonoid fisetin for cancer prevention and treatment. Mol Nutr Food Res 2016; 60(6): 1396-405.
[http://dx.doi.org/10.1002/mnfr.201600025] [PMID: 27059089]

[116] Kunnumakkara AB, Bordoloi D, Padmavathi G, *et al.* Curcumin, the golden nutraceutical: multitargeting for multiple chronic diseases. Br J Pharmacol 2017; 174(11): 1325-48.
[http://dx.doi.org/10.1111/bph.13621] [PMID: 27638428]

[117] Pulido-Moran M, Moreno-Fernandez J, Ramirez-Tortosa C, Ramirez-Tortosa MC. Curcumin and Health. Molecules 2016; 21(3): 264.
[http://dx.doi.org/10.3390/molecules21030264] [PMID: 26927041]

[118] Zhu XX, Ding YH, Wu Y, Qian LY, Zou H, He Q. Silibinin: a potential old drug for cancer therapy. Expert Rev Clin Pharmacol 2016; 9(10): 1323-30.
[http://dx.doi.org/10.1080/17512433.2016.1208563] [PMID: 27362364]

[119] Zi X, Zhang J, Agarwal R, Pollak M. Silibinin up-regulates insulin-like growth factor-binding protein 3 expression and inhibits proliferation of androgen-independent prostate cancer cells. Cancer Res 2000; 60(20): 5617-20.

[PMID: 11059749]

[120] Fontana F, Raimondi M, Marzagalli M, Di Domizio A, Limonta P. The emerging role of paraptosis in tumor cell biology: Perspectives for cancer prevention and therapy with natural compounds. Biochim Biophys Acta Rev Cancer 2020; 1873(2): 188338.
[http://dx.doi.org/10.1016/j.bbcan.2020.188338] [PMID: 31904399]

[121] Shanmugam MK, Rajendran P, Li F, *et al.* Ursolic acid inhibits multiple cell survival pathways leading to suppression of growth of prostate cancer xenograft in nude mice. J Mol Med (Berl) 2011; 89(7): 713-27.
[http://dx.doi.org/10.1007/s00109-011-0746-2] [PMID: 21465181]

[122] Yap WN, Chang PN, Han HY, *et al.* γ-Tocotrienol suppresses prostate cancer cell proliferation and invasion through multiple-signalling pathways. Br J Cancer 2008; 99(11): 1832-41.
[http://dx.doi.org/10.1038/sj.bjc.6604763] [PMID: 19002171]

[123] Seyfried TN, Huysentruyt LC. On the origin of cancer metastasis. Crit Rev Oncog 2013; 18(1 - 2): 43-73.
[http://dx.doi.org/10.1615/CritRevOncog.v18.i1-2.40] [PMID: 23237552]

[124] Hu HJ, Lin XL, Liu MH, Fan XJ, Zou WW. Curcumin mediates reversion of HGF-induced epithelial-mesenchymal transition *via* inhibition of c-Met expression in DU145 cells. Oncol Lett 2016; 11(2): 1499-505.
[http://dx.doi.org/10.3892/ol.2015.4063] [PMID: 26893768]

[125] Chun JY, Tummala R, Nadiminty N, *et al.* Andrographolide, an herbal medicine, inhibits interleukin-6 expression and suppresses prostate cancer cell growth. Genes Cancer 2010; 1(8): 868-76.
[http://dx.doi.org/10.1177/1947601910383416] [PMID: 21442031]

[126] Mir H, Kapur N, Singh R, Sonpavde G, Lillard JW Jr, Singh S. Andrographolide inhibits prostate cancer by targeting cell cycle regulators, CXCR3 and CXCR7 chemokine receptors. Cell Cycle 2016; 15(6): 819-26.
[http://dx.doi.org/10.1080/15384101.2016.1148836] [PMID: 27029529]

[127] Wong C, Sagineedu SR, Lajis NH, Loke SC, Stanslas J. Andrographolide induces cell cycle arrest and apoptosis in PC-3 prostate cancer cells. Afr J Pharm Pharmacol 2011; 5(2): 225-33.
[http://dx.doi.org/10.5897/AJMR10.383]

[128] Wong HC, Wong CC, Sagineedu SR, Loke SC, Lajis NH, Stanslas J. SRJ23, a new semisynthetic andrographolide derivative: *in vitro* growth inhibition and mechanisms of cell cycle arrest and apoptosis in prostate cancer cells. Cell Biol Toxicol 2014; 30(5): 269-88.
[http://dx.doi.org/10.1007/s10565-014-9282-5] [PMID: 25070834]

[129] Okamoto M, Lee C, Oyasu R. Interleukin-6 as a paracrine and autocrine growth factor in human prostatic carcinoma cells *in vitro* . Cancer Res 1997; 57(1): 141-6.
[PMID: 8988055]

[130] Zhang ZR, Al Zaharna M, Wong MMK, Chiu SK, Cheung HY. Taxifolin enhances andrographolide-induced mitotic arrest and apoptosis in human prostate cancer cells *via* spindle assembly checkpoint activation. PLoS One 2013; 8(1): e54577.
[http://dx.doi.org/10.1371/journal.pone.0054577] [PMID: 23382917]

[131] Kumar D, Kumar S, Gorain M, *et al.* Notch1-MAPK Signaling Axis Regulates CD133[+] Cancer Stem Cell-Mediated Melanoma Growth and Angiogenesis. J Invest Dermatol 2016; 136(12): 2462-74.
[http://dx.doi.org/10.1016/j.jid.2016.07.024] [PMID: 27476721]

[132] Vickers NJ. Animal Communication: When I'm Calling You, Will You Answer Too? Curr Biol 2017; 27(14): R713-5.
[http://dx.doi.org/10.1016/j.cub.2017.05.064] [PMID: 28743020]

[133] Rivera JMS, Rivas AL, Reyes YR, *et al.* Abstract 4784: Andrographolide induces metabolic changes and suppresses mitochondrial activity in prostate cancer. Cancer Res 2020; 80(16_Supplement)

(Suppl.): 4784.
[http://dx.doi.org/10.1158/1538-7445.AM2020-4784]

[134] Roque-Reyes YM, Sosa-Rivera J, Sánchez-Vázquez MM, Ayala-Peña S, Torres-Ramos CA, Martínez-Ferrer M. Abstract 2343: Andrographolide treatment results in decreased mtDNA damage and loss of the mitochondrial membrane potential while increasing ROS production in prostate cancer. Cancer Res 2022; 82(12_Supplement) (Suppl.): 2343.
[http://dx.doi.org/10.1158/1538-7445.AM2022-2343]

[135] Jada SR, Matthews C, Saad MS, *et al.* Benzylidene derivatives of andrographolide inhibit growth of breast and colon cancer cells *in vitro* by inducing G $_1$ arrest and apoptosis. Br J Pharmacol 2008; 155(5): 641-54.
[http://dx.doi.org/10.1038/bjp.2008.368] [PMID: 18806812]

[136] Liu Y, Liang RM, Ma QP, *et al.* Synthesis of thioether andrographolide derivatives and their inhibitory effect against cancer cells. MedChemComm 2017; 8(6): 1268-74.
[http://dx.doi.org/10.1039/C7MD00169J] [PMID: 30108837]

[137] Mitra Ghosh T, Kansom T, Mazumder S, *et al.* The Andrographolide analogue 3A.1 synergizes with taxane derivatives in aggressive metastatic prostate cancers by upregulation of heat shock proteins and downregulation of MAT2A-mediated cell migration and invasion. J Pharmacol Exp Ther 2022; 380(3): 180-201.
[http://dx.doi.org/10.1124/jpet.121.000898] [PMID: 34949650]

[138] Ansbaugh N, Shannon J, Mori M, Farris PE, Garzotto M. Agent Orange as a risk factor for high□grade prostate cancer. Cancer 2013; 119(13): 2399-404.
[http://dx.doi.org/10.1002/cncr.27941] [PMID: 23670242]

CHAPTER 10

Andrographolide and its Analogs in the Treatment of Lung Cancer: An Update

Vinod K. Nelson[1,#, *]**, Juturu Mastanaiah**[2,#]**, Nazemoon Reddy**[3,†]**, Manohar Reddy**[4,†]**, P. Divya Bargavi**[5,‡]**, Sheik Nasar Ismail**[6,‡]**, Ravishankar Ram Mani**[7]**, Vinyas Mayasa**[8]**, Hari Hara sudan**[1]**, Nem Kumar Jain**[9]**, Alagusundaram Muthumanickam**[9] **and Kranthi Kumar Kotha**[10,*]

[1] *Centre for Global Health Research, Saveetha Medical College and Hospital, Saveetha Institute of Medical and Technical Sciences, Chennai 602105, Tamil Nadu, India*

[2] *Department of Pharmacology, Balaji College of Pharmacy, Anantapur, Andhra Pradesh, India*

[3] *Bharat Institute of Technology, Magalpalli, Ibrahimpatnam, Hyderabad, Telangana 501510, India*

[4] *Department of Pharmacology, P. Rami Reddy Memorial College of Pharmacy, Kadapa, Andhra Pradesh, India*

[5] *Department of Pharmacognosy, JSS College of Pharmacy, JSS Academy of Higher Education and Research, Ooty, Nilgiris, Tamil Nadu, India*

[6] *Department of Pharmacology, East Point College of Pharmacy, East Point Group of Institutions, Jnana Prabha Campus, Bengaluru, India*

[7] *Faculty of Pharmaceutical Sciences, UCSI University, Cheras, Kuala Lumpur 56000, Malaysia*

[8] *Department of Pharmacology, GITAM School of Pharmacy, Gandhi Institute of Technology and Management Deemed to be University, Hyderabad, Telangana, India*

[9] *Department of Pharmaceutics, School of Pharmacy, ITM University, Gwalior, Madhya Pradesh, India*

[10] *Department of Pharmaceutics, College of Pharmaceutical Sciences, Dayananda Sagar University, Bengaluru, Karnataka 560078, India*

Abstract: Lung cancer refers to the changes in the lung tissue and cells that lead to cancer growth due to gene mutations and cellular changes that result in uncontrollable cell growth and division. However, the exact pathophysiology of lung cancer is not yet fully understood. It is a significant cause of mortality worldwide and can be divided

* **Corresponding authors Vinod K. Nelson and Kranthi Kumar Kotha:** Centre for Global Health Research, Saveetha Medical College and Hospital, Saveetha Institute of Medical and Technical Sciences, Chennai 602105, Tamil Nadu, India; E-mail: vinod.kumar457@gmail.com
Department of Pharmaceutics, College of Pharmaceutical Sciences, Dayananda Sagar University, Bengaluru, Karnataka 560078, India; E-mail: kranthikumarkotta@gmail.com
# These authors share the first authorship of this work.
† These authors share second authorship to this work.
‡ These authors share third authorship to this work

into two main types: small-cell lung cancer (SCLC) and non-small-cell lung cancer (NSCLC). The specific subtypes of NSCLC are adenocarcinoma, large-cell carcinoma, and squamous cell carcinoma. Risk factors for lung cancer include exposure to radon, smoking, air pollution, and a family history of lung cancer. Symptoms may include shortness of breath, chest pain, coughing, and weight loss. Early detection and proper treatment, including chemotherapy, radiation therapy, surgery, and targeted therapy, can improve the prognosis and survival rates. However, the deaths and the cases of lung cancer are constantly rising. This increases the need for potential drug treatment for lung cancer. Among the various available sources for identifying novel therapies for multiple diseases, such as cancer, medicinal plants and plant-derived compounds play a significant role. In addition, several studies revealed that *Andrographis paniculata* and its derived compounds have shown various pharmacological effects, including anti-cancer effects. Recently, andrographolide and its structural analogs have also gained attention in lung cancer due to their unique potential. Studies have shown that andrographolide and its analogs can restrict the development of lung cancer cells *via* the induction of apoptosis, a programmed cell death. They have also been shown to target specific signaling pathways that play a role in the development and progression of lung cancer, including the NF-kB and MAPK pathways. Additionally, andrographolide and its analogs have been shown to exhibit low toxicity, making them attractive as potential therapeutic agents for the treatment of lung cancer. Additional investigations are required to thoroughly understand these compounds' mechanisms of action and potential clinical applications in lung cancer treatment. In summary, andrographolide and its structural analogs have shown promising results in both *in vitro* and *in vivo* studies as potential therapeutic agents for lung cancer treatment. Their anti-cancer properties, including inhibition of cancer cell growth and induction of apoptosis, make them of significant interest for further research.

Keywords: Analogs, Andrographolide, Current treatments, Lung cancer, Risk factors, Targets.

INTRODUCTION

The battle against cancer is an enormous challenge. One of the deadliest and most prevalent malignant tumors around the globe is lung cancer [1]. Lung cancer is divided into two types: Small-cell lung cancer (SCLC) and non-small cell lung cancer (NSCLC) [2]. SCLC constitutes 10 to 15 percent of all instances of lung cancer; it is characterized by an elevated rate of proliferation and rapid metastatic spread and is strongly associated with the use of products containing tobacco. One-third of SCLC patients are identified with limited-stage illness. Still, most patients suffering from SCLC exhibit extensive-stage (ES-SCLC) metastatic disease (stage IV); SCLC primarily responds extraordinarily well to chemotherapy, which is platinum-based, due to which few patients live for more than a few years. Still, the resistance to that develops quickly [3]. The remaining 85% of cases are affected by NSCLC. The three pathologic subtypes of NSCLC include adenocarcinoma, the most common kind, giant cell carcinoma, and squamous cell carcinoma. NSCLC is typically accompanied by generally poor outcomes and a high significance of tumor recurrence [4]. In most nations, the most predominant neoplasm is lung cancer, which affects both men and women. According to Globocan 2020, across the globe, lung cancer holds 2nd place as a common type in terms of its incidence and the primary reason for mortality, with 22 lakh newly diagnosed cases and a mortality of 1.8 million [5]. Every day, approximately 350 individuals are killed by lung cancer, which accounts for 2.5 folds higher than colorectal cancer (CRC), as well as the death rate among lung cancer patients is higher than breast, pancreatic, and prostate cancers combined. It is anticipated that around 105,840 deaths, *i.e.*, 81 percent of 130,180 lung cancer deaths in 2022, are attributed to smoking, with an additional 3650 mortalities due to passive smoking. It will become the 9th most common cause of cancer-related deaths if an extra 20,700 deaths related to non-smoking-related lung cancer are included separately [6]. While rates of localized-stage lung cancer grew by 4.5% every year, the incidence of advanced illness continued to fall dramatically. Localized-stage diagnoses increased from 17% in the early 2000s to 28% in 2018, and 3-year comparative long-term survival increased to 31% from 21% in 2018 [7]. Further, studies also projected that by 2030, the incidence of cancer is predicted to rise by 50%, with low-and middle-income nations bearing most of the burden [8].

The search for novel therapies and early disease diagnosis in oncology remains imperative despite recent scientific developments that have created new diagnostic and therapeutic techniques. Surgery, radiation, chemotherapy, targeted therapy, anti-microbial peptides (AMPs), immunotherapy, and combinations of these treatments are available for treating lung cancer. While chemotherapy is still the conventional first- and second-line treatment for lung cancer, significant advancements in the therapy and control of lung cancer were made by immunotherapy. Numerous researches have shown that the QOL and overall survival of patients with both preliminary and advanced lung cancer are improved by the usage of chemotherapy, either alone or in addition to other kinds of therapies. Despite the lack of general acceptance for surgery in SCLC, it is an option for tiny biopsy-proven tumors (very restricted disease). A tiny SCLC is most frequently discovered after a lung lesion of uncertain origin has been surgically removed. Surgery was not recommended in a systematic study for certain types of SCLC. Because SCLC spreads quickly and widely throughout the body, it is typically impossible to remove it through surgery. There are several adverse effects after surgery, with pain being the most significant constraint. The standard treatment for LD-SCLC, which aims to cure the disease, involves platinum-doublet chemotherapy of four cycles along radiotherapy. Even in elderly individuals, the overall survival rate is improved when using this treatment compared to chemotherapy. While the previous phase 3 trials preferred radiotherapy twice daily, a large number of patients did not meet the criteria for the therapy as a result of comorbidity and status of performance. Lots of patients do not meet the requirements for twice-daily, even though once-daily radiation therapy is still the standard in most centers due to logical concerns. Radiation therapy has several limitations, one of which is a high prevalence of adverse effects brought on by nonspecific targeting. Another disadvantage of radiation therapy is that it is expensive. Normal cells harmed by radiation treatment generally recover within a few months. However, some people may experience adverse effects that may not improve. Certain side effects may appear years or months after the radiation therapy is completed. These are known as late effects. Even though chemotherapy and other invasive approaches have significantly increased the survival rate of patients, it has some drawbacks, including an elevated degree of adverse events brought on by nonspecific targeting, poor effectiveness, and a relatively short overall survival time when compared to targeted therapy or immunotherapy [9]. The earliest known instance of immunotherapy was the successful use of bacterial toxins by William Coley to treat an incurable sarcoma in 1910. Following Coley's success, scientists have worked hard to control host immune responses for cancer immunotherapy since the late 1990s. Examples include lymphokine-induced killer cells, interleukin-2 (1-2), tumor-infiltrating lymphocytes (TILs), and the first therapeutic prostate cancer vaccination. However, the below-par efficiency, severe toxicity at high dosages, and the inflated treatment burden prevent these medicines from being employed in various clinical settings. Due to the efficiency of chimeric antigen receptor T-cells and immune checkpoint inhibitor drugs against various cancers, immunotherapy was the scientific breakthrough published in the Science Journal in 2013. Immunotherapy (IO) development, notably for NSCLC, has altered how many malignancies are treated. Immune-checkpoint inhibitors (ICI) have enhanced the prognoses of NSCLC subjects in various circumstances, from vigorously spreading disease to locally progressed and treatable disease. They were evaluated in single-agent therapy, in combination with other ICI and IO drugs, and in conjunction with chemotherapy (CT). Several monoclonal antibodies that target the programmed cell death protein 1 (PD-1) or its ligand (PD-L1) are currently approved for use in patients with advanced NSCLC who have not yet received treatment or who have had treatment in the past [10]. More clinical treatments with lower toxicity and higher efficacy are still urgently needed. Patients with advanced NSCLC may be treated with therapies specifically targeted to their condition. Gefitinib, afatinib, and erlotinib are examples of small-molecule EGFR inhibitors, whereas osimertinib specifically targets T790M. The small molecule inhibitor crizotinib inhibits ALK, ROS1, and MET. The IGF-1 and ALK receptors are the focus of the small-molecule pharmacological inhibitor ceritinib. Alectinib, a small molecule inhibitor, goes after ALK and RET. These proteins are the targets. Oral TKIs include osimertinib, erlotinib, gefitinib, afatinib, crizotinib, ceritinib, and gefitinib. Additionally, more specifically tailored treatments are currently being developed [11]. Resistance in its many varied manifestations, toxicity, and the increased prices of these targeted drugs, which block access for all NSCLC patients, are the primary obstacles that stand in the way of expanding the use of these compounds to reach a cure for advanced NSCLC [12].

These contemporary treatments for cancer have some success, but they have ample adverse side effects. Therefore, research concentrates on plants and substances produced from plants to create powerful medications to treat cancer. Various disorders are treated and prevented using medicinal characteristics found in many plant species. However, it is believed that 50–60% of cancer patients in the US use alternative therapies that are derived from plants [13]. Historically, Herbs have been a critical component of cancer treatment in several nations, mainly in Europe and the Middle East. The World Health Organization has released several reports indicating that several countries have legalized using natural products to treat lung cancer. Approximately 5–15% of the herbs used to treat cancer are thought to have undergone research on their anticancer effects [14]. There is reason to be optimistic about using plant preparations as a potential option for the creation of more efficient techniques for chemotherapy and chemoprevention. Researchers are also looking for alternative anticancer drugs that decrease the establishment of resistance by chemotherapies to inhibit and decrease cancer incidence. According to their mode of action, two-thirds of cancer medicines are made from natural products, especially herbs [2].

The main bioactive component of one such scientifically significant *Andrographis paniculata*, employed extensively in alternative medicine, particularly in India, China, and Southeast Asia, is andrographolide (AGP). The substance holds multiple therapeutic benefits, including anti-inflammatory and anticancer effects. AGP's structural changes have been made several times to increase its potency and selectivity. Several attempts have been undertaken to increase the structural variability of AGP and increase bioavailability. AGP also offers a useful adjustable pharmacophore for a variety of pharmacological activities. Improved bioavailability and increased therapeutic efficacy have been seen in some analogs. By inhibiting the growth of several types of cancer through various modes of action, research investigations have recognized AGP and some of its analogs as possible chemotherapeutic drugs. Because of its notable pharmacological properties and promising preclinical data, andrographolide has been evaluated for effectiveness in lung cancer therapy alone and in addition to capecitabine (NCT01993472). It was also examined in a clinical trial as a chemosensitizer for CRC. The inclusion of AGP in clinical investigations demonstrated its promising potential. This current chapter highlights the critical highlights of lung cancer and describes the role of AGP and its analogs in treating LC.

Risk Factors for Lung Cancer

Several risk factors accompany the occurrence of lung cancer. Age and cigarette smoking are the main risk factors. Radon exposure, occupational exposure, HIV, other lifestyle factors, second-hand smoke exposure, electronic cigarettes, tobacco use, and cannabis use are other common factors. Some probable risk factors and causes include a history of infectious or non-infectious respiratory disorders, a history of contagious respiratory diseases, and inherited genetics.

Tobacco Smoking

Unquestionably, smoking is the most significant and common cause of lung cancer. Amongst the earliest diseases to be causally associated with smoking tobacco, albeit it was a rare condition before the commencement of the 20th century. Lung cancer mortality and incidence both grew in the US over most of the 20th century. According to the research, smoking cigarettes causes men's lung cancer. More than 4,000 compounds containing at least 69 known cancer-causing substances and other poisonous substances linked to severe illnesses are found in tobacco smoke. Online tools that evaluate risk utilizing demographic information, such as smoking history and magnitude, are commonly accessible [15].

Exposure to Second-hand Smoke

An implicit carcinogenic exposure caused by the smoking of products made of tobacco is known as side-stream smoke. Second-hand smoke exposure among people who never smoked in the US considerably decreased from 87.5% to 25.2% between 1988 and 2014, thanks to tobacco control initiatives and smoke-free workplaces and public place rules [16]. Nitrosamines, aromatic amines, and polycyclic aromatic hydrocarbons have all been identified as carcinogens in second-hand smoke. Studies have demonstrated that when non-smokers are exposed to second-hand smoke, their urine contains nicotine, its metabolite cotinine, and DNA adducts from tobacco carcinogens. There is no degree of exposure to side-stream smoke that is safe. The evidence supports the hypothesis that lifetime non-smokers' exposure to second-hand smoke causes lung cancer [15].

Electronic Cigarettes

Electronic nicotine delivery systems (ENDS) can be used to deliver nicotine to the lung epithelium, commonly identified as electronic cigarettes. Even though a patent for this kind of device was initially granted in 1965, it was not until 2003 that e-cigarettes began to be produced in large quantities and were readily accessible in the U S by 2005. Over 460 brands and 7,700 flavors are available in the US, and the occurrence of e-cigarette use in adults is thought to range between 2.6% and 4.5% [17, 18]. Teenagers are especially at risk for using e-cigarettes; according to the National Youth Tobacco Survey in 2017, 3.3% and 11.7% of middle school and high school students have used e-cigarettes in a month, respectively. After a year, e-cigarette use was reported by 20.8% of students in high school and 4.9% of students in middle school, reflecting increases of 78% and 48%, respectively [19]. The studies showed that the vapors from the two primary solvents, propylene glycol and vegetable glycerine, used in e-cigarettes include hazardous and cancer-causing carbonyl chemicals such as acetaldehyde, formaldehyde, acrolein, and acetone. Studies have also revealed that using electronic cigarettes is linked to an increase in oxidative stress. Human bronchial and lung epithelial cells exposed to e-cigarettes experience oxidative stress, leading to undesirable transitional events such as cytotoxicity, inflammation, and intensified permeability of endothelial cells. Additionally, research has shown that using e-cigarettes has an immediate negative impact on lung function. Data taken together indicate that vapor from e-cigarettes may include potentially dangerous substances and hurt human health. Although studies have suggested e-cigarettes may be a safer option than regular cigarettes, at this time, there are no estimates available for long-lasting cancer risk associated with even low levels of exposure to the identified carcinogens.

Other Tobacco Use

While cigarettes remain a widely used nicotine product in the US, different other kinds of tobacco products, including cigarettes, pipes, and hookahs, are commonly used and are connected to the potential risk of LC as well as an increased death rate. The regular consumers of tobacco with the highest risk of death were those who smoked cigarettes (12.7 times augmented risk), followed by those who smoked cigars (4.2 times augmented risk), and last, the ones who smoked pipes (1.7 times augmented risk). A meta-analysis of 287 epidemiologic studies found that smoking pipes alone was connected to a 3.3 times rise in augmented risk of developing malignancy. At the same time, the use of cigars alone was linked to a 2.95-times higher risk [15, 20, 21].

Cannabis

Cannabis is the general phrase that covers cannabinoids, marijuana, and hemp, which are extracted from the *Cannabis sativa* plant, even though the terms are sometimes used interchangeably. Cannabis holds 2nd place as a product that is widely inhaled in the US, below tobacco, with roughly 7,000 new consumers every day [22]. As of the beginning of 2019, many states have outlawed personal marijuana possession. Columbia and 20 other states have allowed its medicinal use. The chemical poisons and carcinogens found in smoked cannabis, however, are like those found in tobacco smoke. These include acrolein, acetaldehyde, carbon monoxide, ammonia, formaldehyde, nitrosamines, polycyclic aromatic hydrocarbons, and phenols. In addition to this, consuming cannabis regularly has the same negative consequences on the respiratory system as smoking cigarettes. Although there is proof of harmful biological outcomes, there is currently insufficient data to link cannabis use to a grown risk of LC conclusively. However, according to a pooled analysis of 2,159 individuals of LC and 2,985 controls from the International Lung Cancer Consortium, there was an elevated risk of LC among long-term or chronic cannabis users [23].

Radon

Subsidiary factors contributing to lung cancer are typically given a lower priority than leading causes since the use of tobacco is a significant and ubiquitous risk factor. Other exposures are, nevertheless, causally linked to the chance of developing tumors. The radioactive decay of thorium and uranium naturally produces radon; it is found in soil and is a radioactive gas with no taste or smell. Exposure to radon is linked to anywhere between 3% and 14% of lung cancer cases worldwide; the range is due to regional variations in radon levels and the calculating method.

Occupational Exposures

According to estimates, 5% to 10% of lung malignancies are caused by occupational exposure to carcinogens; historically, the most common in this kind is asbestos exposure [24, 25]. In the marketplace, "asbestos" refers to a class of organically formed mineral silicate fibers comprising chrysotile and amphiboles. Although the molecular pathways that play a crucial role in asbestos-related cancer are critical and not wholly understood, fibrosis, oxidative damage, cellular toxicity, persistent inflammation, as well as genetic and epigenetic modifications are all probably involved in the occurrence of the disease. A lot of occupational exposures are connected to lung cancer in humans, including chromium, arsenic, cadmium, beryllium, diesel exhaust, and particular occupations such as coke production, gasification of coal, steel founding, iron and underground hematite mining, painting, rubber production, and aluminum manufacturing [15].

History of Non-infectious Respiratory Disorders

Emphysema and chronic bronchitis are both types of chronic inflammatory illness known as chronic obstructive pulmonary disease (COPD), which causes permanent constriction of the small airways and damage to the alveolar wall. Since the chronic inflammatory response in the bronchi is complemented by a continuous cycle of damage and restoration, it may be crucial. The primary lung cancer risk factor for COPD is tobacco use. A prevalent childhood illness, asthma, affects 300 million individuals globally [26]. Chronic lung inflammation that manifests as airway hyper-reactivity, increased mucus production, and breathing obstruction is what defines asthma. Since inflammation is a significant factor in the etiology of disease, asthma has been assumed as a possible risk factor [15].

Respiratory Illnesses with an Infectious History

"pneumococcal illness" refers to various disorders brought on by multiple organisms, with varying signs and aftereffects. The *Streptococcus pneumoniae* bacteria, which most frequently causes bacteremia and pneumonia, is the source of pneumococcal illness (meningitis). Through several potential processes from arbitrators of persistent local inflammation, such as enhanced ROS that can induce somatic mutations and DNA damage, increased angiogenesis, and antiapoptotic signaling, pneumonia is a prospective risk factor for disease. LC can cause a compromised immune system, leading to pulmonary infections. The most prevalent intracellular bacterial infection that causes sinusitis, pharyngitis, and pneumonia is *Chlamydia pneumoniae*. It spreads through secretions produced by the respiratory system and may raise the threat of lung cancer due to inflammatory moderators that are like those hypothesized for pneumonia [15].

HIV

Multiple variables, including HIV-related immunosuppression, make it challenging to control inflammatory mediators, infections, and coinfection due to oncogenic viruses such as hepatitis B and C. People with HIV have an elevated risk of developing a variety of malignancies.

Other Aspects of Lifestyle

Additionally, there is convincing evidence that other variables, such as malnutrition and a lesser BMI, may contribute to an enhanced risk of bronchogenic carcinoma in both non-smokers and smokers.

Genetic Inheritance

As the human genome has been thoroughly analyzed, searching for connections involving hereditary SNPs (single nucleotide polymorphisms) and diseases in individuals is feasible. With varied degrees of association evidence, GWA studies have effectively found genetic variables connected strongly to bronchogenic carcinoma susceptibility. Specific locations were narrowed to given subgroups, like smoking status, ethnicity, histologic subtypes, and sex. Polygenic risk scores, determined by the set of SNPs that produces the most effective prediction model, might be developed using the data from these extensive GWA investigations.

Menopause

Smoking significantly modifies the relationship between menopause and the risk of disease, which may not be proportional. Smoking appears to be the primary factor between bronchogenic carcinoma and early menopause, as evidenced by the elevated risk of disease among women who had it early (< 45 years).

Drugs Targets in Lung Cancer

Several proteins that have changed amounts in lung cancer have recently been identified, serving as new and promising disease markers and therapeutic targets. Lung cancer remains fatal, even though advances have made it feasible to extend the time until tumor recurrence considerably. So, it is crucial to look for new targets to combat this disease [27]. Oncogene changes bring on most NSCLCS, and in recent years, the mortality rate from NSCLC has significantly decreased because of the development of targeted medicines [28]. Patients who have actionable mutations in BRAF (V-raf murine sarcoma viral oncogene homolog B), ALK (anaplastic lymphoma kinase), MET (mesenchymal-epithelial transition factor), EGFR (epidermal growth factor receptor), NTRK (neurotrophic tyrosine receptor kinase), and ROS1 (c-Ros oncogene 1) have access to a variety of targeted drugs that have FDA approval. Some of the novel targets have been briefed below.

Tyrosine Kinase and the Epidermal Growth Factor Receptor (EGFR) (TKs)

It is a type of tyrosine kinase receptor. In Western society, 15% of individuals with NSCLC possess EGFR mutations, but in the Asian community, this figure jumps to 35% [29]. Furthermore, non-smokers showed a greater frequency of EGFR mutations. FDA has approved drugs like erlotinib, gefitinib, dacomitinib, osimertinib, and afatinib for their application as first-line treatments for individuals with rapidly spreading NSCLC who have tumors with EGFR exon 19 deletions or mutations of exon 21 L858R. Furthermore, afatinib was beneficial against NSCLC tumors with unusual EGFR mutations, such as Leu861Gln, Gly719Xaa, and Ser768Ile, but less effective against other mutation types.

The RET gene encodes an RTK from the RET family. KIF5B is the most prevalent fusion partner in NSCLC patients with RET rearrangements. Targeting RET fusion-driven NSCLCs multi-targeted TKIs (MKIs) like lenvatinib, vandetanib, sunitinib, and cabozantinib, which have been tested. NSCLC with HER2 mutations is currently thought to be a unique molecular subgroup. In NSCLC, HER2 activation occurs by three mechanisms: gene mutation (1%-4% of cases), gene amplification (2%-5%), and protein overexpression (2%-30%), with varying prognostic and predictive consequences. Hence, HER2 is also a potent target in lung cancer [30].

ALK (Anaplastic Lymphoma Kinase)

The EML4-ALK novel fusion oncogene was created by the inversion of the two genes located on chromosome 2's short arm, EML4 and ALK. NSCLC, inflammatory myofibroblastic tumors, and anaplastic large cell lymphomas all include rearrangements of chromosome segments involving the ALK, making it a potential target. ALK signaling dysfunction results in "oncogene addiction" and increased susceptibility to ALK inhibitors [31]. The foremost accepted targeted therapy for advanced NSCLC with an ALK-positive mutation is crizotinib.

ROS1

ROS1 alteration affects around 1-2% of NSCLC cases, primarily in younger adults who did not previously smoke [32]. Tyrosine kinase receptor encoding is produced by the ROS1 gene, which is situated on chromosome 6. Cricotinib was approved in March 2016 for the treatment of metastatic ROS1-positive NSCLC.

The Neurotrophic Tropomyosin Receptor Kinase (NTRK)

NTRK gene fusions, which can arise in several tumor types, involve either NTRK1, 2, or 3. NTRK gene fusion has been found as an oncogenic driver of many solid tumors, and it is uncommon in NSCLC, arising at a rate of less than 1%. Even though approximately 1% of NTRK gene fusions are seen in NSCLC patients, its identification has become increasingly important after the discovery of such TRK inhibitors [33]. Larotrectinib was the first oral TKI for NRTK to receive approval.

BRAF V600E Mutations

BRAF is the name of a gene as well as a protein. The BRAF protein regulates cell development. When the BRAF gene is mutated, an aberrant protein is produced that transmits signals that lead to uncontrolled cell multiplication and cancer. To regulate cell development, the BRAF protein collaborates with another protein called MEK. The BRAF gene encodes the V-Raf, which is essential for cell signaling, development, and survival. Alterations in the BRAF gene lead to the advancement and succession of disease. BRAF has many variants, but the one with FDA-approved therapy in lung cancer is BRAF V600E. This mutation is a variant of the BRAF protein. BRAF may always activate the MEK protein in cells with this mutation. BRAF mutations are frequent among females, non-smokers, and aggressive histological forms of NSCLC, accounting for 1%-2% of adenocarcinoma. Traditional treatment is ineffective in BRAF-mutated NSCLC patients [34].

KRAS Mutation as Target

Approximately thirty percent of adenocarcinomas of the lungs have an alteration in the gene that encodes the Kirsten rat sarcoma virus oncogene homolog (KRAS), making it the most common carcinogenic promotor in advanced NSCLC. More than 80% of KRAS oncogene mutations start at codon 12, where different amino acids take the place of glycine molecules resulting in genomic variations in KRAS mutant tumors. Roughly thirteen percent of individuals with pulmonary adenocarcinoma have mutant KRAS glycine to cystine modifications, which make up 44% of all mutations of the KRAS gene in NSCLC [35].

Antibody-drug Conjugates

A specific antibody of EGFR-cMet called JNJ-372 showed activity in NSCLC with EGFRm. A phase 1 trial included individuals who had progressed EGFRm NSCLC, including those who had advanced on the 3rd generation EGFR Exon 20 and EGFR TKI disease. An antibody-drug combination that targets the protein tyrosine kinase, called PTK7PF-06647020 (PF-7020), was evaluated in end-stage solid tumors in phase I clinical trials. The results of the antibody-drug combination demonstrate a respectable safety record and encouraging results.

Receptors Involved in Immunotherapy

Active immunotherapy, which uses vaccines to encourage the immune system to confront tumor cells, and passive immunotherapy, which uses checkpoint inhibitors to activate the immune system, both involve the activation of the body's defense mechanism. Nivolumab was the foremost drug for immunotherapy of metastatic NSCLC to receive approval. It is an antibody that blocks the human IgG4 PD-1 immune-checkpoint. It adheres to the PD-1 receptor and blocks malignant PD-L1 from connecting to T cells, reinstating the immune response against the malignancy.

Current Treatment Strategies and Side Effects

Lung cancer can be healed with chemotherapy, radiation, surgery, TDDS, anti-microbial peptides (AMPs), immunotherapy, and combinations of these therapies. We have seen significant advancements in its therapies over the last few decades. Even though the advancements in this area have not been as rapid as those in molecular targeted therapy and immune-oncology, chemotherapy is still a crucial component in the treatment of pulmonary adenocarcinoma, irrespective of mutational subtype, immunologic status, stage, and histology. In comparison to the standard of care, the advent of new therapeutic approaches—such as preservation therapy, NDDS, and combinations with several different types of anti-neoplastic medications have clearly improved survival and/or toxicity. Chemoimmunotherapy has shown encouraging results, and it can be a novel first-line treatment for NSCLC that is not oncogene-dependent. Overall, in this epoch of precision medicine, chemotherapy is still effective [9].

Surgery entails removing all or a tissue of the lung. This process is frequently accomplished by thoracotomies and minimally invasive surgery. The decision is based on the surgeon's experience and the size, location, and stage of the lung tumor. The four surgical methods employed are lobectomy, segmentectomy, wedge resection, and pneumonectomy. Lung cancer surgery is a big procedure with the potential for serious side effects, so it is not recommended for everyone. After lung cancer surgery, recovery usually takes a few weeks to several months [15].

Radiation therapy for lung cancer comes in two primary forms: radiotherapy using an external beam and brachytherapy (internal radiation therapy). In radiotherapy, 2 radiation types are commonly used: electromagnetic and particle radiation. X-rays and γ-rays are components of the first, whereas electrons, protons, and neutrons belong to the second. While radiotherapy has many different impacts on the body, it mostly works by destroying tumor cells and impairing their capacity to proliferate. These events can come from direct cellular damage to DNA or other vital molecules (most frequently described in the context of particle radiation from protons, electrons, or alpha particles) or indirect cellular damage that follows the generation of free radicals [36]. The standard treatment for LD-SCLC is four rounds of platinum-doublet chemotherapy as well as radiation to cure the illness. Even in elderly individuals, this form of therapy enhances the chance of survival when contrasted with chemotherapy alone. While once-daily radiation remains the standard in most facilities due to practical concerns, even if prior phase 3 studies recommended twice-daily radiotherapy, the majority of patients do not match the criteria due to comorbidity and performance status. Radiation therapy has several drawbacks, such as a high prevalence of adverse effects brought on by nonspecific targeting. Vomiting, nausea, and fatigue are frequent side effects in lung cancer patients. Appetite loss, weight loss, mild redness to blistering, peeling of the skin in the area being treated, and hair loss at the site of radiation exposure are the negative effects that persist even after the therapies have been completed.

One of the most crucial treatments for patients with cancer is chemotherapy. NSCLC collaborative research group conducted a meta-analysis in 1995 and found that platinum-based chemotherapy considerably improves overall survival. Furthermore, as contrasted with non-platinum-based regimens or solo drugs, the platinum doublet was more effective. In a prospective study, the Eastern Cooperative Oncology Group (ECOG) E1594 examined four platinum-based doublets for terminal stages of NSCLC and found a significant correlation between longer life and improved performance level (ECOG 0 or 1). Pemetrexed, a novel chemotherapeutic medication with proven therapeutic efficiency in pulmonary cancer therapy, was introduced in the early 2000s. Pemetrexed showed a significant clinical advantage over squamous cells in the phase 3 JMDB study, supporting the idea that histology is important for lung cancer treatment. The therapeutic advantage of pemetrexed in non-squamous cell cancer was later demonstrated by the phase 3 study. Those who received pemetrexed maintenance medication following a 4-cycle platinum doublet had a considerably higher median overall survival (OS) than patients who did not get maintenance therapy. Bevacizumab and innovative drug delivery technologies like nanoparticle albumin-bound paclitaxel are utilized for treating cancer. The new standard of care for NSCLC that is not oncogene-dependent is chemoimmunotherapy, in particular, because of its optimistic results.

First-line systemic therapy for metastasized SCLC: Chemotherapy-sensitive SCLC typically responds quickly to treatment. Platinum-based chemotherapy is now the 1st-line therapy for ED-SCLC, comprising 4-6 treatments of platinum with irinotecan in Japan as well as etoposide with cis-platin in Europe and the US. Because of its equivalent efficacy and lesser toxicity, carboplatin is frequently used over cisplatin in medical procedures. However, most patients observe recurrence during the 1st year of therapy; some of them are affected while receiving therapy (platinum-resistant), some do so within three months of treatment cessation (platinum-refractory), and others do so more than 90 days after therapy has ended (platinum-sensitive). Carboplatin and cisplatin are examples of platinum-based medicines used in first-line chemotherapy for NSCLCs, along with docetaxel, paclitaxel, and gemcitabine [37]. Topotecan is the only medication officially licensed as a 2nd line treatment for SCLC, and it continues to be the gold standard of care [38].

Chemotherapy can have terrible side effects. However, most of them will fade away after the treatment, and many of them can be treated or prevented. Most of them will go away once you finish your course of treatment. Feeling tired all the time is among the common side effects of chemotherapy. A substantial number of patients undergoing chemotherapy will experience periods during which they feel nauseous or vomit. Medication that treats or prevents motion sickness is often known as an antiemetic. Constipation, indigestion, trouble sleeping (insomnia), and headaches are some of the adverse reactions that might occur after taking anti-nausea medication. In virtually all cases, the hair loss is just temporary. As soon as the therapy is complete, your hair should begin the process of growing back. Chemotherapy can impair the effectiveness of the immune system, making it harder for the body to respond to infections. Because of this, your risk of contracting infections that could lead to serious illness is increased. Chemotherapy can reduce the RBC count in the body, which can result in anemia. Chemotherapy can occasionally cause the lining of the mouth to become inflamed and uncomfortable. This condition is referred to as mucositis. A loss of appetite is a common side effect of chemotherapy. Certain chemotherapy medications have been linked to the development of transient skin and nail abnormalities. During chemotherapy, some patients experience difficulties with their ability to concentrate as well as their attention span and short-term memory. Another potential side effect is sleeplessness. During chemotherapy, many patients report that they have a loss of interest in sexual activity. A few days after beginning chemotherapy, you may experience diarrhea or constipation. The chemotherapy treatment process can be extremely discouraging, taxing, and upsetting [39].

As a substitute to chemotherapy for NSCLC, the molecular targeted treatment of EGFR TKI has emerged as the first-line therapeutic. TKI resistance, which can be caused by several different processes, typically makes it difficult to maintain targeted therapy in the clinic. For instance, the majority of individuals receiving gefitinib therapy for NSCLC with an EGFR mutation will eventually acquire resistance to medication as a result of mutations in EGFRT790M. Olga et al. described a therapy technique to inhibit four different classes of EGFR-TKIs by various siRNAs utilizing liposomal paclitaxel altered by LHRH decapeptide. The pulmonary adenocarcinoma cells with variable sensitivity to the drug were used to test the liposomes *in vitro*. Inhaled delivery was also used to evaluate them in an orthotopic A549 cancer cell mouse model. Both models demonstrated that liposomes had favorable organ dispersion and an anticancer impact [40, 41].

For patients suffering from metastasized NSCLC, whose tumor consisted of exon 21 L88R mutations or EGFR exon 19 deletions, the following were the foremost legalized drugs for treatment: dacomitinib, erlotinib, gefitinib, osimertinib, and afatinib. Among these, afatinib exhibited better anticancer in tumors that presented rare mutations of EDFR, including Leu861Gln, Gly719Xaa, and Ser768Ile. Osimertinib enhanced survival without progression to 18.9 months in a phase 3 clinical study. Osimertinib is now the preferred front-line treatment for individuals with end-stage NSCLC who possess an EGFR gene mutation since it is more effective, has less severe side effects, and can reach the central nervous system. Stomatitis, maculopapular rash, and diarrhea were the side effects that occurred the most frequently. After taking EGFR TKIs, some individuals get a reduced white blood cell number, upper respiratory tract infection, decreased neutrophil number, vomiting, and diarrhea [42 - 45]. For the management of ALK-positive progressive NSCLC, the first targeted drug to be approved was crizotinib [46]. Its descendants, ALK blockers, have become more potent than their predecessors and can overcome resistance. Other medications that have received regulatory approval include ceritinib, alectinib, brigatinib, and lorlatinib. Lorlatinib is a third-generation inhibitor of ALK and ROS. The symptoms of hypercholesterolemia, hypertriglyceridemia, edema, and peripheral neuropathy were the most often reported side effects. Oral entrectinib is a TKI that inhibits gene fusions involving ROS1, ALK, and NTRK [47, 48]. Some individuals experience TEAEs of grades 3/4, while the majority of patients only experience grade 1 TEAEs. Capmatinib and tepotinib are examples of very selective MET inhibitors. Capmatinib was administered to patients having end-stage NSCLC who carried mutations in MET that bypassed exon 14 or MET amplification in a phase 2 clinical trial, where it was found that those patients were suitable for first-line therapy with tepotinib. Peripheral edema, diarrhea, nausea, and asthenia were the TEAEs that occurred the most frequently. Some patients are forced to stop treatment with TEAEs because they have adverse effects, including nausea and diarrhea in one patient and interstitial lung disease in another [49 - 51].

AMG510 is a relatively small molecule with a lot of potential. It suppresses KRAS G12C in a selective manner by barring it in a dormant GDP-bound form. Nausea, diarrhea, vomiting, increased creatinine, decreased appetite, and raised liver enzymes were typical adverse effects of treatment with TEAEs. Fatigue, decreased appetite, and dyspnoea were the symptoms of toxicity graded as grade 3. M6620 is an ATR inhibitor that is selective in its action. Monotherapy with M6620 is well tolerated but exhibited only little antitumor efficacy. Fatigue, neutropenia, anemia, and thrombocytopenia were the kind of TEAEs that were reported the most frequently. Bemcentinib, a predominantly specific blocker of the AXL tyrosine kinase, can be taken by mouth. The EGFR-cMet bispecific antibody JNJ-372 displayed efficacy in EGFRm NSCLC. The TEAE that was reported the most frequently was fatigue, and it was the only TEAE that was a grade 3 [52].

The CTLA and anti-PD-1/PD-L1 pathway are not the only immunotherapy approaches that have been investigated for progressed or metastatic NSCLC. Immunotherapy that stimulates the immune response *via* additional pathways, for instance, CD40, LAG-3, IDO, TIM, and CD122, shows promise as a treatment option. In this patient population, researchers are also evaluating experimental therapies such as an antibody-drug combination and a neoantigen vaccination. Immunotherapy, which uses antibodies like anti-PDL-1 or anti-PD-1, was employed as an advanced therapy for NSCLC and has proven to be incredibly clinically beneficial. A human anti-PD-1 monoclonal antibody called nivolumab is the first PD-1/PD-L blocking drug for secondary treatment of end-stage NSCLC. Other anti-PD-1/PD-L1 antibody medicines authorized by the FDA for treating pulmonary cancer in recent years include pembrolizumab and atezolizumab [53].

The possibility that immune checkpoint inhibition (ICI) can be used to treat SCLC is a topic of great interest. The soaring mutational liability of this tumor, along with its potential for heightened immunogenicity, is the justification for adding immunotherapy with chemotherapy in SCLC. Chemotherapy can increase the expression of tumor-specific antigens, setting up the tumor to respond to checkpoint inhibitor therapy [38]. Combinational approaches with additional anti-neoplastic agents include combining them with immunotherapy, targeted therapy, and angiogenesis inhibitors [52].

Immunotherapy may have minor, moderate, or even fatal side effects. Minor negative effects of therapy will probably continue if you experience only minor side effects, and your symptoms will be closely watched for any changes. Consequences range from mild to severe. To reduce the immune system activity, your doctor may suspend the course of therapy and prescribe a corticosteroid drug class (such as prednisone or others). Other medicines may be delivered after a corticosteroid injection. Immune cells regularly assault both immune cells and healthy body tissues as immune checkpoint blockers have adverse effects. This is referred to as inflammation. The side effects of immune checkpoint blockers have an impact on various physiological systems given below. Skin issues and digestive system issues are the most frequent adverse reactions of immune checkpoint inhibitors. These include colitis, a type of colon inflammation that typically causes diarrhea. Other less frequent adverse effects include pain in the upper abdomen, difficulty swallowing, nausea, vomiting, joint swelling, discomfort like arthritis, and cramping in the skeleton and muscles. Neuropathy is a major adverse effect of immunotherapy, and it can also cause blood levels to plummet, resulting in bleeding, anemia, and other complications. Immune checkpoint blockers can cause pneumonitis, a lung inflammation that can cause a cough or difficulty in breathing. Although rare, pneumonitis is deadly.

Inflammation of the eye's tissues is a rare side effect but may be more prevalent in patients who take a combination of immune checkpoint inhibitors. Immunotherapy may have an impact on fertility or the capacity to conceive [54 - 56].

Importance of Medicinal Plants and Phytocompounds in Lung Cancer

According to the research studies, plants are essential in the battle against various cancer cell lines. The secondary metabolites in the plant extracts were shown to inhibit cancer cells through damage to DNA and activate apoptosis-inducing enzymes in *in vitro* tests. Research on the *in vivo* actions of plants produced astounding findings in the prevention of cancer in *in vivo* models. Plant-based medicines were identified as one of the appealing strategies for pulmonary adenocarcinoma treatment since they were evaluated to be effective and useful in sensitizing cancer-causing factors, promoting patient survival time, reducing side effects of chemotherapy, and improving the QOL in the subjects. Toxicology reduction, symptom relief from cancer-related conditions, and stimulation of defense mechanisms were the main goals of using natural items as supplemental medicine for the treatment. Cancer cells are induced to undergo apoptosis using plant-derived metabolites [57]. A lot of laboratory-made alternatives and herbal products are still in use, including the two semi-synthetic products of the naturally found substance epipodophyllotoxin, known as clinically effective medications etoposide and teniposide, and the vinca alkaloids like vinblastine and vincristine. Flavopiridol and combretastatin A4 are two more promising drugs that are now in the developmental stage. Additionally, many substances derived from plants or other living things are still investigated using *in vitro* models to ascertain how they interact with lung cancer cells [58]. Here are some plant chemicals that have been utilized to treat lung cancer.

Gallic acid, which has been determined as the active ingredient in *Phaleria macrocarpa* fruit extract, was involved in the stimulation of apoptosis in lung cancer. A significant medicinal plant species of the Lamiaceae family is *Scutellaria barbata*, commonly known as the barbed skullcap, which is used to treat cancer and inflammatory illnesses. It contains significant secondary metabolites, such as polysaccharides, alkaloids, flavones, and steroids in abundance. This species exhibited favorable action against lung cancer in *in vitro* experiments. One of the key anticancer plants, *Wedelia chinensis*, is native to China, South-East Asia, and India. It belongs to the Asteraceae family and is abundant in secondary metabolites such as flavonoids, tannin, and phenols. In an *in vitro* investigation, lung cancer was positively affected by *W. chinensis* essential oils. Two significant constituents, carvacrol and trans-caryophyllene, were detected by the GC-MS study [57]. In China, the root of *Scutellaria baicalensis* is added during chemotherapy for lung cancer. Recently, three substances—baicalin, baicalein, and wogonin—were linked to its activity. Subamolide A, which was isolated from *Cinnamomum subavenium,* caused the demise of lung cancer cells by generating ROS, which then caused mitotic catastrophe and apoptosis. Terpinen-4-ol, a monoterpene found in the essential oils of various aromatic plants, caused the mitochondrial apoptotic pathway to be involved in the antitumor effect it had on NSCLC cells. The primary active component of *Davallia divaricata*, an herb that was historically used by Taiwanese folks for treating lung cancer, is davallic acid [58].

Osthole, a specific nutrient that may be extracted from the medicinal herb *Cnidium monnieri*, has been shown in numerous studies to be effective in a variety of pulmonary cancer cell lines. Numerous studies have demonstrated that osthole can stop various cancer cells from migrating and proliferating in lung tissues (e.g., A549 cells of lungs).

Etoposide, teniposide, and etoposide phosphate, which are derived from *Podophyllum* plants, are employed as anticancer chemotherapeutic agents. Aryltetralin-lignan PTOX has significant cytotoxic potential. The compounds of podophyllotoxin are antiproliferative against small cell and nonsmall cell lung malignancies as well as germ cell tumors [59].

Taxol, also known as paclitaxel, was the primarily extracted chemical from the bark of *Taxus brevifolia* Nutt. (Taxaceae). Several *Taxus* species have been employed for their anticancer properties, including *T. canadensis* Marshall, *T. baccata* L., and *T. brevifolia*. The leaves contain paclitaxel, a chemical component of the *Taxus* species. Baccatins are a large source and main class of medications that are used to treat lung cancer [59].

6-Shogaol, an active substance extracted from ginger, showed promise in animal studies. It was shown to slow down the growth of cancer cells in an experimental model of mice. Significantly lower proliferation and higher activation of apoptosis were related to the growth inhibition of NSCLC [2]. In mice given B16F10 melanoma cells, the potent ginger compound [6]-gingerol demonstrated antiangiogenic action both *in vitro* and *in vivo* and decreased the number of lung metastases. Embelin, an active ingredient found in the fruits of the *Embelia ribes* plant, has demonstrated a lot of medicinal benefits, including antitumor action against lung cancer cells [58].

New technologies have also been used to study herbal extracts. In cell line A549, the ethanolic extract of *Polygala senega* (EEPS) triggered apoptosis. Its poly-(lactic-co-glycolic) acid (PLGA) nanoparticle-encapsulated version, which was more effective than EEPS at inhibiting lung cancer cell growth, improved cellular entrance and bioavailability. The most researched Euphorbiaceae species include *Croton macrostachys, Euphorbia fischeriana, Euphorbia ingens,* and *Euphorbia esula,* all of which exhibit anticancer efficacy against lung cancer models. Extracts have been identified as promising phyto-therapeutic adjuvants in enhanced lung cancer therapy, according to recent research findings. This can result in more advantages and safety for everyone, improving access to medical treatment and the quality of life for lung cancer patients as a result. However, various preclinical and clinical research have demonstrated that herbal extracts have anticancer potential against lung cancer [58].

Andrographolide and its Analog's Role in Lung Cancer

Andrographolide [Structure 1], the principal bioactive chemical element of the *Andrographis paniculata* plant, is a bicyclic diterpenoid lactone with significant anticancer activity. Previous studies have indicated that AGP has anticancer potential in lung cancer, which was expressed through multiple methods that will be described briefly here.

Andrographolide's anti-lung cancer activity was investigated and evidenced in different *in vitro* and *in vivo* models. Exposure to 100 M andrographolide significantly reduced the cell viability of A549, whereas 25 M andrographolide had no impact. Furthermore, 100 M andrographolide dramatically raised the proportion of cells in the subG1 population, but 25 M andrographolide had no impact. These findings imply that the cytotoxic effects of andrographolide grow in proportion to concentration. A549 cell death can be caused by andrographolide at high concentrations at different time points. With raised concentration, the cytotoxic effects become more pronounced [60]. Treating nude mice with cell line (CL1) in combination with andrographolide (4 mg/kg) decreased tumor volume and weight considerably [61]. In a mouse model, results demonstrated that andrographolide dramatically decreased VEGF expression in Clara cells relative to the control group. In the same way, transcriptional and translational expression of Cyclin A&B, Cyclin B, EGFR, and VEGF was inhibited by andrographolide, leading to the blockade of tumor development. These findings suggest that andrographolide-induced VEGF overexpression can inhibit cell cycle progression and produce lung cancers in transgenic mice [62].

AGP's antiangiogenic potential is related to its capacity to suppress the upregulation of hypoxia-inducible factor-1 (HIF-1), a vital modulator of hypoxic cells that contribute to angiogenesis and cancer by persistent suppression of PI3/AKT pathway [63]. Additionally, this study also discovered that AGP increased the proteolytic degradation of HIF-1 *via* PHD2 signaling pathways, which decreased VEGF transcriptional expression. These studies uncovered

AGP's unique involvement in reducing HIF-1 and VEGF production, which may be critical for lung tumor angiogenesis and metastasis, as well as the signaling molecules that underlie this control. When treated with AGP at concentrations less than 5 mM, another cell line, H3255, with a mutation in EGFR, demonstrated reduced DNA fragmentation, protein kinase C activity, and Na+ - K+ -ATPase, as well as lowered TGF-b1 and VEGF levels [64].

Aside from inhibiting angiogenesis, AGP (5mM) has been proven to block the migration and spread of A549 cells [65]. The results demonstrated that andrographolide inhibited MMP-7 activity as well as mRNA and protein levels, but not MMP-9 or MMP-2. MMP-7 expression appears to be decreased by AGP *via* activator protein-1 (AP-1). These findings showed that andrographolide might limit MMP-7 production by blocking PI3K/Akt/AP-1 signaling, resulting in reduced invasiveness of cancer. In yet another investigation, AGP (1, 5 and 10 mM) was reported to reduce cell proliferation in H3255 lung cancer cells, as well as downregulation of eMMP-9 mRNA expression and blockage of change in location of NF-kB p65 subunit *via* repression of IkB phosphorylation [66]. Andrographolide, on the other hand, decreased MMP-2 expression and changed the expression of 939 genes in NSCLC, resulting in blockage of cell cycle and apoptotic death. In a SCLC cell line (NCI H358), it also boosted the expression of the tumor suppressor protein HLJ1 and blocked its multiplication and spread [61]. AGP's anticancer action may potentially be shown through immunomodulatory effects. AGP elevated IFN-g production by activated NKs and NK-mediated NSCLC cell destroying membrane-bound IL-21 and CD137L modified K562 cells [67].

Furthermore, AGP has also been shown to exhibit synergistic anticancer activity when given with other chemotherapeutics like cisplatin and paclitaxel. When compared to cisplatin alone, the combination of cisplatin and AGP may have delayed tumor progression, reduced the frequency of lung metastases, and improved renal tubular damage [68]. An *in vivo* investigation, including the injection of 100 mg/kg AGP with 20 mg/kg paclitaxel to an A549 NSCLC xenograft, revealed synergistic antitumor efficacy. Despite the fact that the fundamental molecular basis of this anticancer synergy is undetermined, AGP has been shown to improve paclitaxel-mediated antiproliferative and cell death by apoptosis in NSCLC cells by increasing intracellular ROS production and cell cycle arrest in the G2/M phase [69].

Due to various AGP's remarkable antitumor effects, several researchers created synthetic and semisynthetic analogs to examine anticancer effects towards lung cancer and identified a few molecules. In a novel route, a variety of 3,19-O-acetal variants of AGP were produced by preserving hydroxyls at C-3 and C-19. When compared to AGP, among all the derivatives, 3,19-O-ethylidene andrographolide [Structure 2] was 4 times more significantly cytotoxic towards A549 (IC50 2.43 g/mL). SAR demonstrated that cytotoxicity reduced as the length of the aliphatic carbon chain rose on acetal activity from ethylidene to n-pentylidene [Structures 2-5]. Furthermore, as compared to AGP, in A549 (IC50 4.07 g/mL) cell lines, the benzylidene acetal variant [Structure-7] was twice as cytotoxic [70]. These findings suggest that protecting andrographolide's 3,19- 10 hydroxyl groups with an appropriate ethylidene/benzylidene moiety caused considerable cytotoxicity. The cytotoxic impact of lead compound (3) was altered by acetylating or dehydrating its 14-hydroxyl. The epoxidation of [Structure-3] at the C-8 site had no effect on its overall cytotoxicity. Docking studies indicated the binding affinity of the investigated compounds on recognized anticancer targets EGFR and α, β-tubulin.

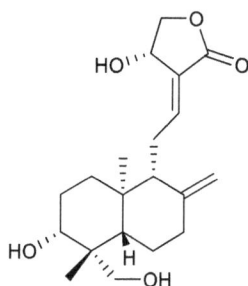

[1] Andrographolide

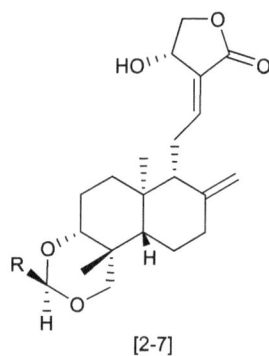

[2-7]

R=methyl [2], ethyl [3], n-propyl [4], n-butyl [5], n-pentyl [6], phenyl [7]

By inserting different aromatic (or heteroaromatic) substituents into C-12 or 14-OH, several new thioether andrographolide derivatives were produced. A total of 38 AGP derivatives were synthesized, among which, only compound [Structure-8] with heteroaromatic thioether substitution possessed substantial cytotoxic effect towards A549 lung cancer cell lines with IC50 of 9μM [71].

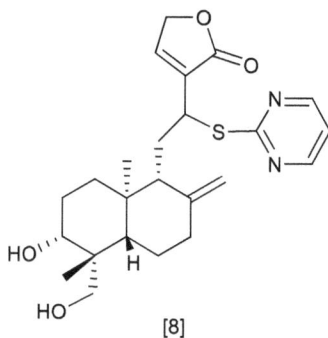

[8]

Similarly, another study modified the C-12 position to obtain 14-deox-
-andrographolide derivatives and assessed their cytotoxic potential in small cell
lung cancer cell line HOP-92. Two analogs, novel 12-phenyl thio and 12-aryl
amino -14-deoxy-andrographolide derivatives [Structures 9&10], exhibited
superior activity and selectivity towards HOP-92 with an inhibition range of 55-
90%. The SAR analyses revealed that compounds with the following
functionalities at C-12 had potent activity: Alkyl amine < benzylamine <
substituted aryl amino/phenyl thio [72].

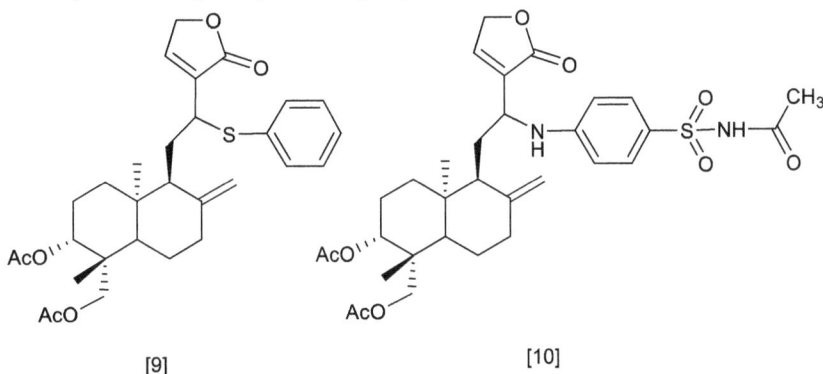

[9]   [10]

Nuclear factor-κB nuclear binding in the A549 non-small cell lung cancer cell line
is inhibited by SRS06 [Structure 11] (3,14,19- tripropionylandrographolide), the
latest semi-synthetic derivative of andrographolide with enhanced anticancer
potential and specificity. SRS06 was discovered to have powerful growth
inhibitory effects on various cancer cell lines in the NCI screening, with a 10-fold
reduced 50% inhibition of growth (GI 50) compared to AGP. The chemical was
also discovered to specifically target melanoma, CNS, kidney, colon, and ovarian
cancer cell lines, as well as NSCL cancer cell lines. The DNA fragmentation
assay demonstrated that the predominant cause of cell death in SRS06-treated
A549 cells was apoptosis. At 5 mol/l, the chemical reduced NF-κB protein
expression and significantly reduced nuclear p65 DNA binding activity [73].

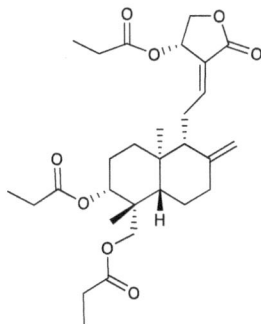

SRS06 [11]

Similarly, one of the andrographolide derivatives, 3,19-diacetyl-14-deoxy-1-,12-didehydro-Andrographolide [Structure 12], also efficiently repressed NF-kB nuclear translocation in A549 cells. In an ovalbumin (OVA)-induced asthma model in female BALB/c mice, there was reduced pulmonary eosinophilia, inflammatory cytokines in BAL fluid, production of serum immunoglobulin (Ig)-E production, mucus hypersecretion, and inflammatory mediators expression in lung tissues [74].

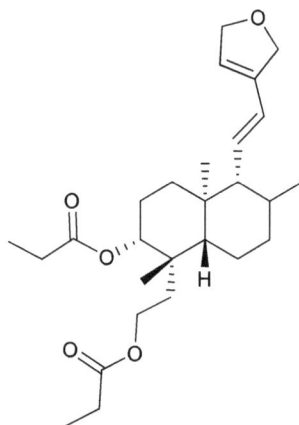

[12]

CONCLUSION

Lung cancer is one of the most lethal and extremely frequent malignant tumors on the planet. It is caused mostly by genetic mutations and cellular alterations, which result in unregulated cell growth and division. However, the specific etiology of lung cancer is still unknown. Because of its possible anti-cancer capabilities, andrographolide and its structural counterparts have received interest in the field of lung cancer. Andrographolide and its analogs have been demonstrated in studies to suppress the development of lung cancer cells by inducing apoptosis or programmed cell death. They have also been demonstrated to target signaling pathways involved in lung cancer formation and progression, such as the NF-kB and MAPK pathways. Andrographolide and its structural counterparts have shown encouraging results as prospective therapeutic agents for lung cancer therapy in both *in vitro* and *in vivo* trials. Their anti-cancer capabilities, which include suppression of cancer cell proliferation and activation of apoptosis, make them of great interest for future research. More studies are needed to completely understand the mechanisms of action of these substances and their potential therapeutic uses in the treatment of lung cancer.

REFERENCES

[1]   Huang X, Zhang F, Lin J, *et al.* Systematically analyzed molecular characteristics of lung adenocarcinoma using metabolism-related genes classification. Genet Mol Biol 2022; 45(4): e20220121.
        [http://dx.doi.org/10.1590/1678-4685-gmb-2022-0121] [PMID: 36622242]

[2]   Chota A, George BP, Abrahamse H. Potential treatment of breast and lung cancer using *Dicoma anomala,* an African medicinal plant. Molecules 2020; 25(19): 4435.
        [http://dx.doi.org/10.3390/molecules25194435] [PMID: 32992537]

[3]   Chemi F, Pearce SP, Clipson A, *et al.* cfDNA methylome profiling for detection and subtyping of small cell lung cancers. Nat Can 2022; 3(10): 1260-70.
        [http://dx.doi.org/10.1038/s43018-022-00415-9] [PMID: 35941262]

[4]   Soo HL, Quah SY, Sulaiman I, Sagineedu SR, Lim JCW, Stanslas J. Advances and challenges in developing andrographolide and its analogs as cancer therapeutic agents. Drug Discov Today 2019; 24(9): 1890-8.
        [http://dx.doi.org/10.1016/j.drudis.2019.05.017] [PMID: 31154065]

[5]   Sung H, Ferlay J, Siegel RL, *et al.* Global Cancer Statistics 2020: GLOBOCAN estimates of incidence and mortality worldwide for 36 cancers in 185 countries. CA Cancer J Clin 2021; 71(3): 209-49.
        [http://dx.doi.org/10.3322/caac.21660] [PMID: 33538338]

[6]   Islami F, Goding Sauer A, Miller KD, *et al.* Proportion and number of cancer cases and deaths attributable to potentially modifiable risk factors in the United States. CA Cancer J Clin 2018; 68(1): 31-54.
        [http://dx.doi.org/10.3322/caac.21440] [PMID: 29160902]

[7]   Siegel RL, Miller KD, Fuchs HE, Jemal A. Cancer Statistics, 2021. CA Cancer J Clin 2021; 71(1): 7-33.
        [http://dx.doi.org/10.3322/caac.21654] [PMID: 33433946]

[8]   Moodley J, Walter FM, Scott SE, Mwaka AM. Towards timely diagnosis of symptomatic breast and cervical cancer in South Africa. S Afr Med J 2018; 108(10): 803-4.
        [http://dx.doi.org/10.7196/SAMJ.2018.v108i10.13478] [PMID: 30421705]

[9]   Lee SH. Chemotherapy for lung cancer in the era of personalized medicine. Tuberc Respir Dis (Seoul) 2019; 82(3): 179-89.
        [http://dx.doi.org/10.4046/trd.2018.0068] [PMID: 30841023]

[10]   Di Federico A, De Giglio A, Gelsomino F, Sperandi F, Melotti B, Ardizzoni A. Predictors of survival to immunotherapy and chemoimmunotherapy in non-small cell lung cancer: A meta-analysis. J Natl Cancer Inst 2023; 115(1): 29-42.
        [http://dx.doi.org/10.1093/jnci/djac205] [PMID: 36322815]

[11]   Ettinger DS, Wood DE, Aisner DL, *et al.* Non–Small Cell Lung Cancer, Version 5.2017, NCCN Clinical Practice Guidelines in Oncology. J Natl Compr Canc Netw 2017; 15(4): 504-35.
        [http://dx.doi.org/10.6004/jnccn.2017.0050] [PMID: 28404761]

[12]   Rivera-Concepcion J, Uprety D, Adjei AA. Challenges in the Use of Targeted Therapies in Non–Small Cell Lung Cancer. Cancer Res Treat 2022; 54(2): 315-29.
        [http://dx.doi.org/10.4143/crt.2022.078] [PMID: 35209703]

[13]   Gutheil WG, Reed G, Ray A, Anant S, Dhar A. Crocetin: an agent derived from saffron for prevention and therapy for cancer. Curr Pharm Biotechnol 2012; 13(1): 173-9.
        [http://dx.doi.org/10.2174/138920112798868566] [PMID: 21466430]

[14]   Hassan B. Plants and cancer treatment. Med Plants Use Prev Treat Dis 2019; pp. 1-11.

[15]   Schabath MB, Cote ML. Cancer Progress and Priorities: Lung Cancer. Cancer Epidemiol Biomarkers Prev 2019; 28(10): 1563-79.
        [http://dx.doi.org/10.1158/1055-9965.EPI-19-0221] [PMID: 31575553]

[16]   Tsai J, Homa DM, Gentzke AS, *et al.* Exposure to secondhand smoke among nonsmokers - United States, 1988-2014. MMWR Morb Mortal Wkly Rep 2018; 67(48): 1342-6.
[http://dx.doi.org/10.15585/mmwr.mm6748a3] [PMID: 30521502]

[17]   Mirbolouk M, Charkhchi P, Kianoush S, *et al.* Prevalence and distribution of E-cigarette use among U.S. adults: Behavioral risk factor surveillance system, 2016. Ann Intern Med 2018; 169(7): 429-38.
[http://dx.doi.org/10.7326/M17-3440] [PMID: 30167658]

[18]   Jaber RM, Mirbolouk M, DeFilippis AP, *et al.* Electronic cigarette use prevalence, associated factors, and pattern by cigarette smoking status in the United States From NHANES (National Health and Nutrition Examination Survey) 2013-2014. J Am Heart Assoc 2018; 7(14): e008178.
[http://dx.doi.org/10.1161/JAHA.117.008178] [PMID: 30007934]

[19]   Kosmider L, Sobczak A, Fik M, *et al.* Carbonyl compounds in electronic cigarette vapors: effects of nicotine solvent and battery output voltage. Nicotine Tob Res 2014; 16(10): 1319-26.
[http://dx.doi.org/10.1093/ntr/ntu078] [PMID: 24832759]

[20]   Lee PN, Forey BA, Coombs KJ. Systematic review with meta-analysis of the epidemiological evidence in the 1900s relating smoking to lung cancer. BMC Cancer 2012; 12(1): 385.
[http://dx.doi.org/10.1186/1471-2407-12-385] [PMID: 22943444]

[21]   Boffetta P, Pershagen G, Jöckel KH, *et al.* Cigar and pipe smoking and lung cancer risk: a multicenter study from Europe. J Natl Cancer Inst 1999; 91(8): 697-701.
[http://dx.doi.org/10.1093/jnci/91.8.697] [PMID: 10218507]

[22]   Azofeifa A, Mattson ME, Schauer G, McAfee T, Grant A, Lyerla R. National estimates of marijuana use and related indicators - National survey on drug use and health, United States, 2002-2014. MMWR Surveill Summ 2016; 65(11): 1-28.
[http://dx.doi.org/10.15585/mmwr.ss6511a1] [PMID: 27584586]

[23]   Zhang LR, Morgenstern H, Greenland S, *et al.* Cannabis smoking and lung cancer risk: Pooled analysis in the International Lung Cancer Consortium. Int J Cancer 2015; 136(4): 894-903.
[http://dx.doi.org/10.1002/ijc.29036] [PMID: 24947688]

[24]   Alberg AJ, Brock MV, Ford JG, Samet JM, Spivack SD. Epidemiology of lung cancer: Diagnosis and management of lung cancer, 3rd ed: American College of Chest Physicians evidence-based clinical practice guidelines. Chest 2013; 143: e1S-e29S.

[25]   Driscoll T, Nelson DI, Steenland K, *et al.* The global burden of disease due to occupational carcinogens. Am J Ind Med 2005; 48(6): 419-31.
[http://dx.doi.org/10.1002/ajim.20209] [PMID: 16299703]

[26]   Masoli M, Fabian D, Holt S, Beasley R. The global burden of asthma: executive summary of the GINA Dissemination Committee Report. Allergy 2004; 59(5): 469-78.
[http://dx.doi.org/10.1111/j.1398-9995.2004.00526.x] [PMID: 15080825]

[27]   Klett-Mingo JI, Pinto-Díez C, Cambronero-Plaza J, *et al.* Potential therapeutic use of aptamers against HAT1 in lung cancer. Cancers (Basel) 2022; 15(1): 227.
[http://dx.doi.org/10.3390/cancers15010227] [PMID: 36612223]

[28]   Li BT, Smit EF, Goto Y, *et al.* DESTINY-Lung01 trial investigators. Trastuzumab Deruxtecan in *HER2*-mutant non-small-cell lung cancer. N Engl J Med 2022; 386(3): 241-51.
[http://dx.doi.org/10.1056/NEJMoa2112431] [PMID: 34534430]

[29]   Ramalingam SS, Vansteenkiste J, Planchard D, *et al.* FLAURA Investigators. Overall survival with osimertinib in untreated, *EGFR*-mutated advanced NSCLC. N Engl J Med 2020; 382(1): 41-50.
[http://dx.doi.org/10.1056/NEJMoa1913662] [PMID: 31751012]

[30]   Riudavets M, Sullivan I, Abdayem P, Planchard D. Targeting HER2 in non-small-cell lung cancer (NSCLC): a glimpse of hope? An updated review on therapeutic strategies in NSCLC harbouring HER2 alterations. ESMO Open 2021; 6(5): 100260.
[http://dx.doi.org/10.1016/j.esmoop.2021.100260] [PMID: 34479034]

[31]   Shaw AT, Solomon B. Targeting anaplastic lymphoma kinase in lung cancer. Clin Cancer Res 2011; 17(8): 2081-6.
[http://dx.doi.org/10.1158/1078-0432.CCR-10-1591] [PMID: 21288922]

[32]   Shaw AT, Riely GJ, Bang YJ, *et al.* Crizotinib in ROS1-rearranged advanced non-small-cell lung cancer (NSCLC): updated results, including overall survival, from PROFILE 1001. Ann Oncol 2019; 30(7): 1121-6.
[http://dx.doi.org/10.1093/annonc/mdz131] [PMID: 30980071]

[33]   Haratake N, Seto T. NTRK Fusion-positive Non–small-cell Lung Cancer: The Diagnosis and Targeted Therapy. Clin Lung Cancer 2021; 22(1): 1-5.
[http://dx.doi.org/10.1016/j.cllc.2020.10.013] [PMID: 33272813]

[34]   Yan N, Guo S, Zhang H, Zhang Z, Shen S, Li X. BRAF-mutated non-small cell lung cancer: current treatment status and future perspective. Front Oncol 2022; 12: 863043.
[http://dx.doi.org/10.3389/fonc.2022.863043] [PMID: 35433454]

[35]   Veluswamy R, Mack PC, Houldsworth J, Elkhouly E, Hirsch FR. KRAS G12C-mutant non-small cell lung cancer: Biology, developmental therapeutics, and molecular testing. J Mol Diagn 2021; 23(5): 507-20.
[http://dx.doi.org/10.1016/j.jmoldx.2021.02.002] [PMID: 33618059]

[36]   Gianfaldoni S, Gianfaldoni R, Wollina U, Lotti J, Tchernev G, Lotti T. An overview on radiotherapy: From its history to its current applications in dermatology. Open Access Maced J Med Sci 2017; 5(4): 521-5.
[http://dx.doi.org/10.3889/oamjms.2017.122] [PMID: 28785349]

[37]   Wang W, Hao Y, Liu Y, Li R, Huang DB, Pan YY. Nanomedicine in lung cancer: Current states of overcoming drug resistance and improving cancer immunotherapy. Wiley Interdiscip Rev Nanomed Nanobiotechnol 2021; 13(1): e1654.
[http://dx.doi.org/10.1002/wnan.1654] [PMID: 32700465]

[38]   Hiddinga BI, Raskin J, Janssens A, Pauwels P, Van Meerbeeck JP. Recent developments in the treatment of small cell lung cancer. Eur Respir Rev 2021; 30(161): 210079.
[http://dx.doi.org/10.1183/16000617.0079-2021] [PMID: 34261744]

[39]   Lewandowska A, Rudzki G, Lewandowski T, *et al.* Quality of life of cancer patients treated with chemotherapy. Int J Environ Res Public Health 2020; 17(19): 6938.
[http://dx.doi.org/10.3390/ijerph17196938] [PMID: 32977386]

[40]   Nan X, Xie C, Yu X, Liu J. EGFR TKI as first-line treatment for patients with advanced EGFR mutation-positive non-small-cell lung cancer. Oncotarget 2017; 8(43): 75712-26.
[http://dx.doi.org/10.18632/oncotarget.20095] [PMID: 29088904]

[41]   Wu SG, Shih JY. Management of acquired resistance to EGFR TKI–targeted therapy in advanced non-small cell lung cancer. Mol Cancer 2018; 17(1): 38.
[http://dx.doi.org/10.1186/s12943-018-0777-1] [PMID: 29455650]

[42]   Karachaliou N, Fernandez-Bruno M, Bracht JWP, Rosell R. EGFR first- and second-generation TKIs—there is still place for them in *EGFR*-mutant NSCLC patients. Transl Cancer Res 2018; 8(S1) (Suppl. 1): S23-47.
[http://dx.doi.org/10.21037/tcr.2018.10.06] [PMID: 35117062]

[43]   Harvey RD, Adams VR, Beardslee T, Medina P. Afatinib for the treatment of *EGFR* mutation-positive NSCLC: A review of clinical findings. J Oncol Pharm Pract 2020; 26(6): 1461-74.
[http://dx.doi.org/10.1177/1078155220931926] [PMID: 32567494]

[44]   Zhang T, Wan B, Zhao Y, *et al.* Treatment of uncommon *EGFR* mutations in non-small cell lung cancer: new evidence and treatment. Transl Lung Cancer Res 2019; 8(3): 302-16.
[http://dx.doi.org/10.21037/tlcr.2019.04.12] [PMID: 31367543]

[45]   Fu K, Xie F, Wang F, Fu L. Therapeutic strategies for EGFR-mutated non-small cell lung cancer

patients with osimertinib resistance. J Hematol Oncol 2022; 15(1): 173.
[http://dx.doi.org/10.1186/s13045-022-01391-4] [PMID: 36482474]

[46]   Ou SHI, Bartlett CH, Mino-Kenudson M, Cui J, Iafrate AJ. Crizotinib for the treatment of ALK-rearranged non-small cell lung cancer: a success story to usher in the second decade of molecular targeted therapy in oncology. Oncologist 2012; 17(11): 1351-75.
[http://dx.doi.org/10.1634/theoncologist.2012-0311] [PMID: 22989574]

[47]   Ando K, Manabe R, Kishino Y, *et al.* Comparative efficacy of ALK inhibitors for treatment-naïve ALK-positive advanced non-small cell lung cancer with central nervous system metastasis: A network meta-analysis. Int J Mol Sci 2023; 24(3): 2242.
[http://dx.doi.org/10.3390/ijms24032242] [PMID: 36768562]

[48]   Gristina V, La Mantia M, Iacono F, Galvano A, Russo A, Bazan V. The emerging therapeutic landscape of ALK inhibitors in non-small cell lung cancer. Pharmaceuticals (Basel) 2020; 13(12): 474.
[http://dx.doi.org/10.3390/ph13120474] [PMID: 33352844]

[49]   Brazel D, Zhang S, Nagasaka M. Spotlight on tepotinib and capmatinib for non-small cell lung cancer with MET Exon 14 skipping mutation. Lung Cancer (Auckl) 2022; 13: 33-45.
[http://dx.doi.org/10.2147/LCTT.S360574] [PMID: 35592355]

[50]   Desai A, Cuellar S. The Current Landscape for *MET*ex14 skipping mutations in non-small cell lung cancer. J Adv Pract Oncol 2022; 13(5): 539-44.
[http://dx.doi.org/10.6004/jadpro.2022.13.5.8] [PMID: 35910499]

[51]   Wu YL, Smit EF, Bauer TM. Capmatinib for patients with non-small cell lung cancer with MET exon 14 skipping mutations: A review of preclinical and clinical studies. Cancer Treat Rev 2021; 95: 102173.
[http://dx.doi.org/10.1016/j.ctrv.2021.102173] [PMID: 33740553]

[52]   Chen R, Manochakian R, James L, *et al.* Emerging therapeutic agents for advanced non-small cell lung cancer. J Hematol Oncol 2020; 13(1): 58.
[http://dx.doi.org/10.1186/s13045-020-00881-7] [PMID: 32448366]

[53]   Xia L, Liu Y, Wang Y. PD-1/PD-L1 blockade therapy in advanced non-small-cell lung cancer: Current status and future directions. Oncologist 2019; 24(S1) (Suppl. 1): S31-41.
[http://dx.doi.org/10.1634/theoncologist.2019-IO-S1-s05] [PMID: 30819829]

[54]   Luke JJ, Barlesi F, Chung K, *et al.* Phase I study of ABBV-428, a mesothelin-CD40 bispecific, in patients with advanced solid tumors. J Immunother Cancer 2021; 9(2): e002015.
[http://dx.doi.org/10.1136/jitc-2020-002015] [PMID: 33608377]

[55]   Martins F, Sofiya L, Sykiotis GP, *et al.* Adverse effects of immune-checkpoint inhibitors: epidemiology, management and surveillance. Nat Rev Clin Oncol 2019; 16(9): 563-80.
[http://dx.doi.org/10.1038/s41571-019-0218-0] [PMID: 31092901]

[56]   Winer A, Bodor JN, Borghaei H. Identifying and managing the adverse effects of immune checkpoint blockade. J Thorac Dis 2018; 10(S3) (Suppl. 3): S480-9.
[http://dx.doi.org/10.21037/jtd.2018.01.111] [PMID: 29593893]

[57]   Khan T, Ali M, Khan A, *et al.* Anticancer plants: A review of the active phytochemicals, applications in animal models, and regulatory aspects. Biomolecules 2019; 10(1): 47.
[http://dx.doi.org/10.3390/biom10010047] [PMID: 31892257]

[58]   Monteiro LS, Bastos KX, Barbosa-Filho JM, de Athayde-Filho PF, Diniz MFFM, Sobral MV. Medicinal plants and other living organisms with antitumor potential against lung cancer. Evid Based Complement Alternat Med 2014; 2014(1): 604152.
[http://dx.doi.org/10.1155/2014/604152] [PMID: 25147575]

[59]   Regassa H, Sourirajan A, Kumar V, Pandey S, Kumar D, Dev K. A review of medicinal plants of the Himalayas with anti-proliferative activity for the treatment of various cancers. Cancers (Basel) 2022; 14(16): 3898.

[http://dx.doi.org/10.3390/cancers14163898] [PMID: 36010892]

[60]   Zhang J, Li C, Zhang L, *et al.* Andrographolide induces Noxa-Dependent Apoptosis by transactivating ATF4 in human lung adenocarcinoma cells. Front Pharmacol 2021; 12: 680589.
       [http://dx.doi.org/10.3389/fphar.2021.680589] [PMID: 33995110]

[61]   Lai YH, Yu SL, Chen HY, Wang CC, Chen HW, Chen JJW. The HLJ1 -targeting drug screening identified Chinese herb andrographolide that can suppress tumour growth and invasion in non-smal--cell lung cancer. Carcinogenesis 2013; 34(5): 1069-80.
       [http://dx.doi.org/10.1093/carcin/bgt005] [PMID: 23306212]

[62]   Tung YT, Chen HL, Tsai HC, Yang SH, Chang YC, Chen CM. therapeutic potential of andrographolide isolated from the leaves of *Andrographis paniculata* Nees for treating lung adenocarcinomas. Evid Based Complement Alternat Med 2013; 2013: 1-8.
       [http://dx.doi.org/10.1155/2013/305898] [PMID: 23997793]

[63]   Lin HH, Tsai CW, Chou FP, *et al.* Andrographolide down-regulates hypoxia-inducible factor-1α in human non-small cell lung cancer A549 cells. Toxicol Appl Pharmacol 2011; 250(3): 336-45.
       [http://dx.doi.org/10.1016/j.taap.2010.11.014] [PMID: 21134392]

[64]   Luo X, Luo W, Lin C, Zhang L, Li Y. Andrographolide inhibits proliferation of human lung cancer cells and the related mechanisms. Int J Clin Exp Med 2014; 7(11): 4220-5.
       [PMID: 25550934]

[65]   Lee YC, Lin HH, Hsu CH, Wang CJ, Chiang TA, Chen JH. Inhibitory effects of andrographolide on migration and invasion in human non-small cell lung cancer A549 cells *via* down-regulation of PI3K/Akt signaling pathway. Eur J Pharmacol 2010; 632(1-3): 23-32.
       [http://dx.doi.org/10.1016/j.ejphar.2010.01.009] [PMID: 20097193]

[66]   Luo W, Liu Y, Zhang J, Luo X, Lin C, Guo J. Andrographolide inhibits the activation of NF-κB and MMP-9 activity in H3255 lung cancer cells. Exp Ther Med 2013; 6(3): 743-6.
       [http://dx.doi.org/10.3892/etm.2013.1196] [PMID: 24137258]

[67]   Gong C, Ni Z, Yao C, *et al.* High-throughput assay for screening of natural products that enhanced tumoricidal activity of NK Cells. Biol Proced Online 2015; 28;17: 12.
       [http://dx.doi.org/10.1186/s12575-015-0026-6]

[68]   Yuwen D, Mi S, Ma Y, *et al.* Andrographolide enhances cisplatin-mediated anticancer effects in lung cancer cells through blockade of autophagy. Anticancer Drugs 2017; 28(9): 967-76.
       [http://dx.doi.org/10.1097/CAD.0000000000000537] [PMID: 28692436]

[69]   Yuan H, Sun B, Gao F, Lan M. Synergistic anticancer effects of andrographolide and paclitaxel against A549 NSCLC cells. Pharm Biol 2016; 54(11): 2629-35.
       [http://dx.doi.org/10.1080/13880209.2016.1176056] [PMID: 27159496]

[70]   Devendar P, Nayak VL, Yadav DK, *et al.* Synthesis and evaluation of anticancer activity of novel andrographolide derivatives. MedChemComm 2015; 6(5): 898-904.
       [http://dx.doi.org/10.1039/C4MD00566J]

[71]   Liu Y, Liang RM, Ma QP, *et al.* Synthesis of thioether andrographolide derivatives and their inhibitory effect against cancer cells. MedChemComm 2017; 8(6): 1268-74.
       [http://dx.doi.org/10.1039/C7MD00169J] [PMID: 30108837]

[72]   Kandanur SGS, Golakoti NR, Nanduri S, Letters MC. Synthesis and *in vitro* cytotoxicity of novel C-12 substituted-14-deoxy-andrographolide derivatives as potent anti-cancer agents. Bioorg Med Chem Lett 2015; 25(24): 5781-6.
       [http://dx.doi.org/10.1016/j.bmcl.2015.10.053] [PMID: 26561364]

[73]   Lim JCW, Jeyaraj EJ, Sagineedu SR, Wong WSF, Stanslas J. SRS06, a new semisynthetic andrographolide derivative with improved anticancer potency and selectivity, inhibits nuclear factor-κB nuclear binding in the A549 non-small cell lung cancer cell line. Pharmacology 2015; 95(1-2): 70-7.

[http://dx.doi.org/10.1159/000370313] [PMID: 25613753]

[74] Lim JCW, Goh FY, Sagineedu SR, *et al.* A semisynthetic diterpenoid lactone inhibits NF-κB signalling to ameliorate inflammation and airway hyperresponsiveness in a mouse asthma model. Toxicol Appl Pharmacol 2016; 302: 10-22.
[http://dx.doi.org/10.1016/j.taap.2016.04.004] [PMID: 27089844]

CHAPTER 11

Anticancer Potential of Andrographolide and its Analogs in Colorectal Cancer: An Update

Sunkara Surya Lakshmi[1], Geetha Birudala[2], Beda Durga Prasad[3], Praveen Kumar Kusuma[4], Moturi Anvesh Raj[5], Kranthi Kumar Kotha[6], Shaik Shakir Basha[7], Vinyas Mayasa[8], Sandeep Kanna[9,*] and Vinod K. Nelson[7,*]

[1] *Srinivasarao College of Pharmacy, Visakhapatnam, Andhra Pradesh-530041, India*

[2] *Faculty of Pharmacy, Dr. M.G.R. Educational and Research Institute, Velappanchavadi, Chennai, India*

[3] *Department of Pharmaceutical Chemistry, GITAM School of Pharmacy, Hyderabad, Telangana, India*

[4] *Department of Pharmaceutical Chemistry, School of Pharmaceutical Sciences, Govt. of NCT of Delhi, Delhi Pharmaceutical Sciences and Research University (DPSRU), Mehrauli-Badarpur Road, India*

[5] *JSS Academy of Higher Education & Research, Rocklands, Ooty, Nilgiris, Tamil Nadu-643001, India*

[6] *Departement of. Pharmaceutics, College of Pharmaceutical Sciences, Dayananda Sagar University, Bengaluru, Karnataka 560078, India*

[7] *Centre for Global Health Research, Saveetha Medical College and Hospital, Saveetha Institute of Medical and Technical Sciences, Chennai 602105, Tamil Nadu, India*

[8] *Department of Pharmacology, GITAM School of Pharmacy, Gandhi Institute of Technology and Management Deemed to be University, Hyderabad, Telangana, India*

[9] *Department of Pharmaceutics, Chalapathi Institute of Pharmaceutical Sciences, Chalapathi Nagar, Lam - 522034, India*

Abstract: Colorectal cancer (CRC) is a highly prevalent and leading cause of death globally. Though well-developed treatment strategies are available, colorectal cancer is still a challenging health problem in developed and developing countries. Despite advanced treatment methods, all may not exterminate the tumor since most cases of CRCs are diagnosed at the last stage, and treatment-associated drug toxicity and resistance are major concerns. Therefore, it is imperative to discover anticancer drugs with less toxicity and no drug resistance. During the process of new drug discovery, medicinal plants and their derivatives play a significant role. This chapter/review

* **Corresponding authors Sandeep Kanna and Vinod K. Nelson:** Department of Pharmaceutics, Chalapathi Institute of Pharmaceutical Sciences, Chalapathi Nagar, Lam - 522034, India; Centre for Global Health Research, Saveetha Medical College and Hospital, Saveetha Institute of Medical and Technical Sciences, Chennai 602105, Tamil Nadu, India; E-mails: sandeepkanna866@gmail.com; vinod.kumar457@gmail.com

S. Karuppusamy, Vinod K. Nelson & T. Pullaiah (Eds.)
All rights reserved-© 2024 Bentham Science Publishers

explores andrographolides and their derivatives as potential anticancer drug candidates to combat colorectal cancer. This chapter describes the molecular mechanisms of colorectal cancer, potential drug targets in cancer, the anticancer potential of andrographolide derivatives in various malignancies, and its specific function in preventing CRC. This review provides concise information and possible clues for researchers to develop andrographolides, their derivatives and anticancer drugs to treat colorectal cancer.

Keywords: Anticancer agents, Andrographolide, Colorectal cancer, Potential targets.

INTRODUCTION

Cancer is an unpleasant disease among non-communicable disorders, and it rapidly deteriorates a person's health. Colorectal cancer (CRC) is a primary cause of death and ranks 3rd among various cancers globally. CRC develops in the inner lining layers of the colonic and rectal mucosa or musculature [1]. Different types of cancers are involved in colo-rectum, like mucus-producing cell adenocarcinoma, gastrointestinal stromal tumors, and carcinoid tumors. The Cancer Survey 2018 reports that CRC in males is 12.8%, and in females, it is 11.3%, which accounts for 700,000 deaths globally. The surveys have predicted that the incidence of CRS will be 3.2 million by 2040 [2]. The United States of America and China recorded the maximum number of CRC cases in 2020, with anticipated new cases increasing by 64% by 2040. However, in India, the incidence of CRC is minimal compared to other countries [3]. Recent WHO reports point out that the increasing speed of CRC occurrence has been an atrocious concern worldwide in the past decade; the triggering factors of this scenario are changing lifestyle factors like dietary habits [4]. The prevalence rate of CRC in Western countries is higher than in Asian countries and least in African countries [5]. The key risk factors involved in developing CRC include inflammatory bowel disease, decreased physical activity, obesity, consumption of alcohol and a diet with low fiber, vegetables, and fruits, and poor gut microflora maintenance. The additional contributory factors, including low socio-economic status, age, and race, determine a role in the progress of CRC [6].

Though well-developed treatment strategies are available, cancer is still a considerable health problem in both urbanized and underdeveloped countries [7]. The foremost action patterns of CRC include chemotherapy, immunotherapy, and surgeries. 5-Fluorouracil (5-FU) is used as an individual drug or combined with other anticancer medications like cisplatin, irinotecan, and capecitabine [8]. These treatment methods may not exterminate the tumor since most cases of CRC are diagnosed at the last stage with significant spread, which increases the mortality rate and economic burden on the families. Despite the advanced drugs available to treat CRC, treatment-associated drug toxicity and drug resistance are primary concerns [9]. Therefore, it is imperative to discover anticancer drugs with less toxicity and no drug resistance; nevertheless, alternative therapies were explored less for such compounds.

Humans have been associated with plants and their derived materials for treating diseases since ancient times. Ethno-pharmacological reports on various medicinal plants are encouraged to investigate the suitable method of plant selection, isolation of its active principle, and calculation of therapeutic dose to establish and accomplish the benefits of these medicinal plants [10]. Several plant sources, secondary metabolites, and animal and microbial sources confirmed their essential medicinal properties and potential anticancer agents. They are being used in the current treatment strategies for CRC [11 - 13]. With the availability of a unique chemical library and insignificant toxicity, the medicinal plant and its metabolites promise a better alternative drug discovery source for treating dreadful diseases like cancer [14]. FDA disclosed that 40% of drugs have derived from natural origin or its derivative compounds; among those, 74% are merely approved for cancer treatment [15].

Andrographis paniculata (AP) is an inhabitant medicinal plant in India, Bangladesh, China, and Sri Lanka. It is widely practiced in alternative Indian Medicinal systems like Ayurveda, Siddha, and Unani to treat various ailments. *Andrographis paniculata* is called King of Bitters or Kalmegh and is prominent for its traditional or folklore uses, including as a bitter tonic, antipyretic, and febrifuge. It also treats malaria and various gastrointestinal disorders. Traditional Chinese medicine uses *Andrographis paniculata* to treat fever and as a detoxifying agent. At the same time, in Europe, the treatment of common flu is used as a home remedy [16 - 19]. Andrographolides and their derivatives are diterpenoid and terpenoid glycoside compounds of *Andrographis paniculata* with diverse biological actions, including anticancer activity. Chemically, the andrographolide is 3-alfa, 14, 15, 18-tetrahydroxy-5beta, 9beta H, 10α-lambda-8, γ12-dien-16-oic acid γ-lactone with a 350.4 g/mol of molecular weight. Among the identified molecules from AP andrographolide, deoxy andrographolide, 14-deoxy-11, 12-didehydroandrographolide, and neoandrographolide and their derivatives abide by pharmacological actions [20]. The important pharmacological activities of andrographolides include anticancer, bone metabolism, anti-inflammatory, immunomodulatory, anti-viral, anti-hepatitis effects, anti-arthritis, and neuroprotective actions [21 - 23]. The anticancer mechanisms of andrographolides are well-reported. These compounds can arrest the cell cycle and inhibit cytokine, NF-$\kappa\beta$, and angiogenesis [24].

Similarly, andrographolides exhibit anticancer potential in colorectal cancer cells by inducing apoptosis through free radicals production and stimulation of the mTOR- caspase-3 mediated pathway [25]. Earlier studies reveal that andrographolides and their derivatives show significant anticancer activity in colon, cervical, liver, leukemia, breast, and non-small cell lung cancer [26]. Besides, andrographolides and their derivatives are potential anticancer agents in modulating multiple signaling pathways. The present review intends to discuss the importance of andrographolide and its structural analogs in colorectal cancer.

ANTICANCER EFFECT OF ANDROGRAPHOLIDE AND ITS DERIVATIVES

Andrographolide is the chief and biologically active metabolite of *Andrographis paniculata*, available at a high concentration of 1.84% of the total extract. The structural analogs of andrographolide such as 14-deoxy andrographolide, deoxy andrographiside , homo andrographolide, neo andrographolide, andrographian, stigmasterol, andrographosterin, andrographon, and 14-deoxy andrographolide belong to diterpenoids and diterpenoid glycosides. Together with these phytocompounds, it contains other flavonoid compounds like 7-O-methyl wogonin, 5-hydroxy-7, 8, 2'-trimethoxy flavones, and dimethoxy flavones [27]. The chemical structure is essential for andrographolides' biological activity. Alfa β-unsaturated γ- butyro lactone ring and olefin bonds at $\Delta 8$ and $\Delta 12$ positions with hydroxyl groups C-3, C-14, and C-19 positions are responsible for possessing the anticancer action of andrographolide and their analogs [28].

Andrographolide demonstrates anticancer effects in the HCT 116 colorectal cancer cell line by increasing IL-8. The activation of TNF-α linked IL-8 is increased, and the effect is concentration-dependent and suppressed angiogenesis in the tumor microenvironment [29]. The previous reports suggest that andrographolides exhibit anticancer effects by inducing apoptosis *via* activation of caspases, Bax, p53, and JNK pathway proteins [30]. Andrographolide effectively suppresses tumor growth by the ERK1/2 protein pathway [31, 32]. Dai *et al.* revealed that increased doses of andrographolide have an anticancer effect in SGC7901 cells by hampering the G2/M2 and G1/M cell cycle. Similarly, the proposed mechanism of action was stimulating cyclin B1, Timp-1/2, p-Cdc2, and Bax pathway and inhibiting anti-apoptosis protein Bcl-2 and MMP-2/9 proteins [33]. The apoptosis-inducing capacity of andrographolides in AGS, SNU638, and SNU601 cells by interacting with TRAIL (tumor necrosis factor-related apoptosis-inducing ligand), which activates the downstream caspase-3/caspase-8 signaling pathways [34]. Andrographolide derivative 19-triisopropyl andrographolide produces its anticancer effect in MKN-45 and AGS cells by inducing apoptosis. The proposed mechanism was down-regulating DNA topoisomerase-Iα protein expression *via* up-regulating DNA damage marker γ-H2A.X protein and caspase3 expression [28]. TRAIL receptors are the critical drug targets for anticancer drugs. TRAIL-induced apoptosis is a widely accepted drug target for many anticancer molecules. Andrographolide shows a potent anticancer effect evident by Annexin V/PI staining assay, up-regulation of death receptor four, and augmented p53 protein, which help produce free radicals in the cells and are the ultimate cause of death of malignant cells [35].

Another mechanism proposed for the anticancer activity of andrographolide in PC-3, DU145, and LNCaP *via* down-regulating IL-6 cytokines and their mediated pathways includes JAK/STAT and MAPK [36]. Identical results are observed in DU145-induced tumors in the mice xenograft model, where it additionally activates apoptotic signals such as caspases, Bcl-2, and poly-ADP ribose polymerase proteins (PARP) (33). SRJ23 (3, 19-(3-Chloro-4-fluorobenzylidene) andrographolide) and SRJ11 (3, 19-(2- chlorobenzylidene) andrographolide) are semi-synthetic derivatives of andrographolide with considerable anticancer activity by modulating cell cycle. These derivatives suppress cyclin-dependent kinase (CDK) 1 alone with no effect on CDK 4 and cyclin D, whereas the same compound inhibits CDK4 and cyclin D1 levels in DU145 and LNCaP cells [37].

Luo *et al.*, in their study of C57BL/6 mice with Lewis lung carcinoma, find significant protection against lung cancer [20]. Gao *et al.* found that andrographolide is effective in anticancer activity in the same C57BL/6 mice against radiation-induced lung injury. The proposed anticancer mechanism was hampering interferon-inducible protein-2 inflammasomes, preventing them from translocating into the nucleus to sense DNA damage. This effect further suppresses inflammation, acute pneumonia, and chronic fibrosis induced by radiation in rats [38]. In the same way, in transgenic animals with pulmonary cancer induced by the over-expression of hVEGF-A165, andrographolide treatment was found to hamper the expression of hVEGF-A165 along with suppressing the activation of signaling molecules like EGFR, VEGF, Cyclin A, and Cyclin B at both mRNAs as well as protein levels [39]. Andrographolide exerted its anticancer effect in A549 cells by inhibiting the levels of MMP-7, which was evidenced by the suppression of the PI3K/AKT/AP-1 signaling mechanism [40]. Breast cancer is a life-threatening cancer. Natural and semi-synthetic andrographolide derivatives effectively mitigate breast cancer in cell lines and animal models. Andrographolide effectively arrested breast cancer cell (MDA-MB-23) propagation by enhancing the production of ROS and stimulation of caspase-9 and caspase-3 with Bcl-2 and Bcl-xL expression inhibition, and it was further evidenced by Annexin V staining assay [41]. The isolated andrographolides induce apoptosis in breast cancer cells (TD-47) by enhancing the expression of Bax, caspase-3, p53, and down-regulating expression of Bcl-2

[42]. Andrographolide in liposomal form prevents cancer in female BALB/c nude mice and 4T1 breast cancer cell line. It significantly arrests lung tumor growth by involving the VEGF pathway to prevent angiogenesis [43]. A semi-synthetic derivative of andrographolide 3,19-(2-bromobenzylidene) andrographolide (SRJ09) also accounts for its significant antitumor activity in breast cancer cells by apoptosis-induced cell death and cell cycle arrest at G1 phase. Additionally, it expresses its mechanism by enhancing extrinsic apoptotic pathways and freeing Bcl-2 and p53 activity modulation [44]. 14-deoxy-11,12-didehydroandro-ra-pholide, an andrographolide derivative, possesses anticancer activity in T-47D breast carcinoma cells by increasing the cytosol calcium concentration to altering mitochondrial membrane potential and increases the endoplasmic reticulum stress [45].

Similarly, andrographolide and its derivatives were effective in hepatic carcinomas. AG demonstrates anticancer outcomes in andrographolide Hep3B cells as well as in diethylnitrosamine-induced liver cancer in the experimental animals by inducing apoptosis and activation of the tissue-based antioxidant system like increasing superoxide dismutase, reduced glutathione, glutathione--transferase and decreasing the level of malondialdehyde and nitric oxide [46]. In another study, andrographolide possesses an anti-cancer effect by activating autophagy-mediated cell death in hepatocarcinoma cells. It was supported by increasing the mitochondrial permeability, potential, and generation of free radicals [47]. Further, andrographolide hinders the growth of Hep3B and SMCC7721 malignant cells by altering the expression of micro RNAs such as miR-222-3p, miR-30b-5p, miR-106b-5p, and miR-23a-5p and the similar results was observed in xenografted mouse model [48]. Additionally, there was evidence that andrographolide and its analogs were efficient in facilitating the multiplication of oral cancer. According to data from animal studies, andrographolide effectively inhibits the NF-κB, cyclin, and D c-Myc activity proteins in oral cancer provoked by DMBA in hamsters [26, 49]. Andrographolide derivative dehydroandrographolide accounted for potential anti-cancer effects in oral malignant cells by activating autophagy-associated cell death by up-regulating JNK 1/2 and down-regulating Akt and p38 expression [50]. 3, 19-isopropylidene, andrographolide, another semi-synthetic derivative of AP with anticancer activity in human papillomavirus-16 positive cervical cancer cells, exerts anticancer activity by p53-associated apoptosis induction [51]. 14-deoxy andrographolide has the anticancer effect by inhibiting cell growth at the G_0/G_1 phase and also by increasing cytochrome c and expression of Bax, along with decreasing the BCL-2 expression in HL-60 cells [52]. Nevertheless, andrographolide and its derivatives bear distinguished protection against various malignancies, and promising andrographolides are potential drug molecules to combat cancer. Table **1** gives the list of compounds from andrographolides showing potent anticancer effects.

Table 1. Compounds from *Andrographis paniculata* showing potent anticancer effect.

S. No	Compound	Structure	Cancer Model	References
1	Andrographolide		PC-3, DU145, and LNCaP cell lines. C57BL/6 mice against radiation-induced lung injury	[38, 53]
2	14-deoxy-11,12-didehydroandrographolide		T-47D breast carcinoma cells	[45]
3	3,19-isopropylidene andrographolide		HPV16-positive cervical cancer cell lines	[51]
4	14-deoxyandrographolide		HL-60 cell line	[52]

POTENTIAL DRUG TARGETS IN COLORECTAL CANCER

CRC is a highly prevalent and leading cause of death among malignancies. The presently available therapeutic approaches include surgery, immunotherapy, and chemotherapy. Considering the severity of the disease, there is an imperative need to discover a novel treatment for colon cancer [54]. Targeted therapy is a novel approach to treat colorectal cancer patients to improve their life span. In recent days, potential drug targets have been identified in colorectal cancer with the help of novel technology and external agents. Such targets' modulation has helped develop a safe and potential drug molecule for colorectal cancer. This therapy unswervingly impacts the malignant cells by controlling their growth, adaptation, and migration and modulating the cancer cell environment, like blood vessels and immune cell formation linked with the tumor [55]. Many small molecules from plant and animal sources were developed as potential anticancer agents targeting various proteins and biomolecules in colon cancer. These molecules include cyclin-dependent kinases, PARP, and proteasomes; they have become the potential target for anticancer drugs *in vitro* and *in vivo* [56]. As mentioned above, many potential drug targets in colorectal cancer have been identified, and few of them serve as ideal drug targets for newly discovered and clinically used drugs. Some mechanisms involved that regulate the growth, differentiation, and metastasis in colorectal cancer include Wnt/β-catenin, Notch, Hedgehog, and transforming growth factor-β (TGF-β)/suppressor of mothers against decapentaplegic (SMAD) and its corresponding downstream signaling molecules such as PI3K/AKT or Rat sarcoma (RAS)/rapidly accelerated fibrosarcoma (RAF) [57]. The other significant mechanisms both in the progression of the disease and as a potential drug target include VEGF (vascular endothelial growth factor) and its receptor, epidermal growth factor and its receptor (EGFR), hepatocyte growth factor (HGF), mesenchyme-epithelial transition factor, IGF/ IGF-1R, and transforming growth factor. EGFR is usually over-expressed in cancer cells. Some factors like mutation and truncation in various proteins or interlinked pathways trigger it. Mutation in the epidermal growth factor directs the overexpression of downstream pro-oncogenic signaling pathways that include mitogen-activated protein kinase (MAPK), RAS/RAF/MEK/ERK, and AKT/PI3K/mTOR signaling mechanism. Activating these pathways facilitates the proliferation of carcinoma cells and the progression of the cell cycle [58]. Such mutations in EGFR activate a proto-oncogene c-RAS/RAF by engaging the son of seven fewer homologs (SOSs), which activates MAP kinase to ERK (activate extracellular signal-related kinase). The ERK translocates into the nucleus to promote the transcription of c-FOS and ELK1, which are essential for activating the RAS and RAF pathways. RAS kindles the formation of active factors like A-Raf, B-Raf, and C-Raf (protein-serine/threonine protein kinases) by a complex process, which is essential for activating the MAPK cascade. Activated A-RAF, B-RAF, and C-RAF phosphorylate MEK1 and MEK2 to activate MAP/ERK kinase. Further, the activated MAP/ERK kinase activates PI3K to assist the conversion of the second messenger inositol-bisphosphate (PIP2) into inositol-trisphosphate (PIP3) *via* phosphorylation. The phosphorylated PIP3 triggers Akt to bind to its sulfhydryl domain of serine/threonine kinase to inactivate the transcription of FOXO, which regulates the downstream signals *via* phosphorylation and finally upholds the survival, growth, and proliferation of malignant cells [59]. PI3K/Akt/mTOR signals regulate critical cellular events like cell proliferation, growth, metabolism, apoptosis, and autophagy. However, abnormal activation of these pathways is essential for cancer development. mTORC1 is a sensitive marker activated by nutrients, growth factors, hypoxia, and DNA damage. It also gets activated by over-expression of PI3K and AKT. PI3K stimulates Akt to convert inositol bisphosphate to inositol triphosphate, which further triggers the release of intracellular Ca+2 releases, ultimately leading to carcinogenesis [60]. Activating growth factors and the PI3K/AKT pathway inhibit apoptosis and favor cancer cell growth. Hence, PI3K/Akt/mTOR signals become a significant drug-target molecule in developing novel anticancer molecules.

Angiogenesis is another vital mechanism engaged in the progression of CRC. The existing reports say that the VEGF and its receptors are essential angiogenic factors involved in several malignancies, including CRC, and are also connected with the metastases of cancers [61]. VEGF binds to its receptors (VEGFR-1/2), primarily expressed in malignant cells, to promote cellular functions like cell differentiation and migration of epithelial cells during angiogenesis. Furthermore, it activates downstream signals like PI3K/AKT and MAPK/ERK1, releasing inflammatory cytokines like TNF-α, IL-6, IL-1β, and IL-8 to play an important role in colorectal cancer [8]. Hence, targeting the VEGF and its associated pathway becomes a potential drug target tool for colorectal cancer.

Another vital signaling mechanism in CRC progression is the Wnt/β-catenin pathway (canonical Wnt pathway). It helps in protecting gut homeostasis. The stimulation of the Wnt/β-catenin pathway involves the hyperproliferation of gastrointestinal mucosa, leading to colorectal cancer. PI3K/Akt/mTOR and canonical Wnt pathway are interconnected to be involved in CRC. Under normal cellular physiology, a tumor inhibitor gene called adenomatous polyposis coli (APC) binds to β-catenin. Nevertheless, mutation or deletion of the APC gene triggers continuous stimulation of the Wnt/β-catenin pathway to induce hyperproliferation of the intestinal cells. Wnt/β-catenin signaling mechanism is also linked with other molecules, such as Hippo/YAP, EGFR, nuclear factor kappa-B (NF-κB), Sonic Hedgehog, Notch, and PI3K/Akt pathway, to play a significant role in colon cancer development. Hence, any drug molecule that targets the Wnt/β-catenin and its downstream signaling pathways will be a better therapeutic agent in CRC [62].

ANDROGRAPHOLIDE AND ITS DERIVATIVES IN COLORECTAL CANCER

Derivatives of andrographolide with structural similarities were well-known anticancer agents in animal and *in vitro* models. These compounds exert their anticancer effect through various mechanisms, including immunomodulation, ROS/JNK-dependent mechanisms, PI3K/AKT signaling pathway, *etc.* Andrographolide possesses anticancer activity by activating the Wnt/β-catenin pathway, and it is an important drug target for anticancer agents. 17-epoxy andrographolide, 19-O-triphenyl methyl andrographolide, and 19-tes- -butyldiphenylsilyl-8exert anticancer effects in HT-29, HCT116, and SW480 cells by down-regulating the Wnt/β-catenin pathway *via* the GSK-3 β-dependent pathway [63, 64]. A vital drug target is the anticancer mechanism, which induces apoptosis in malignant tumors. Andrographolides also exhibit their anticancer action by apoptosis-inducing mechanism in colorectal cancer cells. Natural andrographolide exhibits its anticancer effect in different CRC cells by increasing TRAIL-induced apoptosis by activating the death receptor (DR5) [34]. Zhang *et al.* observed that andrographolide represses propagation and induces apoptosis in SW620 cells by inhibiting TLR4/MyD88/NF-κB/MMP-9 signaling mechanism [24]. 19-triisopropyl andrographolide, an andrographolide derivative, shows its anticancer effect by inducing DNA damage by attenuating the expression of DNA topoisomerase IIα and activating cleaved PARP-1 and caspase-3 to initiate the apoptosis process in MKN-45 and AGS cells without inhibiting the p53 gene [65]. Similarly, a semi-synthetic derivative of andrographolide 3, 19-(2 bromobenzylidene) andrographolide also possesses an anticancer effect by arresting the G1 phase of cell cycle along with apoptosis induction (p53 independent and Bcl-2 inhibition) in HCT-116 cells xenograft mice [66].

Another proposed mechanism to elicit the andrographolide anticancer effect was inducing the endoplasmic reticulum-induced stress to initiate apoptosis in various cell lines, including HCT-116, T84, and COLO 205 [25]. Besides, andrographolide significantly reduces the 5-fluorouracil-induced drug resistance. Concomitant treatment with andrographolide enhances the anticancer potential by the cellular-mesenchymal to epithelial transition factor pathway [67]. The additional support of the anticancer effect of andrographolide in colorectal cancer is by down-regulating the TNF-α associated release of different inflammatory cytokines. In the same way, a 15-benzylidene substituted derivative of andrographolide (andrographolide-9) and andrographolide-26b (12α-isomer) exhibits a potential anticancer drug candidate in cancer cell lines and zebrafish acting through VEGF/VEGFR2/AKT signaling pathway, which deals with growth, multiplication, migration, and capillaries formation in the tumor. These are more potential anticancer agents than parent andrographolide [68, 69].

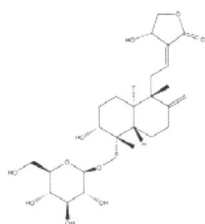

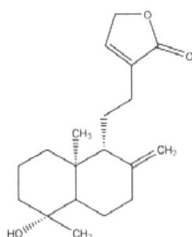

Androgrophoside   **Andrograpanin**   **Andrographidine**

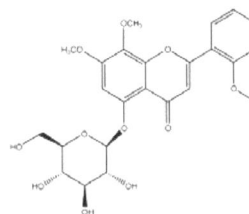

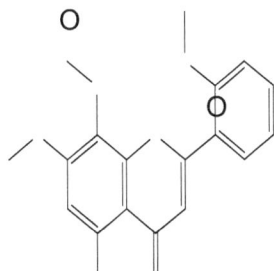

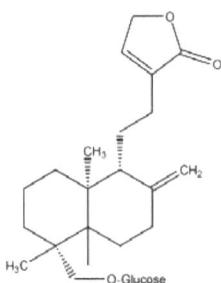

Neoandrographolide

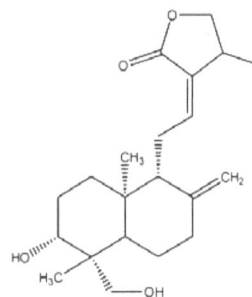

Isoandrographolide

Andrographin

Structures of derivatives of andrographolide

CONCLUSION

CRC is a highly prevalent and leading cause of death globally. The currently available treatment options, including surgery, chemotherapy, immunotherapy, and radiotherapies, were mainly associated with several potential side effects. Hence, it requires a possible source for identifying ideal drug candidates with minimal toxicity for colon cancer. Evidence suggests medicinal plants and their secondary metabolites as a source of promising anticancer candidates against colorectal cancer. Taking into account the prevalence and severity of colorectal cancer, it is required to develop an ideal treatment or drug molecule with the desired characteristics to treat colorectal cancer patients. Andrographolides are traditionally critical components in complementary and alternative medicinal systems with multiple biological and anticancer activity, including anticancer activity. The chapter comprehensively presents the possible and significant mechanism of action of andrographolides and their derivatives on colorectal cancer by modulating various signaling molecules *in vitro* and *in vivo*. These molecules and their derivatives possess the anticancer effect through death receptor modulation, Wnt/β-catenin pathway, PI3K/AKT/mTOR signaling pathway, and apoptosis-induced cell death. Considering that andrographolide derivatives have proven to be prospective new drug molecules to combat colorectal cancer, these compounds may develop into a potential drug choice along with the current therapies.

REFERENCES

[1]   Esmeeta A, Adhikari S, Dharshnaa V, *et al.* Plant-derived bioactive compounds in colon cancer treatment: An updated review. Biomedicine & pharmacotherapy = Biomedecine & pharmacotherapie. 2022; 153: 113384.

[2]   Xi Y, Xu P. Global colorectal cancer burden in 2020 and projections to 2040. Transl Oncol 2021; 14(10): 101174.
[http://dx.doi.org/10.1016/j.tranon.2021.101174] [PMID: 34243011]

[3]   Mohandas KM. Colorectal cancer in India: controversies, enigmas and primary prevention. Indian J Gastroenterol 2011; 30(1): 3-6.
[http://dx.doi.org/10.1007/s12664-010-0076-2] [PMID: 21222189]

[4]   Haggar F, Boushey R. Colorectal cancer epidemiology: incidence, mortality, survival, and risk factors. Clin Colon Rectal Surg 2009; 22(4): 191-7.
[http://dx.doi.org/10.1055/s-0029-1242458] [PMID: 21037809]

[5]   Arnold M, Sierra MS, Laversanne M, Soerjomataram I, Jemal A, Bray F. Global patterns and trends in colorectal cancer incidence and mortality. Gut 2017; 66(4): 683-91.
[http://dx.doi.org/10.1136/gutjnl-2015-310912] [PMID: 26818619]

[6]   Keum N, Giovannucci E. Global burden of colorectal cancer: emerging trends, risk factors and prevention strategies. Nat Rev Gastroenterol Hepatol 2019; 16(12): 713-32.
[http://dx.doi.org/10.1038/s41575-019-0189-8] [PMID: 31455888]

[7]   Sankaranarayanan R. Screening for cancer in low- and middle-income countries. Ann Glob Health 2014; 80(5): 412-7.
[http://dx.doi.org/10.1016/j.aogh.2014.09.014] [PMID: 25512156]

[8]   Xie YH, Chen YX, Fang JY. Comprehensive review of targeted therapy for colorectal cancer. Signal Transduct Target Ther 2020; 5(1): 22.
[http://dx.doi.org/10.1038/s41392-020-0116-z] [PMID: 32296018]

[9]   Majidinia M, Mirza-Aghazadeh-Attari M, Rahimi M, *et al.* Overcoming multidrug resistance in cancer: Recent progress in nanotechnology and new horizons. IUBMB Life 2020; 72(5): 855-71.
[http://dx.doi.org/10.1002/iub.2215] [PMID: 31913572]

[10]   Jaradat NA, Al-Ramahi R, Zaid AN, Ayesh OI, Eid AM. Ethnopharmacological survey of herbal remedies used for treatment of various types of cancer and their methods of preparations in the West Bank-Palestine. BMC Complement Altern Med 2016; 16(1): 93.
[http://dx.doi.org/10.1186/s12906-016-1070-8] [PMID: 26955822]

[11]   Harvey A. Natural products in drug discovery. Drug Discov Today 2008; 13(19-20): 894-901.
[http://dx.doi.org/10.1016/j.drudis.2008.07.004] [PMID: 18691670]

[12]   Nelson VK, Sahoo NK, Sahu M, Sudhan HH, Pullaiah CP, Muralikrishna KS. In vitro anticancer activity of *Eclipta alba* whole plant extract on colon cancer cell HCT-116. BMC complementary

medicine and therapies. 2020; 20(1):355.

[13] Pullaiah CP, Nelson VK, Rayapu S, G v NK, Kedam T. Exploring cardioprotective potential of esculetin against isoproterenol induced myocardial toxicity in rats: *in vivo* and *in vitro* evidence. BMC Pharmacol Toxicol 2021; 22(1): 43.
[http://dx.doi.org/10.1186/s40360-021-00510-0] [PMID: 34266475]

[14] Choudhari AS, Mandave PC, Deshpande M, Ranjekar P, Prakash O. Phytochemicals in cancer treatment: From preclinical studies to clinical practice. Front Pharmacol 2020; 10: 1614.
[http://dx.doi.org/10.3389/fphar.2019.01614] [PMID: 32116665]

[15] Newman DJ, Cragg GM. Natural Products as Sources of New Drugs from 1981 to 2014. J Nat Prod 2016; 79(3): 629-61.
[http://dx.doi.org/10.1021/acs.jnatprod.5b01055] [PMID: 26852623]

[16] Hossain MS, Urbi Z, Sule A, Rahman KMH. *Andrographis paniculata* (Burm. f.) Wall. ex Nees: a review of ethnobotany, phytochemistry, and pharmacology. ScientificWorldJournal 2014; 2014: 1-28.
[http://dx.doi.org/10.1155/2014/274905] [PMID: 25950015]

[17] Nelson VK, Pullaiah CP, Saleem TS M, *et al.* Natural products as the modulators of oxidative stress: An herbal approach in the management of prostate cancer. Adv Exp Med Biol 2022; 1391: 161-79.
[http://dx.doi.org/10.1007/978-3-031-12966-7_10] [PMID: 36472822]

[18] De S, Paul S, Manna A, *et al.* Phenolic phytochemicals for prevention and treatment of colorectal cancer: A critical evaluation of *in vivo* studies. Cancers (Basel) 2023; 15(3): 993.
[http://dx.doi.org/10.3390/cancers15030993] [PMID: 36765950]

[19] Badavenkatappa gari S, Nelson VK, Peraman R. *Tinospora sinensis* (Lour.) Merr alkaloid rich extract induces colon cancer cell death *via* ROS mediated, mTOR dependent apoptosis pathway: "an *in-vitro* study". BMC Complementary Medicine and Therapies 2023; 23(1): 33.
[http://dx.doi.org/10.1186/s12906-023-03849-5] [PMID: 36737760]

[20] Luo W, Jia L, Zhang JW, Wang DJ, Ren Q, Zhang W. Andrographolide against lung cancer-new pharmacological insights based on high-throughput metabolomics analysis combined with network pharmacology. Front Pharmacol 2021; 12: 596652.
[http://dx.doi.org/10.3389/fphar.2021.596652] [PMID: 33967748]

[21] Kumar G, Singh D, Tali JA, Dheer D, Shankar R. Andrographolide: Chemical modification and its effect on biological activities. Bioorg Chem 2020; 95: 103511.
[http://dx.doi.org/10.1016/j.bioorg.2019.103511] [PMID: 31884143]

[22] Nelson VK, Paul S, Roychoudhury S, *et al.* Heat shock factors in protein quality control and spermatogenesis. Adv Exp Med Biol 2022; 1391: 181-99.
[http://dx.doi.org/10.1007/978-3-031-12966-7_11] [PMID: 36472823]

[23] Dutta N, Ghosh S, Nelson VK, *et al.* Andrographolide upregulates protein quality control mechanisms in cell and mouse through upregulation of mTORC1 function. Biochimica et biophysica acta General subjects. 2021;1865(6):129885.
[http://dx.doi.org/10.1016/j.bbagen.2021.129885]

[24] Zhang R, Zhao J, Xu J, *et al.* Andrographolide suppresses proliferation of human colon cancer SW620 cells through the TLR4/NF-κB/MMP-9 signaling pathway. Oncol Lett 2017; 14(4): 4305-10.
[http://dx.doi.org/10.3892/ol.2017.6669] [PMID: 28943944]

[25] Banerjee A, Banerjee V, Czinn S, Blanchard T. Increased reactive oxygen species levels cause ER stress and cytotoxicity in andrographolide treated colon cancer cells. Oncotarget 2017; 8(16): 26142-53.
[http://dx.doi.org/10.18632/oncotarget.15393] [PMID: 28412728]

[26] Islam MT, Ali ES, Uddin SJ, *et al.* Andrographolide, a diterpene lactone from *Andrographis paniculata* and its therapeutic promises in cancer. Cancer Lett 2018; 420: 129-45.
[http://dx.doi.org/10.1016/j.canlet.2018.01.074] [PMID: 29408515]

[27] Altemimi A, Lakhssassi N, Baharlouei A, Watson DG, Lightfoot DA. Phytochemicals: Extraction, isolation, and identification of bioactive compounds from plant extracts. Plants (Basel, Switzerland). 2017; 6(4).

[28] Kim Y, Sengupta S, Sim T. Natural and synthetic lactones possessing antitumor activities. Intern J Mol Sci. 2021; 22(3).
[http://dx.doi.org/10.3390/ijms22031052]

[29] Yuan M, Meng W, Liao W, Lian S. Andrographolide antagonizes TNF-α-Induced IL-8 *via* inhibition of NADPH oxidase/ROS/NF-κB and Src/MAPKs/AP-1 Axis in human colorectal cancer HCT116 cells. J Agric Food Chem 2018; 66(20): 5139-48.
[http://dx.doi.org/10.1021/acs.jafc.8b00810] [PMID: 29672044]

[30] Lee SY, Debnath T, Kim SK, Lim BO. Anti-cancer effect and apoptosis induction of cordycepin through DR3 pathway in the human colonic cancer cell HT-29. Food Chem Toxicol 2013; 60: 439-47.
[http://dx.doi.org/10.1016/j.fct.2013.07.068] [PMID: 23941773]

[31] Farooqi AA, Attar R, Sabitaliyevich UY, *et al.* The Prowess of andrographolide as a natural weapon in the war against cancer. Cancers (Basel) 2020; 12(8): 2159.
[http://dx.doi.org/10.3390/cancers12082159] [PMID: 32759728]

[32] Tohkayomatee R, Reabroi S, Tungmunnithum D, Parichatikanond W, Pinthong D. Andrographolide exhibits anticancer activity against breast cancer cells (MCF-7 and MDA-MB-231 Cells) through suppressing cell proliferation and inducing cell apoptosis *via* inactivation of ER-α receptor and PI3K/AKT/mTOR signaling. Molecules 2022; 27(11): 3544.
[http://dx.doi.org/10.3390/molecules27113544] [PMID: 35684480]

[33] Dai L, Wang G, Pan W. Andrographolide inhibits proliferation and metastasis of SGC7901 gastric cancer cells. BioMed Res Int 2017; 2017: 1-10.
[http://dx.doi.org/10.1155/2017/6242103] [PMID: 28194420]

[34] Lim SC, Jeon HJ, Kee KH, Lee MJ, Hong R, Han SI. Andrographolide induces apoptotic and non-apoptotic death and enhances tumor necrosis factor-related apoptosis-inducing ligand-mediated apoptosis in gastric cancer cells. Oncol Lett 2017; 13(5): 3837-44.
[http://dx.doi.org/10.3892/ol.2017.5923] [PMID: 28529596]

[35] Zhang X-S, Wei R-J, He DL. Andrographolide sensitizes prostate cancer cells to TRAIL-induced apoptosis. Asian J Androl 2018; 20(2): 200-4.
[http://dx.doi.org/10.4103/aja.aja_30_17] [PMID: 28869219]

[36] Chun JY, Tummala R, Nadiminty N, *et al.* Andrographolide, an herbal medicine, inhibits interleukin-6 expression and suppresses prostate cancer cell growth. Genes Cancer 2010; 1(8): 868-76.
[http://dx.doi.org/10.1177/1947601910383416] [PMID: 21442031]

[37] Soo HL, Quah SY, Sulaiman I, Sagineedu SR, Lim JCW, Stanslas J. Advances and challenges in developing andrographolide and its analogs as cancer therapeutic agents. Drug Discov Today 2019; 24(9): 1890-8.
[http://dx.doi.org/10.1016/j.drudis.2019.05.017] [PMID: 31154065]

[38] Gao J, Peng S, Shan X, *et al.* Inhibition of AIM2 inflammasome-mediated pyroptosis by Andrographolide contributes to amelioration of radiation-induced lung inflammation and fibrosis. Cell Death Dis 2019; 10(12): 957.
[http://dx.doi.org/10.1038/s41419-019-2195-8] [PMID: 31862870]

[39] Tung YT, Chen HL, Tsai HC, Yang SH, Chang YC, Chen CM. Therapeutic potential of andrographolide isolated from the leaves of *Andrographis paniculata* Nees for treating lung adenocarcinomas. Evidence-based Complem Altern Med : eCAM. 2013;2013:305898.

[40] Lee YC, Lin HH, Hsu CH, Wang CJ, Chiang TA, Chen JH. Inhibitory effects of andrographolide on migration and invasion in human non-small cell lung cancer A549 cells *via* down-regulation of PI3K/Akt signaling pathway. Eur J Pharmacol 2010; 632(1-3): 23-32.

[http://dx.doi.org/10.1016/j.ejphar.2010.01.009] [PMID: 20097193]

[41] Banerjee M, Chattopadhyay S, Choudhuri T, *et al.* Cytotoxicity and cell cycle arrest induced by andrographolide lead to programmed cell death of MDA-MB-231 breast cancer cell line. J Biomed Sci 2016; 23(1): 40.
[http://dx.doi.org/10.1186/s12929-016-0257-0] [PMID: 27084510]

[42] Sukardiman H, Widyawaruyanti A, Sismindari, Zaini NC. Apoptosis inducing effect of andrographolide on TD-47 human breast cancer cell line. Afr J Tradit Complement Altern Med 2007; 4(3): 345-51.
[PMID: 20161898]

[43] Kang X, Zheng Z, Liu Z, *et al.* Liposomal codelivery of doxorubicin and andrographolide inhibits breast cancer growth and metastasis. Mol Pharm 2018; 15(4): 1618-26.
[http://dx.doi.org/10.1021/acs.molpharmaceut.7b01164] [PMID: 29498868]

[44] Sharma V, Sharma T, Kaul S, Kapoor KK, Dhar MK. Anticancer potential of labdane diterpenoid lactone "andrographolide" and its derivatives: a semi-synthetic approach. Phytochem Rev 2017; 16(3): 513-26.
[http://dx.doi.org/10.1007/s11101-016-9478-9]

[45] Tan HK, Muhammad TST, Tan ML. 14-Deoxy-11,12-didehydroandrographolide induces DDIT3-dependent endoplasmic reticulum stress-mediated autophagy in T-47D breast carcinoma cells. Toxicol Appl Pharmacol 2016; 300: 55-69.
[http://dx.doi.org/10.1016/j.taap.2016.03.017] [PMID: 27049118]

[46] Thoppil RJ, Bishayee A. Terpenoids as potential chemopreventive and therapeutic agents in liver cancer. World J Hepatol 2011; 3(9): 228-49.
[http://dx.doi.org/10.4254/wjh.v3.i9.228] [PMID: 21969877]

[47] Chen W, Feng L, Nie H, Zheng X. Andrographolide induces autophagic cell death in human liver cancer cells through cyclophilin D-mediated mitochondrial permeability transition pore. Carcinogenesis 2012; 33(11): 2190-8.
[http://dx.doi.org/10.1093/carcin/bgs264] [PMID: 22869602]

[48] Lu B, Sheng Y, Zhang J, Zheng Z, Ji L. The altered microRNA profile in andrographolide-induced inhibition of hepatoma tumor growth. Gene 2016; 588(2): 124-33.
[http://dx.doi.org/10.1016/j.gene.2016.05.012] [PMID: 27182051]

[49] Malik Z, Parveen R, Parveen B, *et al.* Anticancer potential of andrographolide from *Andrographis paniculata* (Burm.f.) Nees and its mechanisms of action. J Ethnopharmacol 2021; 272: 113936.
[http://dx.doi.org/10.1016/j.jep.2021.113936] [PMID: 33610710]

[50] Li W, Fan M, Chen Y, *et al.* Melatonin induces cell apoptosis in AGS cells through the activation of JNK and P38 MAPK and the suppression of Nuclear Factor-Kappa B: A novel therapeutic implication for gastric cancer. Cell Physiol Biochem 2015; 37(6): 2323-38.
[http://dx.doi.org/10.1159/000438587] [PMID: 26645893]

[51] Ekalaksananan T, Sookmai W, Fangkham S, *et al.* Activity of andrographolide and its derivatives on HPV16 pseudovirus infection and viral oncogene expression in cervical carcinoma cells. Nutr Cancer 2015; 67(4): 687-96.
[http://dx.doi.org/10.1080/01635581.2015.1019630] [PMID: 25837567]

[52] Cheung HY, Cheung SH, Li J, *et al.* Andrographolide isolated from *Andrographis paniculata* induces cell cycle arrest and mitochondrial-mediated apoptosis in human leukemic HL-60 cells. Planta Med 2005; 71(12): 1106-11.
[http://dx.doi.org/10.1055/s-2005-873128] [PMID: 16395645]

[53] Wang S, Li H, Chen S, *et al.* Andrographolide induces apoptosis in human osteosarcoma cells *via* the ROS/JNK pathway. Int J Oncol 2020; 56(6): 1417-28.
[http://dx.doi.org/10.3892/ijo.2020.5032] [PMID: 32236589]

[54] Mishra J, Drummond J, Quazi SH, *et al.* Prospective of colon cancer treatments and scope for combinatorial approach to enhanced cancer cell apoptosis. Crit Rev Oncol Hematol 2013; 86(3): 232-50.
[http://dx.doi.org/10.1016/j.critrevonc.2012.09.014] [PMID: 23098684]

[55] Cerrito MG, Grassilli E. Identifying Novel Actionable Targets in Colon Cancer. Biomedicines 2021; 9(5): 579.
[http://dx.doi.org/10.3390/biomedicines9050579] [PMID: 34065438]

[56] Siddiqui AJ, Jahan S, Singh R, *et al.* Plants in anticancer drug discovery: From molecular mechanism to chemoprevention. BioMed Res Int 2022; 2022: 1-18.
[http://dx.doi.org/10.1155/2022/5425485] [PMID: 35281598]

[57] Koveitypour Z, Panahi F, Vakilian M, *et al.* Signaling pathways involved in colorectal cancer progression. Cell Biosci 2019; 9(1): 97.
[http://dx.doi.org/10.1186/s13578-019-0361-4] [PMID: 31827763]

[58] Wee P, Wang Z. Epidermal growth factor receptor cell proliferation signaling pathways. Cancers (Basel) 2017; 9(5): 52.
[http://dx.doi.org/10.3390/cancers9050052] [PMID: 28513565]

[59] Roskoski R Jr. Targeting oncogenic Raf protein-serine/threonine kinases in human cancers. Pharmacol Res 2018; 135: 239-58.
[http://dx.doi.org/10.1016/j.phrs.2018.08.013] [PMID: 30118796]

[60] Prossomariti A, Piazzi G, Alquati C, Ricciardiello L. Are Wnt/β-Catenin and PI3K/AKT/mTORC1 Distinct Pathways in Colorectal Cancer? Cell Mol Gastroenterol Hepatol 2020; 10(3): 491-506.
[http://dx.doi.org/10.1016/j.jcmgh.2020.04.007] [PMID: 32334125]

[61] Lopez A, Harada K, Vasilakopoulou M, Shanbhag N, Ajani JA. Targeting angiogenesis in colorectal carcinoma. Drugs 2019; 79(1): 63-74.
[http://dx.doi.org/10.1007/s40265-018-1037-9] [PMID: 30617958]

[62] Zhao H, Ming T, Tang S, *et al.* Wnt signaling in colorectal cancer: pathogenic role and therapeutic target. Mol Cancer 2022; 21(1): 144.
[http://dx.doi.org/10.1186/s12943-022-01616-7] [PMID: 35836256]

[63] Reabroi S, Chairoungdua A, Saeeng R, *et al.* A silyl andrographolide analogue suppresses Wnt/β-catenin signaling pathway in colon cancer. Biomedicine & pharmacotherapy = Biomedecine & pharmacotherapie. 2018;101:414-21.

[64] Reabroi S, Saeeng R, Boonmuen N, *et al.* The anti-cancer activity of an andrographolide analogue functions through a GSK-3β-independent Wnt/β-catenin signaling pathway in colorectal cancer cells. Sci Rep 2018; 8(1): 7924.
[http://dx.doi.org/10.1038/s41598-018-26278-8] [PMID: 29784906]

[65] Monger A, Boonmuen N, Suksen K, *et al.* Inhibition of topoisomerase IIα and induction of apoptosis in gastric cancer cells by 19-Triisopropyl Andrographolide. Asian Pac J Cancer Prev 2017; 18(10): 2845-51.
[PMID: 29072435]

[66] Wong CC, Lim SH, Sagineedu SR, Lajis NH, Stanslas J. SRJ09, a promising anticancer drug lead: Elucidation of mechanisms of antiproliferative and apoptogenic effects and assessment of *in vivo* antitumor efficacy. Pharmacol Res 2016; 107: 66-78.
[http://dx.doi.org/10.1016/j.phrs.2016.02.024] [PMID: 26940565]

[67] Su M, Qin B, Liu F, Chen Y, Zhang R. Andrographolide enhanced 5-fluorouracil-induced antitumor effect in colorectal cancer *via* inhibition of c-MET pathway. Drug Des Devel Ther 2017; 11: 3333-41.
[http://dx.doi.org/10.2147/DDDT.S140354] [PMID: 29200829]

[68] Gong C, Xu C, Ji L, Wang Z. A novel semi-synthetic andrographolide analogue A5 inhibits tumor angiogenesis *via* blocking the VEGFR2-p38/ERK1/2 signal pathway. Biosci Trends 2013; 7(5): 230-6.

[http://dx.doi.org/10.5582/bst.2013.v7.5.230] [PMID: 24241173]

[69] Huang B, Peng Y, Li J, *et al.* An andrographolide derivative AGP-26b exhibiting anti-angiogenic activity in HUVECs and zebrafish *via* blocking the VEGFA/VEGFR2 signaling pathway. Mol Biosyst 2017; 13(3): 525-36.
[http://dx.doi.org/10.1039/C6MB00641H] [PMID: 28098292]

CHAPTER 12

Andrographolide and its Analogs as Cardioprotective Agents

Chitikela P. Pullaiah[1], Vinod K. Nelson[2,*], T.S. Mohamed Saleem[3], Sasikala Chinnappan[4], Ravishankar Ram Mani[4], Srilakshmi Bada Venkatappa Gari[5], S.P. Preethi Priyadharshni[6], K. Balaram Kumar[6] and Jamal Basha Dudekula[7]

[1] *Department of Pharmacology, Siddha Central Research Institute, Central Council for Research in Siddha, Ministry of AYUSH, Chennai, 600106, India*

[2] *Centre for Global Health Research, Saveetha Medical College and Hospital, Saveetha Institute of Medical and Technical Sciences, Chennai 602105, Tamil Nadu, India*

[3] *College of Pharmacy, Riyadh ELM University, Riyadh, Kingdom of Saudi Arabia*

[4] *Faculty of Pharmaceutical Sciences, UCSI University, Cheras, Lumpur 56000, Malaysia*

[5] *Faculty of Pharmaceutical Sciences, Jawaharlal Nehru Technological University Anantapur (JNTUA), Anantapur, Andhra Pradesh, India*

[6] *Department of Pharmaceutical Analysis, School of Pharmacy, College of Health and Medical Science (CHMS), Haramaya University, Harar, Ethiopia*

[7] *Department of Pharmacognosy, Amity Institute of Pharmacy, Amity University, Gwalior, Madhya Pradesh, India*

Abstract: Myocardial infarction is a sudden and fatal disease that causes a significant number of deaths in the world. The current treatment strategy for MI is only for symptomatic relief and cannot cure or reverse the disease condition. Hence, there is a need to identify novel, definitive, and minimal toxic drugs to treat MI. Phytochemicals always draw attention as an alternative and upgraded choice to combat various ailments. Photochemical compounds are non-nutritive biologically active secondary metabolites abundantly found in plants. Andrographolide and its derivatives obtained from a medicinal herb, *Andrographis paniculata*, are broadly utilized in traditional medicinal systems to treat various diseases, including cardiovascular diseases. In the present chapter, we explore andrographolide and its derivatives for its cardioprotective potential both *in vitro* and *in vivo*. Andrographolides show their cardioprotective potential by demonstrating multiple mechanisms, including ERK1/2 inhibition associated with anti-platelet action, PI3K/Akt pathway-associated inflammation inhibition, and activation of Nrf-2/HO-1pathway-associated antioxidant mechanism. Cardioprotection of andrographolide and its derivatives are shown by various animal models' anti-arrhythmic, antihypertensive, anti-inflammatory, and antioxidant mecha-

* **Corresponding author Vinod K. Nelson:** Centre for Global Health Research, Saveetha Medical College and Hospital, Saveetha Institute of Medical and Technical Sciences, Chennai 602105, Tamil Nadu, India; E-mail: vinod.kumar457@gmail.com

nisms. In this way, andrographolide and its derivatives can offer a better choice for developing a novel therapeutic molecule for myocardial infarction.

Keywords: Andrographolide, Antioxidant, Cardioprotection, Myocardial infarction, Nuclear factor erythroid 2-related factor (Nrf-2).

INTRODUCTION

Myocardial infarction (MI) is one of the foremost causes of death. Cardiovascular diseases (CVS) are responsible for approximately 17.9 million deaths each year, which accounts for 31% of all deaths worldwide [1]. Reasons for the increase in the prevalence and incidence of cardiovascular disease (CVD) in developing countries, particularly in urban areas, include changing lifestyles like the adoption of a Western diet (which is typically rich in saturated fats and refined sugars), alcohol and tobacco consumption, and sedentary lifestyle [2]. MI significantly occurs in young adults in South Asian countries, including India, Sri Lanka, and Bangladesh, than in individuals from other countries [3]. Pre-existing diseases like obesity, hypertension, diabetes mellitus, and dyslipidemia significantly contribute to the progression of myocardial infarction [4].

Myocardial infarction is the result of myocardial ischemia and rupture of atherosclerotic plaque, which is reported as the most common cause of acute MI [5]. In MI, there is an initial imbalance between the oxygen supply and demand, which leads to insufficient blood flow to the myocardium (myocardial ischemia) and a series of metabolic or pathological changes. These changes may cause irreversible damage to the heart muscle, lead to impairment in diastolic and systolic function, and make the patient prone to arrhythmias. The pathogenesis of MI includes hyperlipidemia, oxidative stress, peroxidation of membrane lipids, and loss of plasma membrane integrity.

Myocardial infarction is observed as an acute and chronic condition. In acute myocardial infarction, blood flow to myocardial muscles suddenly decreases due to any blockage, leading to muscle damage and elevation of troponin concentration. Chronic myocardial injury is characterized by persistent elevated troponin concentration due to myocardial necrosis [6].

In the last few decades, there has been a significant development in identifying interventions to protect the heart from myocardial infarction. These include the utilization of beta-blockers, calcium antagonists, and antioxidants and inhibition of the angiotensin-converting enzyme, although preventive therapy may lead to severe side effects or require high doses [7].

Numerous treatment approaches have been developed to prevent, treat, and attenuate the risk of myocardial infarction, but the majority of them have their limitations, like adverse effects [8]. Natural products have high universal demands due to their claimed advantage in terms of safety and efficacy against various diseases, including MI. However, most fail when shifted from the bench to the bedside [1]. Therefore, there is a need to find new drugs that are hostile to MI, can be used as suitable therapeutic candidates, and can be translated to clinical use in the future [9].

Chemical characterization of secondary metabolites or new chemical molecules from plants and animals provides a crucial scientific basis for identifying new drug discovery processes [10 - 12]. These compounds are essential for their physiological maintenance [13 - 15].

Pathophysiology of Myocardial Infarction

In myocardial infarction (heart attack), significant irreversible necrosis of the myocardium occurs due to prolonged ischemia. Events trigger MI increase in myocardial oxygen demand or decrease in oxygen supply to the myocardium. Initially, an imbalance between the supply of blood flow to the myocardium and its demand is the critical factor for the cause of myocardial infarction [16]. During myocardial infarction, erosion or rupture of lipids occurs, with loaded coronary atherosclerotic plaque upon its exposure to various factors, including hemodynamic changes, inflammation, and blood vessel injury [17]. This result in a highly thrombogenic core in circulation, which blocks the arterioles or tiny blood vessels to cause ischemia followed by hypoxia. These events typically lead to ST segment elevated myocardial infarction when the thrombus is occluded totally and non-ST segment elevated myocardial infarction (non-STEMI) or unstable angina if it is partially occluded [18].

During ischemic or hypoxic conditions, cardiac myocytes experience an inability to produce intracellular energy to meet their cellular metabolic requirements and eventually undergo necrosis and death. Inflammation is an essential factor in repairing and remodeling the infarcted heart. Chemokines play a vital role, like leukocyte trafficking, during inflammation and myocardial infarction repair [19]. Chemokines-mediated signaling processes uphold leukocyte integrin activation and promote the adhesion process between leukocytes and endothelial cells, which causes the liberation of inflammatory cells in the infarcted area [20]. The clinical manifestations of myocardial infarction range from mild nonspecific to life-threatening and depend on the severity of the attack and the immediate treatment to be initiated. Risk factors contributing to the development of myocardial infarction include social habits, smoking, alcohol consumption [21], metabolic abnormalities like alterations in lipid profile and diabetes [22], and hypertension [23].

ANDROGRAPHOLIDE AND ITS DERIVATIVES

Andrographis paniculata (AP) is a native medicinal herb of South Asian countries like India and Sri Lanka. It is commonly known as King of Bitters or Kalmeg, and it is widely used in Siddha, Ayurveda, and other alternative Indian medicinal systems to treat various disorders. In Indian Pharmacopoeia, *A. paniculata* is mentioned widely for its traditional or folklore uses, including as a bitter tonic, antipyretic, and febrifuge; it is also used to treat malaria and various gastrointestinal disorders [24]. In Traditional Chinese Medicine (TCM), AP is used to treat fever and as a detoxifying agent, whereas, in European countries, it is used to treat the common cold as a home remedy [25]. AP is reported for its pharmacological activities, including anticancer [15], anti-inflammatory, antioxidant, hepatoprotective, antidiabetic [26], and cardioprotective activity.

The pharmacologically critical chemical constituents of *A. paniculata* are diterpenoid lactones and their derivatives. Among them, Andrographolide (AG), deoxy andrographolide, 14-deoxy-11, 12-didehydroandrographolide, and neoandrographolide [8] possess diverse pharmacological actions. Andrographolide is a principal secondary metabolite of *A. paniculata* with assorted biological actions [27]. Chemically, andrographolide is 3α, 14, 15, 18-tetrahydroxy-5β, 9βH, 10α-labda-8, γ12-dien-16-oic acid γ-lactone. The molecular weight is 350.4 g/mol, and the formula is $C_{20}H_3O_5$.

Cardioprotective Potential of Andrographolide and its Analogs

Andrographolide has been used clinically, and biologically active diterpenoid is safe and effective in inflammatory diseases [28]. Recent studies have reported the cardioprotective potential of andrographolide and its derivatives in both *in vitro* and *in vivo* models.

Andrographolide Cardioprotection in Animal Models

Lin *et al.*, in their recent study, found 50 mg/kg of andrographolide to prevent high-fat diet-induced myocardial damage by inhibiting apoptosis in mice. Further, animal survival capacity against HFD-induced cardiac apoptosis was achieved by suppressing apoptotic proteins Bar and cytochrome c levels and increasing the protein levels of p-IGF-1R, total IGF-1R, and Bcl-2, Bcl-xL. Reduced apoptotic nuclei in terminal deoxynucleotidyl transferase dUTP Nick-End Labeling (TUNNEL) assay further support the cardioprotective effect [29].

Pre-treatment with *A. paniculata* extract inhibited the expression of COX-2, p-IκBα, and NFκB and cardiac hypertrophy biomarker proteins ANP and BNP. In addition, IL-6 and IL-6-associated myocardial inflammatory biomarkers p-MRK5 and STAT3 were reversed by treating *A. paniculata* extract. The proposed mechanism of the cardioprotective potential of *A. paniculata* was by decreasing the expression of p-MRK1/2 and p-JNK in high-fat diet-induced mice. The protection was further confirmed by TUNNEL assay, histopathological changes in H&E staining, and Masson's trichrome staining analysis for collagen accumulation and fibrosis [30, 31].

Cardioprotection by Anti-arrhythmias in Rabbits

Abnormalities in auto rhythmicity of the heart cause sudden cardiac deaths during heart failure conditions. Zeng *et al.*, in their study, reported that andrographolide significantly reduces isoproterenol and high calcium load-induced inward current of Na^+ and Ca^+ without affecting K^+ current and reduced delay after depolarization or triggered activities in isolated left ventricular myocytes and left atrial myocytes. An *in vivo* study on rabbits against aconite-induced ventricular arrhythmias reveals that andrographolide has a significant cardioprotective effect by inhibiting rabbits' Na^+ and Ca^+ ion channels [32].

Cardioprotection of Andrographolides through Anti-hypertensive Mechanism

Left ventricular function capacity against LPS-induced cardiac malfunction in mice was accessed after 12h of exposure. Ventricular systolic function was significantly reduced in LPS-alone treated mice, whereas the same was prevented with pre-treatment of andrographolide. Andrographolide inhibited the over-expression of IL-1β and TNF-α induced by LPS in mice. The inhibition of phosphorylation of IκB is the key step in protecting against cardiac inflammation. Andrographolide significantly inhibited the phosphorylation of myocardial IκB in LPS-induced IκB activation mice. Andrographolide also reversed LPS-induced activation of apoptosis proteins caspase 3/7, which was further confirmed by TUNNEL assay [33].

The cardioprotective effect of 14-deoxy-11, 12- didehydro, an andrographolide active diterpenoid from *A. paniculata*, significantly decreased rat arterial blood pressure. Another mechanism of cardioprotection was potent vasorelaxation in rats' isolated aorta. The proposed mechanism for vasorelaxation was the release of nitric oxide or the inhibition of Ca^+ entry into vascular smooth muscles [34].

Awang *et al.*, in their study, found the cardioprotective potential of different andrographolides from *A. paniculata*, including 14-deoxy-11,12-dihydro andrographolide, 14 deoxy andrographolide, and 14-deoxy-12- hydroxy andrographolide, which significantly caused vasorelaxation by isolating coronary arteries and decreasing coronary perfusion pressure in isolated hearts [35].

Another group of researchers found the cardioprotective potential of andrographolides in mice against left coronary artery ligation-induced MI. The cardioprotective effect was confirmed by a reduction in hemodynamic parameters and end-diastolic pressure, which helps in the restoration of diastolic function of the heart in andrographolide treatment after three weeks of coronary artery ligation along with echocardiography. Andrographolide supplementation alleviates cardiac dysfunction by improving left ventricle (LV) ejection fraction and reducing LV end-systole. Further, andrographolide suppresses myocardial hypertrophy by decreasing the mRNA expression of hypertrophic markers atrial natriuretic peptide, B-type natriuretic peptides, and β-myosin heavy chain when compared to control. Andrographolide treatment attenuated myocardial fibrosis and left ventricular collagen volume [36].

Andrographolide improves left ventricular ejection fraction and decreases cardiomyocyte hypertrophy. Similarly, myocardial fibrosis was reduced by inhibiting TGF-β and p-smad3 in left anterior descending coronary artery ligation in mice. Myocardial infarction-induced inflammation was reversed by the inhibition of the expression of TNF-α, IL-1β, IL-6, and MCP-1 after three weeks of surgery in mice. Andrographolide treatment increased the expression of antioxidant enzymes Gpx, SOD, and NQO1 [37].

According to Yang *et al.*, the cardioprotective effect of andrographolide and neo-andrographolide on rats was due to the potent hypolipidemic effect by reducing total cholesterol, triglycerides LDL, and atherogenesis-induced myocardial infarction and increasing HDL levels. This was further confirmed by reversing the down-regulation of iNOS expression and up-regulation of endothelial nitric oxide synthase (eNOS) expression in the aorta of hyperlipidemic rats [38].

Cardioprotection of Andrographolides by the Regulation Cell Death Mechanism

Several studies reveal that the number of necrotic cells increased in the progression of myocardial infarction [39, 40]. During MI, cardiomyocytes adopt various mechanisms to protect from harmful stimuli or stress [41]. For specific cytokines, insults like IL-1β, IL-6, TNF-α NF-κB, and Toll-like receptor-4 to cardiomyocytes undergo apoptosis, which is evident by significant increase in Bax and caspase-3 reduction in Bcl-2 and Bxl [42].

Andrographolide inhibited LPS-induced inflammatory markers IL-1β and TNF-α over-expression, whereas the nitric oxide levels were increased in heart tissue. In addition, andrographolide shows cardioprotection through an anti-inflammatory and anti-apoptosis mechanism [33].

Another study by Liang *et al.* reveals that andrographolide treatment attenuated myocardial infarction induced by diabetes dose-dependently. The elevation of pro-inflammatory marker NF-κB, pro-apoptotic proteins Bax/Bcl-2 ratio, caspase-3 and 9, and p-Akt determines the severity of apoptosis and cell death. In diabetic cardiomyopathic rats and H9C2 cardiomyoblasts incubated with a high glucose concentration (25 mM) for 48 h, the markers mentioned above were significantly increased. In contrast, pretreatment with andrographolide distinctly attenuated the elevated levels [43].

Cardiac mitochondrial-dependent apoptosis-associated proteins like total insulin-like growth factor-1 receptor (IGF-1R) levels and pro-apoptotic proteins Bcl-2, Bcl-xL levels were downregulated in high-fat diet-induced mice. Treatment with andrographolide notably enhanced the IGF-1R compensatory mechanism to provide enhanced protection against HFD-induced myocardial cell death. Similarly, abnormal increases in apoptotic and TUNEL-stained nuclei were drastically reduced in mice treated with andrographolide (50 mg/kg) [29]. In the H9c2 cell line, andrographolide at the concentration range from 12.5 to 50 μM inhibits the MAPKs ERK1/2, JNK, and P38 to elicit the cardioprotective effect [36]. These studies bring new insight into the fact that andrographolide prevents myocardial infarction by preventing the apoptosis process both *in vitro* and *in vivo*. In addition, other derivatives of AG (Shown in Tables **1** & **2**) show significant cardioprotective effects in various *in vitro* and *in vivo* models.

Table 1. Cardioprotective effect of andrographolide and its derivatives on various animal models.

Animal Model	Animal Type	Intervention and Dose	Mechanism of Action/ Potential Findings	References
Aconite-induced ventricular arrhythmias in rabbits	Adult New Zealand white rabbits	Andrographolides (10 mg/kg)	Inhibiting the Na^+ and Ca^+ ion channels	[32]

Animal Model	Animal Type	Intervention and Dose	Mechanism of Action/ Potential Findings	References
High-fat diet-induced cardiac apoptosis in mice.	C57/BL6 mice	Andrographolides (50 mg/kg)	Increase survival capacity Suppressed the levels of apoptotic proteins Bar and cytochrome *c*. Protein levels of p-IGF-1R, total IGF-1R and Bcl-2, Bcl-xL Reduced apoptotic nuclei in the TUNNEL assay	[29]
High-fat diet-induced cardiac apoptosis in mice.	C57/BL6 mice	*Andrographis paniculata* extract (2 g/kg/day)	COX-2, p-IκBα and NFκB, ANP and BNP p-MRK5 and STAT3 and p-MRK1/2 and p-JNK TUNNEL assay Masson's trichrome staining analysis	[31]
LPS-induced myocardial malfunctions in mice.	Male BALB/c mice	Andrographolides (10 mg/kg)	IL-1β, TNF-α and IκB caspase 3/7 activity TUNNEL assay	[33]
Measurement of blood pressure in normal rats.	Male Wistar rats	Andrographolide, 14-de-oxy-11, 12-didehydro andrographolide, Neoandrographolide (6-60 mg/kg)	Arterial blood pressure Inhibition of Ca^+ entry into vascular smooth muscles Releasing of nitric oxide	[34]
Langendorff-perfused model of isolated rat hearts	Sprague Dawley rats	14-deoxy-11,12-dihydroandrographolide, 14-deoxyandrographolide 14-deoxy-12-hydroxyl andrographolide (1 mg/mL solution)	Coronary arteries relaxation Coronary perfusion pressure	[35]

(Table 1) cont.....

Animal Model	Animal Type	Intervention and Dose	Mechanism of Action/ Potential Findings	References
Aortic banding-induced experimental cardiac hypertrophy in mice	male C57/BL6 mice	Andrographolide (25 mg/kg/day)	End diastolic pressure Left ventricle (LV) ejection fraction Myocardial natriuretic peptides, B-type natriuretic peptides, and β-myosin heavy chain Myocardial fibrosis and collagen volume Down-regulation of MAPKs ERK1/2, JNK, and P38	[36]
Left coronary descending artery ligation-induced MI	male C57/BL6 mice	Andrographolide (25 mg/kg/day)	Anti-fibrosis by TGF-β and p-smad3 TNF-α, IL-1β, IL-6 and MCP-1 Gpx, SOD and NQO1 Nrf-2 and HO-1	[37]
High-fat diet emulsion induces hyperlipidemia in rats and mice	Male Wistar rats Male mice	Andrographolide (20 mg/kg/day) Neoandrographolide(20 mg/kg/day)	Total cholesterol, triglycerides LDL iNOS HDL levels eNOS	[38]
Isoproterenol-induced myocardial infarction in rats.	Male Wistar rats	Andrographolide (20mg/kg)	Troponin I, CK-MB and LDH, Ica current Prevent elevation of QRS complex and ST-segment elevation	[7]

Table 2. Cardioprotective effect of andrographolide and its derivatives against *in vitro* cell line models.

Type of cell line/isolated heart	Intervention and dose	Mechanism of action/ Potential findings	Reference
Left ventricular myocytes (Whole-cell patch-clamp and current clamp techniques)	Andrographolides (5 and 10μM)	The inward current of Na^+ and Ca^+ does not affect the K^+ current. Delayed after depolarization.	[32]
H9c2 cells	Andrographolides (12.5 to 50μM)	Inhibition of MAPKs ERK1/2, JNK, and P38	[36]
Hypoxia-induced H9c2 cells.	Andrographolides (12.5 to 100μM)	Gpx, SOD and NQO1 Nrf-2 and HO-1	-
High glucose-stimulated H9c2 cells	Andrographolides (20μM)	NF-κB, Bax/Bcl-2 ratio, caspase-3 and 9 and p-Akt Intracellular ROS (DCFH-DA), NADPH oxidizes (NOX2, NOX4, and p47phox) Nrf-2 and HO-1	[43]
Neonatal rat cardiomyocytes exposed to ischemic reperfusion injury (H/R)	Andrographolides (20μM)	SOD, catalase, GPX, and GR, Glutamate cysteine ligase system (GCLC and GCLM)	[47]
H9C2 cells against hypoxia-induced oxidative stress	Andrographolides	Pro-fibrotic proteins TGF-β and p-smad3 CD45 and CD68 Nrf2/HO-1	[36]

Cardioprotection of Andrographolide by the Antioxidant Mechanism

An imbalance between producing and eliminating reactive oxygen species (ROS) and other free radicals alters the cellular antioxidant defense system. During cellular metabolism, some ordinary free radicals like hydroxyl radicals (OH^-), superoxide ion (O^-), and hydrogen peroxide (H_2O_2) and some nitrogen radicals, including peroxynitrite (ONOO−), are generated [44]. Higher levels of free radicals cause low levels of superoxide dismutase (SOD), glutathione peroxidase (GPx), and catalase (CAT) and reduce glutathione (GSH) during myocardial infarction, further exacerbating oxidative stress and resulting in lipid peroxidation and damage of DNA.

Nuclear factor erythroid 2-related factor (Nrf-2) is a cytoprotective protein involved in the up-regulation of antioxidant enzymes to combat oxidative stress. In Nrf2 knockout mice, enhanced susceptibility to oxidative stress-related diseases was observed [45]. When the cell undergoes oxidative stress, Nrf-2 detachs from Keap-1 (Kelch-like ECH-associated protein 1) and is translocated into the nucleus to activate the antioxidant response element (ARE) to protect the cell [46].

Liang *et al.* found in their study a marked reduction in SOD and an increase in lipid peroxides in myocardial infarcted rats, and found that andrographolide could reverse it. Similarly, andrographolide offered its cardioprotection by attenuating ROS generation by restoring Nrf2/HO-1 and inactivating the NADPH oxidases in H9C2.

Andrographolide treatment increased the mRNA expression of antioxidant enzymes SOD, GPx, and NQO1 and decreased the transcription of P67 phlox, Gp91, and NOX4 in mice hearts. The cardioprotective effect of andrographolide was further confirmed by the expression of mRNA level and protein expression of HO-1 and Nrf2 in *in vivo* and H9 C2 cells [37].

Andrographolide exerts its cardioprotective potential by increasing the tissue antioxidant system, including SOD, catalase, GPX, and GR in neonatal rats' cardiomyocytes exposed to ischemic reperfusion injury (H/R). Further, it demonstrated cardioprotection by enhancing glutamate cysteine ligase system (GCLC and GCLM) promoter activities after incubation with andrographolide [47].

The cardioprotection in mice was by mitigating pro-fibrotic proteins TGF-β and p-smad3 in infarcted left coronary artery ligation-induced MI mice. It was noted that the expression of inflammatory factory CD45 and CD68 decreased. Andrographolide restored or enhanced the expression of the Nrf2/HO-1 pathway in H9C2 cells against hypoxia-induced oxidative stress [36, 37]. Andrographolide can protect the myocardium against isoproterenol-induced oxidative stress by enhancing the tissue antioxidant enzyme catalase and glutathione peroxidase in rats [7].

Pre-treatment with 14-deoxy andrographolide and 14-deoxy- 11, 12-didehydroandrographolide isolated from *A. paniculata* significantly increases the tissue antioxidant enzyme activity of SOD, CAT, and GSHPx, with a significant decrease in malondialdehyde levels in isoproterenol-induced myocardial infarction in rats at the same time [48].

Cardioprotection of Andrographolide by Inhibition of PI3K/Akt Pathway in Rats

Phosphatidylinositol-3-kinase (PI3K)/Protein kinase B (Akt) signaling pathway plays an essential role in the development of inflammatory diseases and also physiological cardiac hypertrophy [49]. The activated PI3K by GPCR and tyrosine kinase receptors phosphorylates Akt and eventually engages a series of cascade reactions, including protein synthesis, cell proliferation, and survival [50]. The inhibition of the PI3K pathway is a potential therapeutic target for preventing myocardial infarction [31]. Zhang *et al.* stated in their study that treatment with andrographolide reduced mortality rates and enhanced pathological features of cardiomyocytes and the functioning capacity of the heart. Andrographolide treatment significantly reduced cardiac levels of p-PI3K and p-Akt without any change of PI3K and Akt in experimentally induced immune myocarditis in rats. The proposed mechanism for cardioprotection was the attenuation of myocardial inflammation and down-regulation of the PI3K/Akt pathway [50].

Cardioprotection of Andrographolide Against Isoproterenol-induced Myocardial Infarction

Isoproterenol-induced myocardial infarction is one of the widely used animal models to screen test drugs with cardioprotective potential [1]. Elasoru *et al.* found that pre-treatment of andrographolide significantly protects the myocardium in isoproterenol-induced myocardial infarction. The study results reveal that 20mg/kg of andrographolide prevents the elevation of cardiac biomarkers like troponin I, CK-MB, and LDH and electrocardiographic parameters QRS complex and ST-segment elevation. In addition, cardioprotection is supported by decreasing the Ica current and preserving the K current. Andrographolide can protect the myocardium by preventing the morphological changes evident by histopathological changes and, finally, by elevating the tissue antioxidant cascade of enzymes [7].

Cardioprotection of Andrographolide by Inhibiting Platelet Aggregation

Platelet aggregation in coronary arteries is an important and significant event in the development of myocardial infarction. Extracellular signal-regulated kinase (ERK1/2) activation plays a vital role in the stimulation of thrombin, a potent platelet aggregator. Pre-incubation with andrographolide and 14-deoxy-11, 12-didehydroandrographolide has shown potent inhibition of phosphorylation of ERK1/2. The anti-platelet action is further confirmed by inhibiting the thrombin-activated platelet aggregation [51]. Andrographolide and 14-deoxy-11, 12-didehydroandrographolide are potential candidates for preventing cardiovascular diseases, including MI.

CONCLUSION

In summary, myocardial infarction causes around 31% of total deaths in the world. Despite numerous treatment options, they have limitations, like adverse side effects. Therefore, there is a scope for developing new drugs that antagonize

MI and can be used as suitable therapeutic candidates, particularly from natural sources. The present book chapter focused on cardioprotective candidates of andrographolide and its derivatives. The chapter explains the molecular mechanisms involved in exhibiting the cardioprotective potential of andrographolide and its derivatives both *in vitro* and *in vivo*. Cardioprotection of andrographolide and its derivatives is shown by various animal models' anti-arrhythmic, antihypertensive, anti-inflammatory, and antioxidant mechanisms. Moreover, we described in this chapter distinct ways of activating the Nrf-2/H--1pathway, regulating various apoptotic markers to elicit the protective machinery of andrographolides in ameliorating the insults of myocardial infarction. This chapter may provide insight into andrographolide and its derivatives as an alternative therapeutic drug candidate for combating MI.

REFERENCES

[1]   Pullaiah CP, Nelson VK, Rayapu S, G v NK, Kedam T. Exploring cardioprotective potential of esculetin against isoproterenol induced myocardial toxicity in rats: *in vivo* and *in vitro* evidence. BMC Pharmacol Toxicol 2021; 22(1): 43.
        [http://dx.doi.org/10.1186/s40360-021-00510-0] [PMID: 34266475]

[2]   Gersh BJ, Sliwa K, Mayosi BM, Yusuf S. Novel therapeutic concepts: The epidemic of cardiovascular disease in the developing world: global implications. Eur Heart J 2010; 31(6): 642-8.
        [http://dx.doi.org/10.1093/eurheartj/ehq030] [PMID: 20176800]

[3]   Joshi P, Islam S, Pais P, *et al.* Risk factors for early myocardial infarction in South Asians compared with individuals in other countries. JAMA 2007; 297(3): 286-94.
        [http://dx.doi.org/10.1001/jama.297.3.286] [PMID: 17227980]

[4]   Turk-Adawi K, Sarrafzadegan N, Fadhil I, *et al.* Cardiovascular disease in the Eastern Mediterranean region: epidemiology and risk factor burden. Nat Rev Cardiol 2018; 15(2): 106-19.
        [http://dx.doi.org/10.1038/nrcardio.2017.138] [PMID: 28933782]

[5]   Vogel B, Claessen BE, Arnold SV, *et al.* ST-segment elevation myocardial infarction. Nat Rev Dis Primers 2019; 5(1): 39.
        [http://dx.doi.org/10.1038/s41572-019-0090-3] [PMID: 31171787]

[6]   McCarthy CP, Raber I, Chapman AR, *et al.* Myocardial Injury in the Era of High-Sensitivity Cardiac Troponin Assays. JAMA Cardiol 2019; 4(10): 1034-42.
        [http://dx.doi.org/10.1001/jamacardio.2019.2724] [PMID: 31389986]

[7]   Elasoru SE, Rhana P, de Oliveira Barreto T, *et al.* Andrographolide protects against isoproterenol-induced myocardial infarction in rats through inhibition of L-type Ca^{2+} and increase of cardiac transient outward K^+ currents. Eur J Pharmacol 2021; 906: 174194.
        [http://dx.doi.org/10.1016/j.ejphar.2021.174194] [PMID: 34044012]

[8]   Mandal S, Nelson VK, Mukhopadhyay S, *et al.* 14-Deoxyandrographolide targets adenylate cyclase and prevents ethanol-induced liver injury through constitutive NOS dependent reduced redox signaling in rats. Food Chem Toxicol 2013; 59: 236-48.
        [http://dx.doi.org/10.1016/j.fct.2013.05.056] [PMID: 23764359]

[9]   Schreiber T, Salhöfer L, Quinting T, Fandrey J. Things get broken: the hypoxia-inducible factor prolyl hydroxylases in ischemic heart disease. Basic Res Cardiol 2019; 114(3): 16.
        [http://dx.doi.org/10.1007/s00395-019-0725-2] [PMID: 30859331]

[10]   Dutta N, Ghosh S, Nelson VK, *et al.* Andrographolide upregulates protein quality control mechanisms in cell and mouse through upregulation of mTORC1 function. Biochim Biophys Acta, Gen Subj 2021;

1865(6): 129885.
[http://dx.doi.org/10.1016/j.bbagen.2021.129885] [PMID: 33639218]

[11] Ghosh S, Hazra J, Pal K, Nelson VK, Pal M. Prostate cancer: Therapeutic prospect with herbal medicine. Current Research in Pharmacology and Drug Discovery 2021; 2: 100034.
[http://dx.doi.org/10.1016/j.crphar.2021.100034] [PMID: 34909665]

[12] Nelson V, Sahoo NK, Sahu M, Sudhan H, Pullaiah CP, Muralikrishna KS. *In vitro* anticancer activity of *Eclipta alba* whole plant extract on colon cancer cell HCT-116. BMC Complementary Medicine and Therapies 2020; 20(1): 355.
[http://dx.doi.org/10.1186/s12906-020-03118-9] [PMID: 33225921]

[13] Dutta N, Pemmaraju DB, Ghosh S, *et al.* Alkaloid-rich fraction of *Ervatamia coronaria* sensitizes colorectal cancer through modulating AMPK and mTOR signalling pathways. J Ethnopharmacol 2022; 283: 114666.
[http://dx.doi.org/10.1016/j.jep.2021.114666] [PMID: 34592338]

[14] Singh BK, Vatsa N, Nelson VK, *et al.* Azadiradione restores protein quality control and ameliorates the disease pathogenesis in a mouse model of Huntington's disease. Mol Neurobiol 2018; 55(8): 6337-46.
[http://dx.doi.org/10.1007/s12035-017-0853-3] [PMID: 29294248]

[15] Nelson VK, Ali A, Dutta N, *et al.* Azadiradione ameliorates polyglutamine expansion disease in *Drosophila* by potentiating DNA binding activity of heat shock factor 1. Oncotarget 2016; 7(48): 78281-96.
[http://dx.doi.org/10.18632/oncotarget.12930] [PMID: 27835876]

[16] Ahmed R, Tanvir EM, Hossen MS, *et al.* Antioxidant properties and cardioprotective mechanism of Malaysian Propolis in Rats. Evid Based Complement Alternat Med 2017; 2017(1): 5370545.
[http://dx.doi.org/10.1155/2017/5370545] [PMID: 28261310]

[17] Anderson JL, Morrow DA. Acute Myocardial Infarction. N Engl J Med 2017; 376(21): 2053-64.
[http://dx.doi.org/10.1056/NEJMra1606915] [PMID: 28538121]

[18] O'Gara PT, Kushner FG, Ascheim DD, *et al.* 2013 ACCF/AHA guideline for the management of ST-elevation myocardial infarction: a report of the American College of Cardiology Foundation/American Heart Association Task Force on Practice Guidelines. Circulation 2013; 127(4): e362-425.
[http://dx.doi.org/10.1161/CIR.0b013e3182742c84] [PMID: 23247304]

[19] Chen B, Frangogiannis NG. Chemokines in Myocardial Infarction. J Cardiovasc Transl Res 2021; 14(1): 35-52.
[http://dx.doi.org/10.1007/s12265-020-10006-7] [PMID: 32415537]

[20] Legler DF, Thelen M. New insights in chemokine signaling. F1000 Res 2018; 7: 95.
[http://dx.doi.org/10.12688/f1000research.13130.1] [PMID: 29416853]

[21] Prescott E, Hippe M, Schnohr P, Hein HO, Vestbo J. Smoking and risk of myocardial infarction in women and men: longitudinal population study. BMJ 1998; 316(7137): 1043-7.
[http://dx.doi.org/10.1136/bmj.316.7137.1043] [PMID: 9552903]

[22] Piegas LS, Avezum Á, Pereira JCR, *et al.* Risk factors for myocardial infarction in Brazil. Am Heart J 2003; 146(2): 331-8.
[http://dx.doi.org/10.1016/S0002-8703(03)00181-9] [PMID: 12891204]

[23] Stamler J, Stamler R, Neaton JD. Blood pressure, systolic and diastolic, and cardiovascular risks. US population data. Arch Intern Med 1993; 153(5): 598-615.
[http://dx.doi.org/10.1001/archinte.1993.00410050036006] [PMID: 8439223]

[24] Prakash J, Srivastava S, Ray RS, Singh N, Rajpali R, Singh GN. Current Status of Herbal Drug Standards in the Indian Pharmacopoeia. Phytother Res 2017; 31(12): 1817-23.
[http://dx.doi.org/10.1002/ptr.5933] [PMID: 29027278]

[25] Singh RK, Mehta S, Sharma AK. Ethnobotany, pharmacological activities and bioavailability studies

on "King of Bitters" (Kalmegh): A Review (2010-2020). Comb Chem High Throughput Screen 2022; 25(5): 788-807.
[http://dx.doi.org/10.2174/1386207324666210310140611] [PMID: 33745423]

[26] Dai Y, Chen SR, Chai L, Zhao J, Wang Y, Wang Y. Overview of pharmacological activities of *Andrographis paniculata* and its major compound andrographolide. Crit Rev Food Sci Nutr 2019; 59(sup1): S17-29.
[http://dx.doi.org/10.1080/10408398.2018.1501657] [PMID: 30040451]

[27] Islam MT. Andrographolide, a new hope in the prevention and treatment of metabolic syndrome. Front Pharmacol 2017; 8: 571.
[http://dx.doi.org/10.3389/fphar.2017.00571] [PMID: 28878680]

[28] Tan WSD, Liao W, Zhou S, Wong WSF. Is there a future for andrographolide to be an anti-inflammatory drug? Deciphering its major mechanisms of action. Biochem Pharmacol 2017; 139: 71-81.
[http://dx.doi.org/10.1016/j.bcp.2017.03.024] [PMID: 28377280]

[29] Lin KH, Marthandam Asokan S, Kuo WW, *et al.* Andrographolide mitigates cardiac apoptosis to provide cardio-protection in high-fat-diet-induced obese mice. Environ Toxicol 2020; 35(6): 707-13.
[http://dx.doi.org/10.1002/tox.22906] [PMID: 32023008]

[30] Chen CC, Lii CK, Lin YH, *et al. Andrographis paniculata* improves insulin resistance in high-fat diet-induced obese mice and TNFα-treated 3T3-L1 adipocytes. Am J Chin Med 2020; 48(5): 1073-90.
[http://dx.doi.org/10.1142/S0192415X20500524] [PMID: 32668968]

[31] Liu HS, Zhang J, Guo JL, Lin CY, Wang ZW. Phosphoinositide 3-kinase inhibitor LY294002 ameliorates the severity of myosin-induced myocarditis in mice. Curr Res Transl Med 2016; 64(1): 21-7.
[http://dx.doi.org/10.1016/j.retram.2016.01.012] [PMID: 27140596]

[32] Zeng M, Jiang W, Tian Y, *et al.* Andrographolide inhibits arrhythmias and is cardioprotective in rabbits. Oncotarget 2017; 8(37): 61226-38.
[http://dx.doi.org/10.18632/oncotarget.18051] [PMID: 28977859]

[33] Zhang J, Zhu D, Wang Y, Ju Y. Andrographolide attenuates LPS-induced cardiac malfunctions through inhibition of IκB phosphorylation and apoptosis in mice. Cell Physiol Biochem 2015; 37(4): 1619-28.
[http://dx.doi.org/10.1159/000438528] [PMID: 26536571]

[34] Yoopan N, Thisoda P, Rangkadilok N, *et al.* Cardiovascular effects of 14-deoxy-11,-2-didehydroandrographolide and *Andrographis paniculata* extracts. Planta Med 2007; 73(6): 503-11.
[http://dx.doi.org/10.1055/s-2007-967181] [PMID: 17650544]

[35] Awang K, Abdullah NH, Hadi AHA, Su Fong Y. Cardiovascular activity of labdane diterpenes from *Andrographis paniculata* in isolated rat hearts. J Biomed Biotechnol 2012; 2012: 1-5.
[http://dx.doi.org/10.1155/2012/876458] [PMID: 22536026]

[36] Wu QQ, Ni J, Zhang N, Liao HH, Tang QZ, Deng W. Andrographolide protects against aortic banding-induced experimental cardiac hypertrophy by inhibiting MAPKs signaling. Front Pharmacol 2017; 8: 808.
[http://dx.doi.org/10.3389/fphar.2017.00808] [PMID: 29184496]

[37] Xie S, Deng W, Chen J, *et al.* Andrographolide protects against adverse cardiac remodeling after myocardial infarction through enhancing Nrf2 Signaling Pathway. Int J Biol Sci 2020; 16(1): 12-26.
[http://dx.doi.org/10.7150/ijbs.37269] [PMID: 31892842]

[38] Yang T, Shi H, Wang Z, Wang C. Hypolipidemic effects of andrographolide and neoandrographolide in mice and rats. Phytother Res 2013; 27(4): 618-23.
[http://dx.doi.org/10.1002/ptr.4771] [PMID: 22744979]

[39] Adameova A, Goncalvesova E, Szobi A, Dhalla NS. Necroptotic cell death in failing heart: relevance

and proposed mechanisms. Heart Fail Rev 2016; 21(2): 213-21.
[http://dx.doi.org/10.1007/s10741-016-9537-8] [PMID: 26872672]

[40]   Zhao Y, Wang H, Chen W, *et al.* Melatonin attenuates white matter damage after focal brain ischemia in rats by regulating the TLR4/NF-κB pathway. Brain Res Bull 2019; 150: 168-78.
[http://dx.doi.org/10.1016/j.brainresbull.2019.05.019] [PMID: 31158461]

[41]   Linkermann A. Death and fire—the concept of necroinflammation. Cell Death Differ 2019; 26(1): 1-3.
[http://dx.doi.org/10.1038/s41418-018-0218-0] [PMID: 30470796]

[42]   Bocci M, Sjölund J, Kurzejamska E, *et al.* Activin receptor-like kinase 1 is associated with immune cell infiltration and regulates CLEC14A transcription in cancer. Angiogenesis 2019; 22(1): 117-31.
[http://dx.doi.org/10.1007/s10456-018-9642-5] [PMID: 30132150]

[43]   Liang E, Liu X, Du Z, Yang R, Zhao Y. Andrographolide ameliorates diabetic cardiomyopathy in mice by blockage of oxidative damage and NF-κB-mediated inflammation. Oxid Med Cell Longev 2018; 2018(1): 9086747.
[http://dx.doi.org/10.1155/2018/9086747] [PMID: 30046380]

[44]   Pizzino G, Irrera N, Cucinotta M, *et al.* Oxidative Stress: Harms and benefits for human health. Oxid Med Cell Longev 2017; 2017(1): 8416763.
[http://dx.doi.org/10.1155/2017/8416763] [PMID: 28819546]

[45]   Ma Q. Role of nrf2 in oxidative stress and toxicity. Annu Rev Pharmacol Toxicol 2013; 53(1): 401-26.
[http://dx.doi.org/10.1146/annurev-pharmtox-011112-140320] [PMID: 23294312]

[46]   Habtemariam S. The Nrf2/HO-1 axis as targets for flavanones: Neuroprotection by pinocembrin, naringenin, and eriodictyol. Oxid Med Cell Longev 2019; 2019: 1-15.
[http://dx.doi.org/10.1155/2019/4724920] [PMID: 31814878]

[47]   Woo AYH, Waye MMY, Tsui SKW, Yeung STW, Cheng CHK. Andrographolide up-regulates cellular-reduced glutathione level and protects cardiomyocytes against hypoxia/reoxygenation injury. J Pharmacol Exp Ther 2008; 325(1): 226-35.
[http://dx.doi.org/10.1124/jpet.107.133918] [PMID: 18174384]

[48]   Ojha SK, Bharti S, Joshi S, Kumari S, Arya DS. Protective effect of hydroalcoholic extract of *Andrographis paniculata* on ischaemia-reperfusion induced myocardial injury in rats. Indian J Med Res 2012; 135(3): 414-21.
[PMID: 22561631]

[49]   Ghigo A, Li M. Phosphoinositide 3-kinase: friend and foe in cardiovascular disease. Front Pharmacol 2015; 6: 169.
[http://dx.doi.org/10.3389/fphar.2015.00169] [PMID: 26321955]

[50]   Zhang Q, Hu L, Li H, Wu J, Bian N, Yan G. Beneficial effects of andrographolide in a rat model of autoimmune myocarditis and its effects on PI3K/Akt pathway. Korean J Physiol Pharmacol 2019; 23(2): 103-11.
[http://dx.doi.org/10.4196/kjpp.2019.23.2.103] [PMID: 30820154]

[51]   Thisoda P, Rangkadilok N, Pholphana N, Worasuttayangkurn L, Ruchirawat S, Satayavivad J. Inhibitory effect of *Andrographis paniculata* extract and its active diterpenoids on platelet aggregation. Eur J Pharmacol 2006; 553(1-3): 39-45.
[http://dx.doi.org/10.1016/j.ejphar.2006.09.052] [PMID: 17081514]

CHAPTER 13

Phytonanomaterials from *Andrographis* Species and their Applications

V. Soundarya[1], L. Baskaran[1] and N. Karmegam[1,*]

[1] *Department of Botany, Government Arts College (Autonomous), Salem, Tamil Nadu 636007, India*

Abstract: *Andrographis* (Acanthaceae) is a genus of 26 species native to India, mainly used for the treatment of snake bites, diabetes, fever, cholera, dysentery, gonorrhea, and malaria. Medicinal properties of *Andrographis* are attributed to the presence of phytochemicals such as andrographolide, neoandrographolide, 14-deoxy-11,-2-didehydroandrographolide, 14-deoxy andrographolide, isoandrographolide, 14-deoxy andrographolide 19 β-Dglucoside, homoandrographolide, andrographan, andrographosterin, and stigmasterol. Nanotechnology is a technique capable of achieving a high degree of precision in functions. By creating eco-friendly materials that can be applied to nanomedicine, plants have mediated the synthesis and fabrication of materials in nanotechnology. Mostly, silver nanoparticles biosynthesized using *Andrographis* species showed significant pharmacological activities *viz* ., antimicrobial, antioxidant, anti-inflammatory, antidiabetic, mosquito larvicidal, hepatocurative, and anticancer activity.

Keywords: Andrographolide, *Andrographis* species, Phyto-nanotechnology, Medicinal plants, Pharmacological activities.

INTRODUCTION

Nanoparticles are synthesized using various plant parts in phyto-nanotechnology. The simplicity and cost-effectiveness of this method have made it a non-conventional method that is gaining attention. Through the use of plant-mediated approaches to material synthesis and fabrication, eco-friendly nanotechnology has been developed for use in nanomedicine [1]. Solutes in plant materials are extracted using different solvents depending on the polarity of the bioactive molecules responsible for nanoparticle synthesis. Nanotechnology is a technique capable of achieving a high degree of precision in functions. This can be performed by controlling the reaction conditions of the molecules participating in

*** Corresponding author N. Karmegam:** Department of Botany, Government Arts College (Autonomous), Salem, Tamil Nadu 636007, India; E-mail: kanishkarmegam@gmail.com

S. Karuppusamy, Vinod K. Nelson & T. Pullaiah (Eds.)

the synthesis of the nanoparticles [2]. Nanoparticles derived from plants are produced using readily available plant materials. Nanoparticles with applications in biomedicine and the environment can be made from plants because of their non-toxic nature.

It has been thousands of years since people started using plants as medicine without proper guidance and scientific knowledge. There are several natural medicinal systems that use plants as medicine. Medicinal plants are now considered an essential source of treating various kinds of diseases. Each plant consists of several important ingredients that can be used in the field of medicine and can be involved in the discovery of drugs. Medicinal plants contain bioactive substances that have definite physiological effects on humans [3, 4]. Traditional medicinal systems are primarily based on herbal treatments. The healthcare system continues to rely heavily on plant-based traditional medicines. Scientific evidence reveals that every part of plants has medicinal properties, including flowers, roots, stems, leaves, fruits, and seeds [5, 6]. Plants have secondary metabolites called phytochemicals, which are active components with numerous therapeutic potentials (alkaloids, flavonoids, saponins, terpenoids, steroids, glycosides, tannins, volatile oils, and others). Additionally, some plants contain toxic compounds that cause adverse effects on the body, which is one reason why they are unsafe for health [7].

Andrographis (family Acanthaceae) is an important genus of 26 species native to India. The southern part of the Eastern Ghats comparatively possesses important ethno-medicinal plant species such as *Andrographis paniculata*, *A. echioides*, *A. serpyllifolia*, *A. lineata*, *A. glandulosa*, *A. affinis*, *A. viscosula*, *A. alata*, *A. nallamalayana*, *A. neesiana*, *A. stenophylla*, *A. ovata*, *A. elongata,* and *A. beddomei*. Only some species have potential medicinal values; while numerous medical systems use *A. paniculata*, including Ayurveda, Homeopathy, Siddha, Unani, and naturopathy [8]. *A. paniculata* is ethnobotanically used for the treatment of snake bites, bug bites, diabetes, influenza, cholera, swellings, dysentery, gonorrhea, fever, and malaria. The decoction is used as a blood purifier and to cure jaundice [3, 9]. *A. alata* and *A. lineata* are traditionally used for treating snake bites, constipation, skin diseases, and lung diseases. The leaf juice of *A. echioides* is used to cure fevers [10]. Leaves and stems of *A. serpyllifolia* possess potent anti-snake and scorpion venom activity. Its leaf extract has been proven to be a highly effective drug to combat bovine mastitis [11]. The phytochemical compounds present in *Andrographis* spp. exhibit different biological activities (Table **1**).

Table 1. Phytochemicals and biological activities of *Andrographis* spp.

Plant Used	Phytochemicals	Activity	References
A. paniculata	Andrographolide	Anti-diabetic activity	[12 - 14]
A. paniculata	Andrographolide	Anti-oxidant activity	[15 - 17]
A. paniculata	Andrographolide	Antiangiogenic activity	[18]
A. paniculata	Andrographolide	Anticancer Activity	[19]
A. paniculata	Andrographolide	Anti-hepatitis C virus	[16]
A. paniculata	Andrographolide	Cardiovascular activity	[15, 20]
A. paniculata	Andrographolide	Antagonistic activity	[21]
A. paniculata	Andrographolide, 14-deoxy andrographolide, 14 – deoxy 12 -hydroxyandrapholide and neoandrographolide	Quorum quenching activity	[22, 23]
		Anticancer Activity	[24]
A. paniculata	andrographiside	Hepato-protective activity	[25]
A. paniculata	19-O-acetyl-14-deoxy-11,12-didehydroandrographolide	Anti-inflammatory activity	[26]

Phytosynthesis of Nanomaterials from *Andrographis* spp.

Various nanoparticles such as silver, zinc oxide, gold, copper, neodymium oxide, lanthanum oxide, ytterbium oxide, and titanium oxide have been synthesized using the *Andrographis* spp. Pharmaceutics and biomedicines are likely to benefit greatly from these nanomaterials. Among different nanomaterials, silver nanoparticles, in comparison, showed significant pharmacological activities like antimicrobial, antioxidant, antidiabetic, mosquito larvicidal, hepatocurative, anti-inflammatory, and anticancer activity.

Andrographolide

As a dietary supplement widely used in herbal medicine because of its diverse biological activities, andrographolide is most abundant in the leaves and stems of *A. paniculata*. This compound has anti-inflammatory, anti-metastatic, anti-angiogenic, anti-proliferative, neuroprotective, and hepatoprotective effects [27]. An andrographolide crystal is a white square prism or flaky crystal made of ethanol or methanol. The crystal has a bitter taste and no odor. It is almost insoluble in water but soluble in boiling ethanol, methanol, or chloroform. The ester structure of andrographolide makes it easy for the drug to be hydrolyzed, opened, and isomerized in solutions that affect its stability. Low temperature improves andrographolide stability; alkaline conditions make it unstable, and alkaline strength increases its instability. The most stable pH value is 3–5. The stability of andrographolide in chloroform is greater [28].

Andrographolide-assisted Synthesis of Nanomaterials

In order to combat drug-resistant bacteria such as *Burkholderia pseudomallei*, andrographolide-stabilized silver nanoparticles were synthesized from *A. paniculata* [29]. In addition to its powerful anti-parasitic properties, andrographolide also acts as an anti-leishmanial compound derived from the leaf extract of the plant *A. paniculata* [30]. Drug-resistant visceral leishmaniasis was controlled by the andrographolide-engineered gold nanoparticle with low toxicity [31].

Pharmacological Activities of Nanoparticles Synthesized from *Andrographis* spp.

The pharmacological activities studied in *Andrographis* spp. are antimicrobial, antioxidant, anticancer, anti-inflammatory, antidiabetic, antitumor, antiplasmodial, hepatocurative, antifilarial, and mosquito larvicidal activities. Nanoparticles biosynthesized using *Andrographis* spp. revealed significant pharmacological activities (Table **2**). Significantly, the nanoparticles synthesized using the phytochemical andrographolide are effective in specific biomedical applications (Table **3**).

Table 2. Biomedical applications of nanoparticles (NPs) derived from different sources.

Andrographis Species Studied	Extract Used	Type of NPs	Activity Studied	Concluding Remarks	References
A. paniculata	Aqueous	Zinc NPs	Antimicrobial activity	Zn NPs exhibited antibacterial activity against *Pseudomonas* and *Proteus* species.	[41]
A. paniculata	Aqueous	Gold NPs	Antimicrobial	Aqueous extract-mediated Au NPs indicated better antimicrobial potential.	[42]

(Table 2) cont.....

Andrographis Species Studied	Extract Used	Type of NPs	Activity Studied	Concluding Remarks	References
A. paniculata	Aqueous	Gold NPs	*In vivo* biological effect on embryonic zebrafish	When AuNPs are exposed to embryonic zebrafish, cytotoxicity results from increased reactive oxygen species.	[59]
A. paniculata	Aqueous	Silver NPs	Anti-fungal activity	The synthesized Ag NPs have very good antifungal activity.	[60]
A. paniculata	Ethanol	Zinc oxide NPs	Anticancer activity	The negatively charged cellular membrane is capable of absorbing ZnO NPs for efficient intracellular distribution and effective anticancer activity.	[50]
A. paniculata	Aqueous	Silver NPs and copper NPs	Anti-bacterial activity	Various biomedical applications for infection prevention may benefit from cotton bandages biofabricated with Ag and Cu NPs.	[37]
A. paniculata	Aqueous	Zinc oxide NPs	Anti-oxidant anti-diabetic anti-inflammatory	The synthesized ZnO NPs can be used to reduce sugar levels and reduce inflammation.	[53]
A. paniculata	Aqueous	Silver NPs	Hepatocurative activity	Ag NPs with low dose (25 mg/kg BW) were effective in the revival of all biological parameters to normal in all intoxicated groups, indicating the curing effects on CCl_4-induced liver injury.	[57]

(Table 2) cont.....

Andrographis Species Studied	Extract Used	Type of NPs	Activity Studied	Concluding Remarks	References
A. paniculata	Aqueous	Silver NPs	Antifilarial activity	Green NPs showed maximum antifilarial efficacy against adult filarial parasites.	[58]
A. paniculata	Ethanol	Lanthanum oxide NPs	Anticancer activity Anti-bacterial activity	La_2O_3 NPs can be utilized in different biological applications in the food and biomedical industries.	[51]
A. paniculata	Ethanol	Samarium oxide NPs	Anti-bacterial activity Anti-oxidant activity Anti-inflammatory activity	Using different concentrations of standard drugs with bovine serum and egg albumin denaturation assays, the anti-inflammatory activity was detected. Sm_2O_3 NPs with IL assistance had a stronger antioxidant effect than vitamin C.	[61]
A. paniculata	Ethanol	Neodymium oxide NPs	Anti-bacterial, anti-diabetic, anti-cancer, anti-oxidant and anti- inflammatory activities	The NP's activity was pronounced against *S. aureus* and *E. coli*. The anticancer activity of Nd_2O_3 and Nd_2O_3-IL NPs confirmed that the activity was concentration based against MCF-7 breast cancer cells.	[52]

(Table 2) cont.....

Andrographis Species Studied	Extract Used	Type of NPs	Activity Studied	Concluding Remarks	References
A. paniculata	Ethanol	Ytterbium oxide NPs	Antibacterial, anti-diabetic, anti-inflammatory and antioxidant activities	High inhibition of Yb_2O_3 and $ILYb_2O_3$ NPs was found against *E. coli* and *S. aureus*. The antidiabetic assay revealed the biomedical behavior of Yb_2O_3 and IL-Yb_2O_3 NPs on α-amylase. The anti-inflammatory assay showed the potential denaturation of bovine serum albumin by Yb_2O_3 and IL- Yb_2O_3 NPs. The antioxidant assay revealed the potential free radical scavenging behavior of Yb_2O_3 and IL-Yb_2O_3NPs. The MTT assay revealed the biomedical potential action of Yb_2O_3 and IL Yb_2O_3 NPs on the MCF-7 cancer cell line.	[54]
A. paniculata	Aqueous	Silver NPs	Anti-tumor activity	Ag NPs were effective against carcinoma cells *in vitro* and *ex vivo*.	[55]
A. paniculata	Aqueous	Silver NPs	Antioxidant activity	The therapeutic dose possessed antioxidant ability in red cells, which might be due to the counteraction of oxidative stress and lipid peroxidation.	[62]

(Table 2) cont.....

Andrographis Species Studied	Extract Used	Type of NPs	Activity Studied	Concluding Remarks	References
A. paniculata	Chloroform	Silver NPs	Anti-cancer activity	Ag-NPs showed maximum activity against HeLa (Human cervical cancer cells) and Hep-2 (Human liver cancer cells)	[47]
A. paniculata	Aqueous	Silver NPs	Antiplasmodial activity	The parasitic property against *Plasmodium falciparum* was analyzed by (IC_{50}) values.	[56]
A. paniculata	Aqueous	Titanium dioxide NPs	Anti-microbial, anti-oxidant and anti-diabetic activities; Zebrafish embryotoxicity	TiO_2 NPs that showed antibacterial activity reduces pathogenic microorganisms. TiO_2 NPs had a significant impact on the surface of the embryo. The green synthesized TiO_2 NPs using *A. paniculata* leaf extract showed potential toxicity in zebrafish.	[41]
A. paniculata	Methanol	Silver NPs	Anti-cancer activity	The Ag NPs of methanol extract of leaves could be a potential anticancer agent against neuroblastoma cells.	[48]
A. paniculata	Aqueous	Silver NPs	Antibacterial activity	Synthesized Ag NPs from leaf extract showed potential antibacterial activity with various human pathogenic bacteria.	[38]

(Table 2) cont.....

Andrographis Species Studied	Extract Used	Type of NPs	Activity Studied	Concluding Remarks	References
A. paniculata	Aqueous Ethyl acetate	Silver NPs	Antibacterial activity	Ag NPs showed better efficiency as bactericidal agents. The Ag NPs coated with bioactive compounds of the plant material can function as a better alternative to control drug-resistant bacteria in place of synthetic medicines used to control or treat bacterial infection.	[39]
A. paniculata	Aqueous	Silver NPs	Antimicrobial activity Antioxidant activity Anticancer activity	Ag NPs showed different activity of leaf extract, *i.e.* strong antioxidant activity, strong antibacterial, and good anticancer activity.	[40]
A. paniculata	Aqueous	Gallium NPs	Antibacterial activity	Green synthesis of gallium NPs can be used in the treatment of bacterial infections.	[43]
A. paniculata	Aqueous	Magnetite NPs	Antidiabetic activity	The $Zn\text{-}Fe_3O_4$NPs strongly inhibited the alpha (α)-amylase enzyme and proved their therapeutic role. $Zn\text{-}Fe_3O_4$NPs are excellent anti-diabetic agents to control type 2 diabetes mellitus.	[63]

(Table 2) cont.....

Andrographis Species Studied	Extract Used	Type of NPs	Activity Studied	Concluding Remarks	References
A. paniculata	Aqueous	Gold NPs	Antibacterial activity Anticancer activity	The antimicrobial efficiency was tested against *E. coli,* and anticancer activity was observed in HeLa cell lines, which proved that the synthesized NPs showed anti-proliferative effects against cervical cancer.	[64]
A. paniculata	Aqueous	Copper NPs	Antibacterial activity	Copper NPs synthesized from aqueous leaf extract showed significant antibacterial activity against selective bacterial species.	[44]
A. paniculata	Aqueous	Silver NPs	Antibacterial activity	The antibacterial activity of synthesized Ag NPs exhibited effective inhibition zones against tested bacterial strains. Among the bacteria tested, *P. aeruginosa* was found to be most susceptible to the Ag NPs.	[34]
A. paniculata	Aqueous	Nickel oxide	Anticancer activity	The anti-breast cancer activity of the prepared NPs was tested against the MCF-7 cell line.	[65]

(Table 2) cont.....

Andrographis Species Studied	Extract Used	Type of NPs	Activity Studied	Concluding Remarks	References
A. paniculata	Aqueous	Silver NPs	Antibacterial activity	Ag NPs were found to be effective against *P.aeruginosa*, *Bacillus* sp., *Micrococcus* sp., and *S. aureus* isolated from the water sample.	[66]
A. paniculata	Aqueous	Silver NPs	Antimicrobial activity	Ag NPs synthesized by leaf extract can also be used in the agriculture industry for effective control of plant pathogens.	[67]
A. paniculata	Aqueous	Silver NPs	Antimicrobial activity	The NPs showed excellent antimicrobial activity against various bacteria. Moreover, *P. aeruginosa* exhibited the highest sensitivity to NPs, while *B. subtilis* was the least sensitive.	[68]
A. paniculata	Aqueous	Hydroxyethylcellulose NPs	Skin permeation, anti-inflammatory activity	The APHECNPs had improved anti-inflammatory activity and skin permeation. These results are promising for the development of HECNPs as drug carriers in biological systems.	[69]
A. paniculata	Aqueous	Copper NPs	Antimicrobial activity	Leaf extract is optimum for the synthesis of copper NPs and it is also known to have the ability to inhibit the growth of various pathogenic microorganisms.	[70]

(Table 2) cont.....

Andrographis Species Studied	Extract Used	Type of NPs	Activity Studied	Concluding Remarks	References
A. paniculata	Ethanol	Gold NPs	Anticancer activity	The synthesized Au NPs were tested for their effect on HeLa (human cervical cancer) and MCF-7 (human breast cancer) cell lines and found to be nontoxic and biocompatible, which are potential carriers for hydrophobic drugs.	[71]
A. paniculata	Aqueous	Cadmium oxide NPs	Antibacterial activity	The bioengineered CdONPs showed good antibacterial activity (zone of inhibition: *E. coli*-16 mm).	[72]
A. echioides	Aqueous	Silver NPs	Antibacterial activity, anti-cancer activity	*In vitro* anticancer activity indicated good biocompatibility of Ag NPs. The antibacterial activity of Ag NPs might be endorsed by the presence of active ingredients (terpenoids)	[49]
A. alata	Aqueous	Zinc oxide NPs	Antibacterial, antioxidant, antidiabetic and anti-Alzheimer's activity	The phytosynthesized ZnO NPs displayed strong anti-bacterial activities against various pathogenic bacterial strains. Moreover, bio-reduced ZnO NPs also had strong anti-oxidant, anti-Alzheimer, and anti-diabetic potencies with IC_{50} values in microgram ranges.	[73]

(Table 2) cont.....

Andrographis Species Studied	Extract Used	Type of NPs	Activity Studied	Concluding Remarks	References
A. serpyllifolia	Aqueous	Zinc oxide NPs	Antimicrobial activity, antidiabetic activity, antioxidant activity	As-ZnO NPs exhibited potential antioxidant activity and effective antibacterial activity against Gram-positive bacteria. ZnO NPs also have potential anti-diabetic activity *in vivo* (rat model).	[36]
A. serpyllifolia	Aqueous	Silver NPs	Antimicrobial activity, antioxidant activity	The antimicrobial studies on Ag NPs on different bacterial strains show effective antimicrobial activity when compared with the standard antibiotic. The biosynthesized As-Ag NPs also showed excellent antioxidant activity using DPPH, nitric oxide, and hydrogen peroxide methods.	[35]
A. serpyllifolia	Aqueous	Silver NPs	Antibacterial activity, larvicidal activity	The antimicrobial study revealed that the Ag NPs have shown prominent activity against the clinical pathogens. Ag NPs demonstrated prominent bioactivity and were used to control the emerging mosquito population.	[46]

(Table 2) cont.....

Andrographis Species Studied	Extract Used	Type of NPs	Activity Studied	Concluding Remarks	References
A. serpyllifolia	Ethanol	Silver NPs	Antibacterial activity, antioxidant activity, anticancer activity	Ag NPs synthesized from ethanol leaf extracts exhibited effective antioxidant and antibacterial as well as cytotoxic activity against liver cancer cell lines.	[74]

Table 3. Andrographolide mediated nanoparticles – synthesis and activity.

Plant Name	Type of Nanoparticles	Activity Studied	Concluding Remarks	References
Andrographis paniculata	Silver	Antimicrobial activity	Andrographolide-stabilized Ag NPs show excellent antimicrobial activity against *B. pseudomallei*.	[29]
Andrographis paniculata	Silver	Antileishmanial activity	Ag NPs have significant potential to target the infested macrophage cells and have proven to be valuable in the chemotherapy of neglected tropical diseases such as leishmaniasis.	[30]
Andrographis paniculata	Gold	Antileishmanial activity	Macrophage cytotoxicity was significantly lower in Au NPs than in Amphotericin-B. Low toxic andrographolide-engineered Au NPs emerged as promising alternatives in the control of wild and drug-resistant visceral leishmaniasis.	[31]
Andrographis paniculata	Gold	Anti-venom activity	Andrographolide-Au NPs may serve as a supportive therapy in snakebite (against venom-induced local damage, organ toxicity, and inflammatory response)	[75]

Antimicrobial Activity

Bacillus cereus (a Gram-positive bacterium) and *Brevibacterium paucivorans* (a Gram-negative bacterium) are highly susceptible to silver nanoparticles derived from leaf extract of *A. echioides* [32]. Silver nanoparticles derived from leaf extract of *A. paniculata* and *A. echioides* showed the maximum zone of inhibition against the bacterium *Klebsiella pneumoniae* and against the fungus *Candida albicans* [33, 34].

Human pathogens were significantly inhibited by silver nanoparticles biosynthesized from *A. serpyllifolia* leaf extract [35]. *A. paniculata* extract-synthesized silver nanoparticles displayed strong antimicrobial activity [36 - 40]. Drug-resistant bacteria were more sensitive to zinc nanoparticles synthesized from aqueous extracts of *A. paniculata* [41]. It has also been demonstrated that gold nanoparticles synthesized from extracts of *A. paniculata* have antimicrobial properties [42]. The aqueous extract of *A. paniculata*-derived gallium nanoparticles was reported to have antimicrobial activity [43]. An aqueous extract of *A. paniculata* was used to produce copper nanoparticles that demonstrated significant antibacterial activity [44].

Antioxidant Activity

Titanium dioxide nanoparticles taken from the plant extract of *A. paniculata* possessed anti-oxidant activity [41]. The silver nanoparticles from *A. paniculata* displayed antioxidant activity against carbon tetrachloride-induced mice [45].

Antilarvicidal Activity

In a study conducted on the effectiveness of silver nanoparticles that were synthesized from the extract of *A. serpyllifolia* leaves, it was found that they are able to kill mosquito larvae [46].

Anticancer Activity

Silver nanoparticles derived from chloroform extract of *A. paniculata* have the highest anticancer activity against HeLa cells and Hep-2 cells [47]. Methanolic extracts of *A. paniculata* leaves showed better anticancer activity against neuroblastoma cells [48]. Silver nanoparticles synthesized from *A. echioides* aqueous extract showed anti-cancer activity [49].

Researchers investigated the anticancer properties of zinc oxide nanoparticles using ethanol extracts of *A. paniculata* [50]. Lanthanum oxide nanoparticles showed good anti-cancer potentials using ethanol extract of *A. paniculata* [51]. The ethanol extract of *A. paniculata* has been shown to have significant anticancer activity against MCF-7 breast cancer cells when used for the biosynthesis of neodymium oxide nanoparticles [52].

Antidiabetic Activity

Green synthesized zinc oxide nanoparticles showed effective antidiabetic activity using aqueous extract of *A. paniculata* [53]. Muthulakshmi and co-workers reported that ytterbium oxide nanoparticles tested for anti-diabetic activity were significant [54]. Using an aqueous extract of *A. paniculata*, titanium oxide nanoparticles were used to study antidiabetic activity in Zebra fish [41].

Antitumor Activity

Silver nanoparticles synthesized from *A. paniculata* exhibited antitumor activity against carcinoma cells *in vitro* and *ex vivo* [55].

Antiplasmodial Activity

From aqueous extracts of *A. paniculata*, silver nanoparticles were synthesized and tested for antiplasmodial activity [56]. The results exhibited that these nanoparticles can be used to develop antiplasmodial agents.

Hepatocurative Activity

Silver nanoparticles phytosynthesized utilizing *A. paniculata* aqueous leaf extract showed effective hepatocurative activity [57].

Antifilarial Activity

Yadav *et al.* [58] reported significant antifilarial activity against adult filarial parasites using silver nanoparticles synthesized from *A. paniculata*.

CHALLENGES AND PROSPECTS IN THE SYNTHESIS AND APPLICATION OF PHYTO-NANOMATERIALS

It has advanced the treatment of a number of diseases, including cardiovascular diseases, cancer, musculoskeletal conditions, neurodegenerative diseases, bacterial and viral infections, and diabetes, by providing innovative imaging techniques and diagnostic tools, drug delivery systems, tissue-engineered constructs, implants, and pharmaceutical therapeutics [76]. A variety of facile methods are being developed for producing monodispersed spherical nanocrystals that can be controlled in particle size, composition, shape, and magnetic properties. The US Food and Drug Administration has approved iron nanoparticles coated with biomolecules for their enhanced biocompatibility. As a result, iron nanoparticles are routinely applied to MRI, drug delivery for targeted disease, gene therapy, cancer treatments, and *in vitro* diagnostics, among other applications [77]. It is important to ensure that the NPs are uniform. Variations in size, shape, and structure are more prevalent in plant-mediated nanoparticles. A major challenge is the conversion of salt to ions. Salt should be converted to ions as efficiently as possible during plant-mediated synthesis. It is important to elucidate how plant molecules function in NPs synthesis. These molecules act as reducing and stabilizing agents, and the production of nontoxic nanoparticles is an unattainable dream. Plant-mediated metallic nanoparticles may pose a threat to humans and the environment, so proper consideration should be given to the potential for toxicity [78].

CONCLUSION

Nanotechnology is a technique capable of achieving a high degree of precision in the functions. This can be performed by controlling the reaction conditions of the molecules participating in the synthesis of the nanoparticles. *Andrographis* is an important medicinal taxon, containing 26 species native to India, and some of the species are present in Southern Eastern Ghats. Only a few species have potential medicinal values. *A. paniculata*, for instance, is extensively used in several medicinal systems, including Ayurveda, Homeopathy, Siddha, Unani, and Naturopathy. Healthcare systems continue to rely heavily on traditional medicine based on plants. Diterpenoid lactone and andrographolide are bitter-tasting phytochemical compounds. Silver nanoparticles derived from *Andrographis* species exhibited a variety of pharmacological activities, *viz.*, antimicrobial, antioxidant, anti-inflammatory, antidiabetic, larvicidal, hepatocurative, and anticancer activity. Nanoparticles synthesized using andrographolide are also effective in exerting antibacterial and antileishmanial activity.

REFERENCES

[1] Elemike EE, Ibe KA, Mbonu JI, Onwudiwe DC. Phytonanotechnology and synthesis of silver nanoparticles.Phytonanotechnology - Challenges and Prospects. Elsevier 2020; pp. 71-96.
[http://dx.doi.org/10.1016/B978-0-12-822348-2.00005-X]

[2] Husam MK, Adnan H. Phytonanotechnology synthesis and characterization of silver nanoparticles using methanolic extract of *L. inermis:* A study of the effect of temperature, ph on the rate of synthesis and biochemical properties. J Glob Pharma Technol 2018; 10: 883-94.

[3] Boopathi CA. *Andrographis* spp.: A source of bitter compounds for medicinal use. Anc Sci Life 2000; 19(3-4): 164-8.
[PMID: 22556939]

[4] Chen K, Wu W, Hou X, Yang Q, Li Z. A review: antimicrobial properties of several medicinal plants widely used in Traditional Chinese Medicine. Food Quality and Safety 2021; 5: fyab020.
[http://dx.doi.org/10.1093/fqsafe/fyab020]

[5] Alagesaboopathi C. Evaluation of antibacterial properties of leaf and stem extracts of *Andrographis elongata* - An endemic medicinal plant of India. Int J Pharma Bio Sci 2013; 4: 503-10.

[6] Krishnaswamy S, Kushalappa BA. Systematic review and meta-analysis of *Andrographis serpyllifolia* (Rottler ex Vahl) Wight: An ethno-pharmaco- botanical perspective. Pharmacogn J 2018; 10(6s): s14-26.
[http://dx.doi.org/10.5530/pj.2018.6s.3]

[7] Stephen sharon, Thomas T. A review on green synthesis of silver nanoparticles by employing plants of Acanthaceae and its bioactivities. Nanomed Res J 2020; 5: 215-24.

[8] Karmegam N, Nagaraj R, Karuppusamy S, Prakash M. Biological and pharmacological activities of *Andrographis* spp. (Acanthaceae) distributed in Southern Eastern Ghats, India. Int J Curr Res Biosci Plant Biol 2015; 2: 140-53.

[9] Hossain MS, Urbi Z, Sule A, Rahman KMH. *Andrographis paniculata* (Burm. f.) Wall. ex Nees: a review of ethnobotany, phytochemistry, and pharmacology. ScientificWorldJournal 2014; 2014: 1-28.
[http://dx.doi.org/10.1155/2014/274905] [PMID: 25950015]

[10] Mathivanan D, Suseem SR. Phytochemical and pharmacological review of *Andrographis echiodies*. Malaya J Biosci 2015; 2: 91-5.

[11] Krishnaswamy S, Kushalappa BA. Systematic review and meta-analysis of *Andrographis serpyllifolia* (Rottler ex Vahl) Wight: An ethno-pharmaco-botanical perspective. Pharmacogn J 2018; 10(6s): s14-26.
[http://dx.doi.org/10.5530/pj.2018.6s.3]

[12] Zhang C, Gui L, Xu Y, Wu T, Liu D. Preventive effects of andrographolide on the development of diabetes in autoimmune diabetic NOD mice by inducing immune tolerance. Int Immunopharmacol 2013; 16(4): 451-6.
[http://dx.doi.org/10.1016/j.intimp.2013.05.002] [PMID: 23707775]

[13] Chakravarti RN, Chakravarti D. Andrographolide, the active constituent of *Andrographis paniculata* Nees; a preliminary communication. Ind Med Gaz 1951; 86(3): 96-7.
[PMID: 14860885]

[14] Jarukamjorn K, Nemoto N. Pharmacological aspects of *Andrographis paniculata* on health and its major diterpenoid constituent andrographolide. J Health Sci 2008; 54(4): 370-81.
[http://dx.doi.org/10.1248/jhs.54.370]

[15] Woo AYH, Waye MMY, Tsui SKW, Yeung STW, Cheng CHK. Andrographolide up-regulates cellular-reduced glutathione level and protects cardiomyocytes against hypoxia/reoxygenation injury. J Pharmacol Exp Ther 2008; 325(1): 226-35.
[http://dx.doi.org/10.1124/jpet.107.133918] [PMID: 18174384]

[16] Lee JC, Tseng CK, Young KC, *et al.* Andrographolide exerts anti-hepatitis C virus activity by up-regulating haeme oxygenase-1 *via* the p38 MAPK / N rf2 pathway in human hepatoma cells. Br J Pharmacol 2014; 171(1): 237-52.
[http://dx.doi.org/10.1111/bph.12440] [PMID: 24117426]

[17] Lin FL, Wu SJ, Lee SC, Ng LT. Antioxidant, antioedema and analgesic activities of *Andrographis paniculata* extracts and their active constituent andrographolide. Phytother Res 2009; 23(7): 958-64.
[http://dx.doi.org/10.1002/ptr.2701] [PMID: 19142986]

[18] Sheeja K, Guruvayoorappan C, Kuttan G. Antiangiogenic activity of *Andrographis paniculata* extract and andrographolide. Int Immunopharmacol 2007; 7(2): 211-21.
[http://dx.doi.org/10.1016/j.intimp.2006.10.002] [PMID: 17178389]

[19] Saraswat B, Visen P, Patnaik G, *et al.* Effect of andrographolide against galactosamine-induced hepatotoxicity. Fitoter 66, 415–420. Fitoter 1995; 66: 415-20.

[20] Zhang CY, Tan BKH. Mechanisms of cardiovascular activity of *Andrographis paniculata* in the anaesthetized rat. J Ethnopharmacol 1997; 56(2): 97-101.
[http://dx.doi.org/10.1016/S0378-8741(97)01509-2] [PMID: 9174969]

[21] Yadav JS, Singh TP. Phytochemical analysis and antifungal activity of *Andrographis paniculata*. Int J Pharm Res Biosci 2012; 1: 240-63.

[22] Tan Lim AM, Oyong GG, Tan MCS, Chang Shen C, Ragasa CY, Cabrera EC. Quorum quenching activity of *Andrographis paniculata* (Burm f.) Nees andrographolide compounds on metallo--lactamase-producing clinical isolates of *Pseudomonas aeruginosa* PA22 and PA247 and their effect on *lasR* gene expression. Heliyon 2021; 7(5): e07002.
[http://dx.doi.org/10.1016/j.heliyon.2021.e07002] [PMID: 34027192]

[23] Das P, Srivastav AK. Phytochemical extraction and characterization of the leaves of *Andrographis paniculata* for its anti-bacterial, anti-oxidant, anti-pyretic and anti-diabetic activity. Int J Innov Res Sci Eng Technol 2014; 3(8): 15176-84.

[http://dx.doi.org/10.15680/IJIRSET.2014.0308016]

[24]   Mulukuri NVLS, Mondal NB, Prasad MR, Renuka S. Isolation of diterpenoid lactones from the leaves of *Andrographis paniculata* and its anticancer activity. Int J Pharmacogn Phytochem Res 2011; 3.

[25]   Kapil A, Koul IB, Banerjee SK, Gupta BD. Antihepatotoxic effects of major diterpenoid constituents of *Andrographis paniculata*. Biochem Pharmacol 1993; 46(1): 182-5.
[http://dx.doi.org/10.1016/0006-2952(93)90364-3] [PMID: 8347130]

[26]   Chao WW, Kuo YH, Lin BF. Anti-inflammatory activity of new compounds from *Andrographis paniculata* by NF-kappaB transactivation inhibition. J Agric Food Chem 2010; 58(4): 2505-12.
[http://dx.doi.org/10.1021/jf903629j] [PMID: 20085279]

[27]   Chan SJ, Wong WSF, Wong PTH, Bian JS. Neuroprotective effects of andrographolide in a rat model of permanent cerebral ischaemia. Br J Pharmacol 2010; 161(3): 668-79.
[http://dx.doi.org/10.1111/j.1476-5381.2010.00906.x] [PMID: 20880404]

[28]   Yan Y, Fang L-H, Du G-H. Andrographolide. Nat. Small Mol. Drugs from Plants.Singapore: Springer Singapore 2018; pp. 357-62.
[http://dx.doi.org/10.1007/978-981-10-8022-7_60]

[29]   Thammawithan S, Talodthaisong C, Srichaiyapol O, Patramanon R, Hutchison JA, Kulchat S. Andrographolide stabilized-silver nanoparticles overcome ceftazidime-resistant *Burkholderia pseudomallei*: study of antimicrobial activity and mode of action. Sci Rep 2022; 12(1): 10701.
[http://dx.doi.org/10.1038/s41598-022-14550-x] [PMID: 35739211]

[30]   Suvadra Das, Tanmoy Bera, Subhasis Mondol, Arup Mukherjee Andrographolide nanoparticles in leishmaniasis: characterization and in vitro evaluations. Int J NanomedicineDovepresssubmit 2010; pp. 1113-21.

[31]   Das S, Halder A, Mandal S, *et al.* Andrographolide engineered gold nanoparticle to overcome drug resistant visceral leishmaniasis. Artif Cells Nanomed Biotechnol 2018; 46(sup1): 751-62.
[http://dx.doi.org/10.1080/21691401.2018.1435549] [PMID: 29421940]

[32]   Sathish Kumar D, Francis Xavier T. Antibacterial activity, biosynthesis and characterization of Silver nanoparticle from the leaf extract of *Andrographis echioides* (L.) Nees. Asian J Pharm Pharmacol 2018; 5(1): 95-100.
[http://dx.doi.org/10.31024/ajpp.2019.5.1.14]

[33]   Anantharaman S, Rego R, Muthakka M, Anties T, Krishna H. *Andrographis paniculata*-mediated synthesis of silver nanoparticles: antimicrobial properties and computational studies. SN Applied Sciences 2020; 2(9): 1618.
[http://dx.doi.org/10.1007/s42452-020-03394-7]

[34]   Sinha SN, Paul D. Phytosynthesis of silver nanoparticles using *Andrographis paniculata* leaf extract and evaluation of their antibacterial activities. Spectrosc Lett 2015; 48(8): 600-4.
[http://dx.doi.org/10.1080/00387010.2014.938756]

[35]   Palithya S, Kotakadi VS, Pechalaneni J, Challagundla VN. Biofabrication of silver nanoparticles by leaf extract of *Andrographis serpyllifolia* and their antimicrobial and antioxidant activity. Int J Nanodimens 2018; 9: 398-407.

[36]   Kotakadi VS, Gaddam SA, Kotha P, Allagadda R, Rao ChA. D. V. R. SG. Bio-inspired multifunctional zinc oxide nanoparticles by leaf extract of *Andrographis serpilifolia* and their enhanced antioxidant, antimicrobial, and antidiabetic activity—a 3-in-1 system. Particul Sci Technol 2022; 40: 485-99.
[http://dx.doi.org/10.1080/02726351.2021.1966145]

[37]   Senthamarai Kannan M, Hari Haran PS, Sundar K, Kunjiappan S, Balakrishnan V. Fabrication of anti-bacterial cotton bandage using biologically synthesized nanoparticles for medical applications. Prog Biomater 2022; 11(2): 229-41.
[http://dx.doi.org/10.1007/s40204-022-00190-x] [PMID: 35622299]

[38] Saratha V, Subasri S, Usharani S. Synthesis of silver nanoparticles from *Andrographis paniculata* and evaluation of their antibacterial activity. Innovare J Life Sci 2018; 6: 10-4.

[39] Abirami T, Govindarajulu B, Karthikeyan J. Green synthesis of silver nanoparticles using aqueous leaf extract of *Andrographis paniculata* and the evaluation of their antibacterial efficacy. J Pharmacogn Phytochem 2019; 8: 3224-8.

[40] Gowsalya P, Mohanapriya T. Biosynthesis of silver nanoparticles from leaf extract of *Andrographis paniculata* leaf extract and its antimicrobial, antioxidant, anticancer activities. Int J Adv Res Innov Ideas Educ 2022; 8.

[41] Rajeshkumar S, Santhoshkumar J, Jule LT, Ramaswamy K. Phytosynthesis of titanium dioxide nanoparticles using king of bitter *Andrographis paniculata* and its embryonic toxicology evaluation and biomedical potential. Bioinorg Chem Appl 2021; 2021: 1-11.
[http://dx.doi.org/10.1155/2021/6267634] [PMID: 34659389]

[42] Razalli N, Gopinath SCB, Kasim FH, Yaakub ARW, Anbu P. Antimicrobial potential of *Andrographis paniculata* conjugated gold nanoparticle. INNOSC Theranostics and Pharmacological Sciences 2019; 2(1): 17-22.
[http://dx.doi.org/10.26689/itps.v2i1.744]

[43] Monika S, Ponlakshmi SH, Sundar K, Vanavil B. Biological synthesis of gallium nanoparticles using extracts of *Andrographis paniculata.* Int J Eng Sci Adv Comput Bio-Technology 2018; 8: 208-22.

[44] Biswas S, Chakraborty S, Mulaba-Bafubiandi AF. Optimization of copper nanoparticle biosynthesis process using aqueous extract of *Andrographis paniculata.* Afr J Sci Technol Innov Dev 2017; 9(1): 131-8.
[http://dx.doi.org/10.1080/20421338.2016.1269463]

[45] Darbar S, Saha S, Chattopadhyay A. Free radical scavenging potential and antioxidant activity of silver nanoparticle coupled with *Andrographis paniculata* (Ap-Ag NP) against carbon tetrachloride (CCl$_4$) induced toxicity in mice. Innoriginal Int J Sci 2019; 1-6.

[46] Madhankumar R, Sivasankar P, Kalaimurugan D, Murugesan S. Antibacterial and larvicidal activity of silver nanoparticles synthesized by the leaf extract of *Andrographis serpyllifolia* Wight. J Cluster Sci 2020; 31(4): 719-26.
[http://dx.doi.org/10.1007/s10876-019-01679-5]

[47] Dhamodaran M, Kavitha S. *In-vitro* anticancer activity of silver nanoparticle in terpenoid for *Andrographis paniculata* (Ag-Nps TAP) by MTT assay method against Hela &Hep-2. Int J Adv Res Chem Sci 2015; 2: 8-13.

[48] Selvam P, Wadhwani A. Design and synthesis of biogenic silver nanoparticles from *Andragraphis paniculata* as potential anticancer agents. Indian J Pharm Sci 2019; 81: 1.
[http://dx.doi.org/10.4172/pharmaceutical-sciences.1000495]

[49] Elangovan K, Elumalai D, Anupriya S, Shenbhagaraman R, Kaleena PK, Murugesan K. Phyto mediated biogenic synthesis of silver nanoparticles using leaf extract of *Andrographis echioides* and its bio-efficacy on anticancer and antibacterial activities. J Photochem Photobiol B 2015; 151: 118-24.
[http://dx.doi.org/10.1016/j.jphotobiol.2015.05.015] [PMID: 26233711]

[50] Kavitha S, Dhamodaran M, Prasad R, Ganesan M. Synthesis and characterisation of zinc oxide nanoparticles using terpenoid fractions of *Andrographis paniculata* leaves. Int Nano Lett 2017; 7(2): 141-7.
[http://dx.doi.org/10.1007/s40089-017-0207-1]

[51] Veerasingam M, Murugesan B, Mahalingam S. Ionic liquid mediated morphologically improved lanthanum oxide nanoparticles by *Andrographis paniculata* leaves extract and its biomedical applications. J Rare Earths 2020; 38(3): 281-91.
[http://dx.doi.org/10.1016/j.jre.2019.06.006]

[52] Sundrarajan M, Muthulakshmi V. Green synthesis of ionic liquid mediated neodymium oxide

nanoparticles by *Andrographis paniculata* leaves extract for effective bio-medical applications. J Environ Chem Eng 2021; 9(1): 104716.
[http://dx.doi.org/10.1016/j.jece.2020.104716]

[53]   Rajakumar G, Thiruvengadam M, Mydhili G, Gomathi T, Chung IM. Green approach for synthesis of zinc oxide nanoparticles from *Andrographis paniculata* leaf extract and evaluation of their antioxidant, anti-diabetic, and anti-inflammatory activities. Bioprocess Biosyst Eng 2018; 41(1): 21-30.
[http://dx.doi.org/10.1007/s00449-017-1840-9] [PMID: 28916855]

[54]   Muthulakshmi V, Kumar P, Sundrarajan M. Green synthesis of Ionic liquid mediated Ytterbium oxide nanoparticles by *Andrographis Paniculata* leaves extract for structural, morphological and biomedical applications. J Environ Chem Eng 2021; 9(4): 105270.
[http://dx.doi.org/10.1016/j.jece.2021.105270]

[55]   Jiang C, Jiang Z, Zhu S, *et al.* Biosynthesis of silver nanoparticles and the identification of possible reductants for the assessment of *in vitro* cytotoxic and *in vivo* antitumor effects. J Drug Deliv Sci Technol 2021; 63: 102444.
[http://dx.doi.org/10.1016/j.jddst.2021.102444]

[56]   Ponarulselvam S, Panneerselvam C, Murugan K, Aarthi N, Kalimuthu K, Thangamani S. Synthesis of silver nanoparticles using leaves of *Catharanthus roseus* Linn. G. Don and their antiplasmodial activities. Asian Pac J Trop Biomed 2012; 2(7): 574-80.
[http://dx.doi.org/10.1016/S2221-1691(12)60100-2] [PMID: 23569974]

[57]   Suriyakalaa U, Antony JJ, Suganya S, *et al.* Hepatocurative activity of biosynthesized silver nanoparticles fabricated using *Andrographis paniculata*. Colloids Surf B Biointerfaces 2013; 102: 189-94.
[http://dx.doi.org/10.1016/j.colsurfb.2012.06.039] [PMID: 23018020]

[58]   Yadav S, Sharma S, Ahmad F, Rathaur S. Antifilarial efficacy of green silver nanoparticles synthesized using *Andrographis paniculata*. J Drug Deliv Sci Technol 2020; 56: 101557.
[http://dx.doi.org/10.1016/j.jddst.2020.101557]

[59]   Kumari S, kumari P, Panda PK, Pramanik N, Verma SK, Mallick MA. Molecular aspect of phytofabrication of gold nanoparticle from *Andrographis peniculata* photosystem II and their *in vivo* biological effect on embryonic zebrafish (*Danio rerio*). Environ Nanotechnol Monit Manag 2019; 11: 100201.
[http://dx.doi.org/10.1016/j.enmm.2018.100201]

[60]   Kotakadi VS, Gaddam SA, Subba Rao Y, Prasad TNVKV, Varada Reddy A, Sai Gopal DVR. Biofabrication of silver nanoparticles using *Andrographis paniculata*. Eur J Med Chem 2014; 73: 135-40.
[http://dx.doi.org/10.1016/j.ejmech.2013.12.004] [PMID: 24389508]

[61]   Muthulakshmi V, Balaji M, Sundrarajan M. Biomedical applications of ionic liquid mediated samarium oxide nanoparticles by *Andrographis paniculata* leaves extract. Mater Chem Phys 2020; 242: 122483.
[http://dx.doi.org/10.1016/j.matchemphys.2019.122483]

[62]   Gopalakrishnan V, Radha K V, Devasena T. Silver nanoparticles synthesised using *Andrographis paniculata* ameliorates oxidative stress in erythrocyte model. Mater Res Express 2019; 6: 0850b6.
[http://dx.doi.org/10.1088/2053-1591/ab24ea]

[63]   Athithan ASS, Jeyasundari J, Renuga D, Naveena A. Nature inspired synthesis, physico-chemical characterization of Zn doped Fe_3O_4 nanoparticles using *Andrographis paniculata* (Burm. f.) Nees leaf extract and assessment of *in vitro* pancreatic alpha amylase inhibitory activity. Int J Appl Pharm 2020; 229-35.
[http://dx.doi.org/10.22159/ijap.2020v12i6.39278]

[64]   Kamala Priya MR, Iyer PR. Anti-cancer activity in hela cell lines of phytosynthesized gold nanocompounds using *Andrographis paniculata* (Nilavembu) - characterisation, optimization,

Phytochemicalanalysis & antimicrobial study. Indian Hournal Appl Res 2019; 9.

[65]   Karthik K, Shashank M, Revathi V, Tatarchuk T. Facile microwave-assisted green synthesis of NiO nanoparticles from *Andrographis paniculata* leaf extract and evaluation of their photocatalytic and anticancer activities. Mol Cryst Liq Cryst (Phila Pa) 2018; 673(1): 70-80.
        [http://dx.doi.org/10.1080/15421406.2019.1578495]

[66]   Jayashree S, Vani GS. *In vitro* study on antibacterial activity of aqueous extract and silver nanoparticles of *Andrographis paniculata*. Int J Curr Microbiol Appl Sci 2016; 5(5): 400-6.
        [http://dx.doi.org/10.20546/ijcmas.2016.505.041]

[67]   Kalbande B, Yadav A. Potential antimicrobial activity of silver nanoparticles biosynthesized by leaf extract of *Andrographis paniculata*. Int J Adv Sci Res 2021; 2021: 83-90.

[68]   Sudhakar PS, Krishna KBM, Sundar BS. Synthesis and characterization of silver nanoparticles using aqueous extract of *Andrographis paniculata* and their antimicrobial activities. Int J Sci Technol 2014; p. 29.

[69]   Singchuwong T, Chareonviriyaphap T, Leepasert T, Taengphan W, Karpkird T. Anti-inflammatory potential and enhanced skin permeation of *Andrographis paniculata* crude extract-loaded Hydroxyethylcellulose nanoparticles. SSRN Electron J 2022.
        [http://dx.doi.org/10.2139/ssrn.4264154]

[70]   Devasenan S, Hajara Beevi N, Jayanthi S. Synthesis and characterization of copper nanoparticles using leaf extract of *Andrographis paniculata* and their antimicrobial activities. Int J Chemtech Res 2016; 9: 725-30.

[71]   Babu PJ, Saranya S, Sharma P, Tamuli R, Bora U. Gold nanoparticles: sonocatalytic synthesis using ethanolic extract of *Andrographis paniculata* and functionalization with polycaprolactone-gelatin composites. Front Mater Sci 2012; 6(3): 236-49.
        [http://dx.doi.org/10.1007/s11706-012-0175-3]

[72]   Karthik K, Dhanuskodi S, Gobinath C, Prabukumar S, Sivaramakrishnan S. *Andrographis paniculata* extract mediated green synthesis of CdO nanoparticles and its electrochemical and antibacterial studies. J Mater Sci Mater Electron 2017; 28(11): 7991-8001.
        [http://dx.doi.org/10.1007/s10854-017-6503-8]

[73]   Dappula SS, Kandrakonda YR, Shaik JB, *et al.* Biosynthesis of zinc oxide nanoparticles using aqueous extract of *Andrographis alata*: Characterization, optimization and assessment of their antibacterial, antioxidant, antidiabetic and anti-Alzheimer's properties. J Mol Struct 2023; 1273: 134264.
        [http://dx.doi.org/10.1016/j.molstruc.2022.134264]

[74]   Kumar RM, Murugesan S. Biosynthesis of silver nanoparticles using *Andrographis serpyllifolia* (Rottler ex Vahl) Wight leaf extracts there in-Vitro biological properties. Int J Bot Stud 2021; 6: 605-10.

[75]   Ghosh S, Dasgupta SC, Dasgupta AK, Gomes A, Gomes A. Gold nanoparticles (AuNPs) conjugated with andrographolide ameliorated viper (*Daboia russellii russellii*) venom-induced toxicities in animal model. J Nanosci Nanotechnol 2020; 20(6): 3404-14.
        [http://dx.doi.org/10.1166/jnn.2020.17421] [PMID: 31748033]

[76]   Sim S, Wong N. Nanotechnology and its use in imaging and drug delivery (Review). Biomed Rep 2021; 14(5): 42.
        [http://dx.doi.org/10.3892/br.2021.1418] [PMID: 33728048]

[77]   Ali A, Zafar H, Zia M, *et al.* Synthesis, characterization, applications, and challenges of iron oxide nanoparticles. Nanotechnol Sci Appl 2016; 9: 49-67.
        [http://dx.doi.org/10.2147/NSA.S99986] [PMID: 27578966]

[78]   Patil S, Chandrasekaran R. Biogenic nanoparticles: a comprehensive perspective in synthesis, characterization, application and its challenges. J Genet Eng Biotechnol 2020; 18(1): 67.
        [http://dx.doi.org/10.1186/s43141-020-00081-3] [PMID: 33104931]

CHAPTER 14

Cultivation of *Andrographis paniculata* (Burm. f.) Nees

M. Johnson[1,*], **B. Shivananthini**[1], **S. Preethi**[1], **Vidyarani George**[1] and **I. Silvia Juliet**[1]

[1] *Centre for Plant Biotechnology, Department of Botany, St. Xavier's College (Autonomous), Palayamkottai – 627002, Tamil Nadu, India*

Abstract: The present chapter provides different cultivation methods used to propagate *Andrographis paniculata* and other factors that regulate the growth and yield of the bioactive principles of andrographolides. The propagation of the Kalmegh is of two types: vegetative, utilizing stem cuttings, and sexual, through seeds. Much work has been done on the *in vitro* propagation of Kalmegh. The growth and quality of the plant are affected by the following factors: plant geometry, planting density and harvesting time, soil health, fertigation, shading level, endophytes, plant growth regulators, weeding control techniques, different accessions of seeds, plant density, co-cultivation, and aging. The available result revealed plots with 30 × 20 cm, cocopeat-RHA medium, and 50 ppm magnesium composition, and integrated use of chemical fertilizers, biofertilizers, and vermicompost treatments were optimum conditions for better yield. Among different seed cultivars, Pranchiburi cultivars showed a good percentage of germination and growth, and the highest andrographolide content was recorded at 135 DAP in the flowering stage. GA_3 treatment, 25% shading level, and co-cultivation with *Cajanus cajan* exhibited better yield and quality of *A. paniculata*. In dry storage, 1 to 3 months and 25°C temperature were recommended. Further works in vegetative propagation may bring out alternative and rapid multiplication methods for large-scale propagation of *A. paniculata*.

Keywords: *Andrographis paniculata*, Andrographolide content, Growth, Plant growth regulators, Seed cultivars, Vegetative propagation, Yield.

INTRODUCTION

Plant cultivation is accomplished through different propagation methods, *viz* ., sexual propagation and vegetative propagation. Sexual propagation includes seed propagation. It is a cost-effective and satisfactory method of plant propagation. Cuttings, layering, and grafting techniques execute vegetative propagation [1].

* **Corresponding author M. Johnson:** Centre for Plant Biotechnology, Department of Botany, St. Xavier's College (Autonomous), Palayamkottai – 627002, Tamil Nadu, India; E-mail: cpbsxc@gmail.com; ptcjohnson@gmail.com

S. Karuppusamy, Vinod K. Nelson & T. Pullaiah (Eds.)

Hydroponics and aeroponics are recent trends in agriculture technology, where plants are cultivated in soil-less cultures under controlled environmental conditions [2].

About 70,000 species of medicinal and aromatic plants are listed worldwide, of which 3,000 are commercially essential plants in trade. Of these, only 900 species are cultivated, and others are exploited from the wild. Annually, India contributes $ 150 million to the present global trade, which is scanty. India recorded 960 medicinal plants that were traded [3]. Among these, 178 species are needed in high volumes of more than 100 tonnes (dry weight) annual requirement. Out of these, only 36 species were cultivated for use. Medicinal and aromatic plants such as mint, basil, chamomile, isabgol, senna, ashwagandha, and opium poppy are cultivated successfully, and India is the largest producer and exporter of these plants [4].

Andrographis paniculata is a member of Acanthaceae and is commonly known as 'Kalmegh'. Various vernacular names also realize it. In north-eastern India, it is known as 'Maha-tita', which means 'King of bitters'. In Tamil, it is known as '*Nila Vembu*'. Among the 26 species of *Andrographis* distributed in tropical Asia, *A. paniculata* is the most popular medicinal plant. Plenty of work has been done to explore the chemical constituents and biological potentials of *A. paniculata* because of its tremendous medicinal importance. *A. paniculata* is mentioned in several countries, such as Materia Medica, and it was mentioned as a widely used medicinal plant in a WHO monograph intended to monitor quality control and herbal medicine usage [5, 6].

Due to the massive demand for *A. paniculata* and *A. paniculata*-based drugs, it is very important and necessary to conserve and cultivate this medicinal plant for sustainable utilization and future use. The tropical and subtropical plains are best for cultivation, and they require clay loam soil to fertile sandy loam soil and a partially shady environment for better growth and yield [7]. In the case of *A. paniculata* cultivation, seed propagation is the most commonly used technique [7, 8]. Vegetative propagation of *A. paniculata* is poor and done by shoot cuttings [9, 10]. Inter-crop cultivation, co-cultivation, integrated nutrient management, ratooning, and fertigation are different methods adopted for the large-scale cultivation of plants [11 - 13]. However, the quality of the plant product, such as the concentration and composition of its phytochemicals, is controlled and affected by different factors, including plant geography, season, soil type, soil health, microbial flora, plant parts, phenological growth stage, harvesting time, time of planting, density of plant growth, shading level, and weeds [14 - 21]. Hence, the present review aims to summarize and provide an idea about the different cultivation methods (Fig. **1**) used to propagate *A. paniculata* and other factors that regulate the growth and yield of the bioactive principles andrographolides.

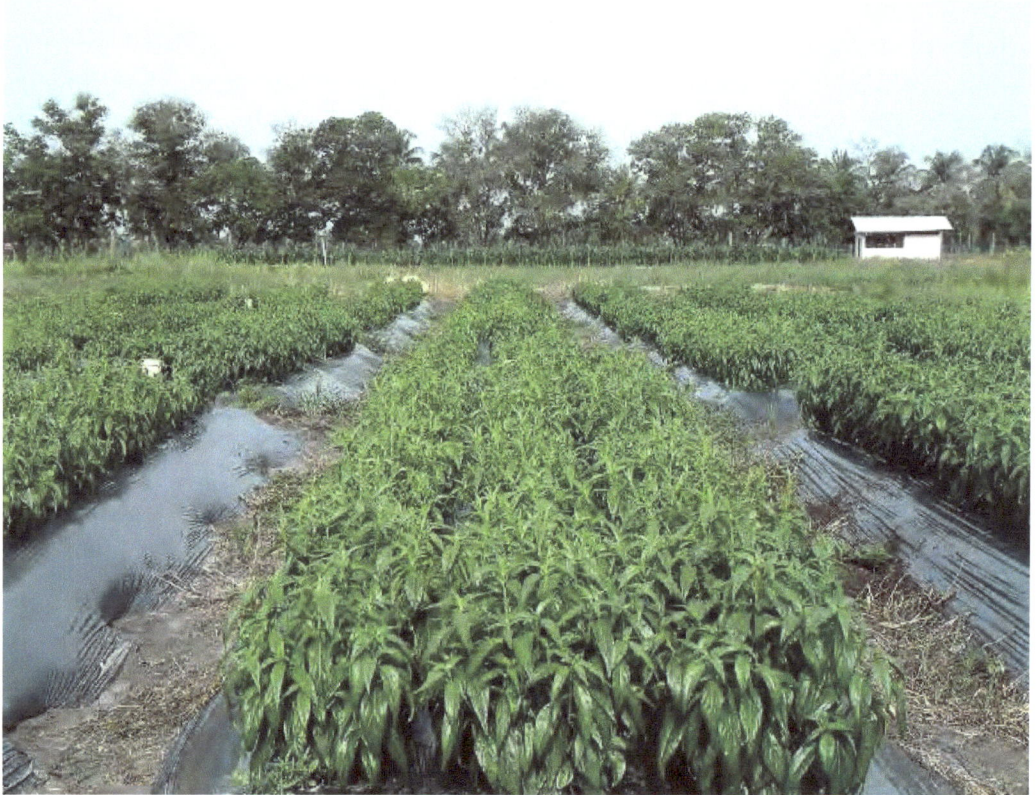

Fig. (1). Cultivation of *Andrographis paniculata* [Source: Global Information Hub on Integrated Medicinehttps://globinmed.com/conservation/hempedu-bumi-79366/].

PROPAGATION OF *ANDROGRAPHIS PANICULATA*

Effect of NAA on the Vegetative Propagation of *A. paniculata*

Hossain and Urbi [9] assessed the effect of NAA on the adventitious rooting in shoot cuttings of *A. paniculata*. The slant cuttings were made, and basal cuttings were soaked in different concentrations of NAA at 0, 0.5, 1.0, 1.5, 2.0, 2.5, and 3.0 mM for 4 seconds without plant growth regulators as control. The cuttings were transferred to the planting tray after 10 minutes of soaking. For each treatment, three replicates were done, and the experiment was repeated twice. The treated cuttings were inoculated into peat moss in the planting tray and further incubated for 15 days under complete shade with temperature ($25 \pm 2°$ C) and relative humidity ($80 \pm 5\%$) for root induction. Water was sprayed once to moisten peat moss. The result showed that root characteristics of *A. paniculata* were significantly (P ≤ 0.05) affected by different concentrations of NAA. Compared to other concentrations and old apical shoots, 2.5 mM of NAA was more productive in induced rooting in young apical shoot cuttings. The researcher concluded that different concentrations of phytohormones and juvenility of plant material affect adventitious rooting, and this technique could be used for commercial propagation of *A. paniculata* (Fig. **2**).

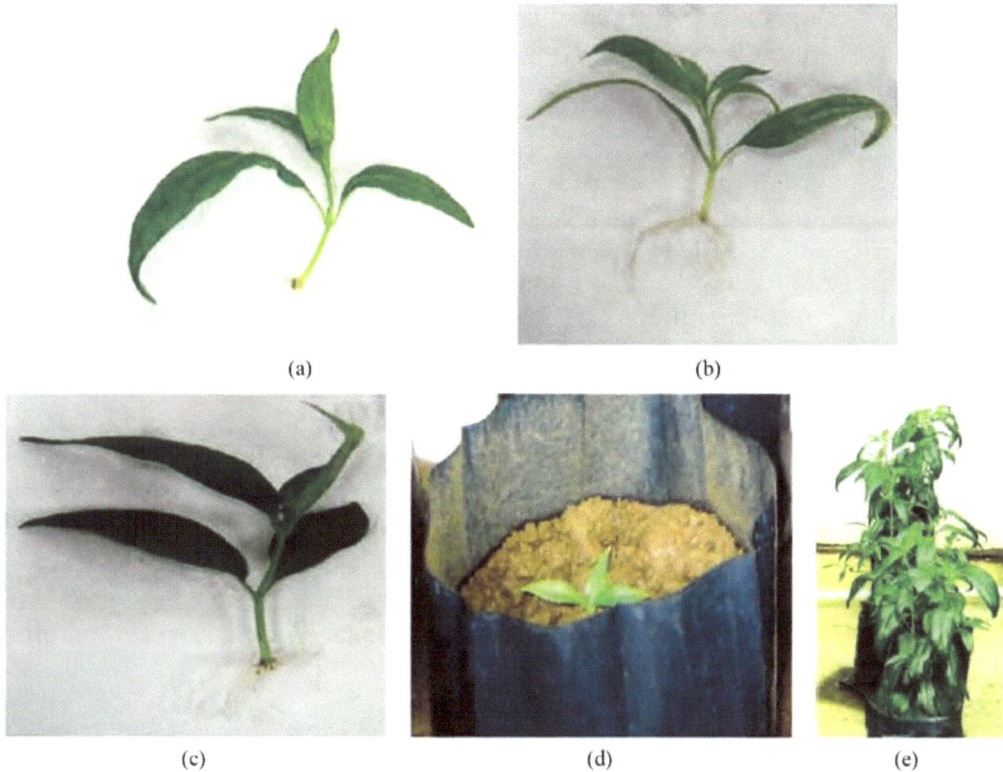

(a)   (b)

(c)   (d)   (e)

Fig. (2). Cultivation of *A. paniculata* from stem cuttings (a-e) (Source: Hossain and Urbi [9],).

An experiment was designed to study the germination, propagation, and selection of *A. paniculata* for future breeding programs. The mother plants were collected from five different populations in Peninsular Malaysia. One hundred viable seeds from mother plants were used for the seed germination test. Matured stems from mother plants were cut slanted within 5 to 7 cm. The bottom of the cutting was dipped into rooting hormone, and stems were planted into the planting bed that contained 100% sand media. The rooted stem cuttings were transferred to different media containing different composition ratios of topsoil, sand, sawdust, coco peat, and CompAcc in the 8" × 8" polybags. The polybags were placed in different growing conditions with open areas and 50% shade. Leaf length, width, number, and collar diameter were recorded. The plants survived and grew well for germplasm conservation and were transferred to a big pot. A quantitative analysis of andrographolide was done to select high-yielding populations. The result of stem cuttings revealed an 80% survival rate. Seed germination results showed a higher percentage at 61% in laboratory conditions than in the nursery, which showed only a 38% germination rate. The survival rate for stem cuttings showed a higher survival rate compared to seed. Hence, stem cuttings were chosen for germplasm establishment. At three months, a maximum number of leaves (14.5 ± 1.73 cm) was obtained while treating CompAcc media in an open area. The andrographolide content was recorded at 9.0 µg/ml in three populations. The author concluded that CompAcc was the best-growing media for cultivating *A. paniculata* [10].

Different Parameters that Affect Seed Germination

Sujatha *et al*. [22] studied seed germination and seedling growth of *A. paniculata* under abiotic stress conditions. Uniform seeds of *A. paniculata* were surface sterilized with 0.1% $HgCl_2$ for 5 min. Afterward, it was rinsed with tap water, followed by soaking seeds in distilled water in case of control, and soaking others in PEG (5%, 10%), $CdSO_4$ (50, 100 µM), and NaCl (25, 50 mM) for 34 hr at 25 ± 2 °C. Seeds were placed on Petri plates lined with two layers of filter paper moistened with PEG, $CdSO_4$, NaCl, and distilled water of the same concentrations and allowed to germinate in the incubator at 25 ± 2 ° C. Root and shoot length, seed vigor index, and seedling fresh weight was measured after 30 days of incubation. The seeds of *A. paniculata* adversely affected the seedling growth in response to different stress conditions such as water deficit (PEG), cadmium treatments (Cd), and salinity (NaCl). The result revealed decreased seed germination at higher cadmium concentrations, and the root length of *A. paniculata* increased with increased concentration in PEG treatment. The result suggested that *A. paniculata* bear drought even at high concentrations.

Seed germination and seedling development of *A. paniculata* was studied by Jayawardhane *et al*. [8]. Seed moisture content employed oven dry method. Dry storage on seed germination, seed germination, and the effect of 500 ppm GA treatment were studied. Different media were used in equal ratios: sand: coir dust: compost, sand: garden soil, sand: coir dust, and sand: compost. Seedlings were transferred to these media and raised for 45 days in a greenhouse. In 7-day intervals, the height of plants and several leaves was measured. Root, shoot, leaf dry, and fresh weight were measured over 45 days. The results of the seed moisture content of *A. paniculata* revealed that it was below 15%. The storage of *A. paniculata* seeds does not require any special conditions. T_{50} value of *A. paniculata* was > 30 days. Thus, *A. paniculata* seeds were dormant. After GA_3

treatment, the germination percentage and dry storage increased above 80%. The result suggested that *A. paniculata* seeds showed non-deep physiological dormancy. The author recommended 1 to 3 months' dry storage for *A. paniculata*. High growth performance was obtained in the sand: garden soil potting medium.

Kumar *et al.* [23] studied the effect of temperature on seed germination parameters in *A. paniculata*. Six constant temperatures, 15°, 20°, 25°, 30°, 35°, and 40° C, were employed for seed germination of *A. paniculata* variety, "CIM-Megha', combined with 16 hr light and 8 hr dark photoperiod. The percentage of germination and germination energy recorded was 23.6 and 94.6 at 25° C, which was considered a suitable temperature. The higher temperature, 40° C, showed a detrimental effect on germination with 0%. The temperatures of 15°, 20°, 30°, and 35° C showed significant decreases in germination energy and germination percentage compared to 25°C. For seed germination of *A. paniculata*, 5-6 days and 7-9 days were ideal for the first and final count.

A study was carried out to determine the effect of seed deterioration on the viability of *A. paniculata* by accelerated aging under 100% relative humidity and 45° C temperature for ten days. Moisture content, seedling vigor index I & II, germination percentage, and biochemical parameters, such as electrical conductivity were recorded. The result revealed decreased speed and rate of germination, and it confirmed the effects of seed aging on seed quality parameters. Increased electrical conductivity, moisture content, and aging period (7, 8, 9, and 10 DAA) showed a decreased percentage of normal seedlings. The lengthening aging period led to detrimental effects on both seed viability and germination potential [24].

Talei *et al.* [25] conducted dormancy breakage and seed germination studies on *A. paniculata*. The experiment included identifying the best physical or chemical agents that improved seed germination and identifying any substance that hindered seed germination in a controlled growth chamber. The first experiment was conducted in a randomized complete block with two factors and three replications. The genetics of the plant were based on two different accessions, and the scarification method was based on 12 different chemical and physical agents, which were the two factors involved in the first experiment. The second experiment was laid out in a randomized complete block design with five treatments and three replications. Seed coat protein extract (SCPE), boiled SCPE, seed protein extract (SPE), boiled SPE, and distilled water were used as treatments. Seeds scarified with sandpaper recorded the highest and fastest germination percentage among the different physical and chemical scarification methods. 72.7% seed germination was obtained after three days of the scarification, and further, it was increased to 90.4% after 15 days. The mean germination time was noted at (MGT $_{a15}$) 4 days. The other physical and chemical treatments failed to reduce (MGT $_{a15}$) but showed moderate effects on germination, with GP15 ranging from 7% to 64%.

Impact of Plant Geometry

The role of weed control techniques and plant geometries on the growth and herbage yield of *A. paniculata* was studied by Semwal *et al.* [20]. The experiment was carried out at MRDC of G.B. Pant University of Agriculture and Technology, Pantnagar (Uttarakhand), India, during the interval of the 2014 and 2015 kharif seasons. The experiment employed three planting geometries, and the measurements of these were as follows: P1 = 30 x 20 cm, P2 = 40 x 25 cm, and P$_3$ = 50 x 30 cm. The experiment was designed in a split-plot manner with main plots with planting geometries and subplots with weed control practices with three replications. The researcher applied six levels of weed control treatment that includes Pendimethalin treatment at 30 E.C. PE @ 1 kg q.i./ha followed by mechanical weeding by hand hoe at 30-35 DAT, Quizalofop ethyl treatment at 5 E.C. PoE @ 50 g a.i./ha at 3-5 leaves stages of weeds followed by mechanical weeding by hand hoe at 30-35 DAT, combined treatment of both Quizalofop ethyl 5 E.C. PoE @ 50 g a.i./ha at 3-5 leaves stages of weeds and Pendimethalin 30 E.C. PE @ 1 kg q.i./ha followed by with and without mechanical weeding by hand hoe at 30-35 DAT, weedy check and weed free. SIM-Megha variety of *A. paniculata* was used for sowing in the nursery. The result revealed that maximum plant height was observed in plot 1 with 30 × 20 cm and weed-free conditions in both years. All the herbicidal treatments showed a significant increase in plant height. P$_3$ with 50 × 30 cm showed more branches than all the other planting geometries during both years and showed wider plant spread and a higher leaf area index significantly. They produced higher dry matter accumulation by crop at harvest during both years. Weed-free and wider rows in plant geometries increase the number of branches significantly. Combined treatment with both Pendimethalin 30 E.C. PE @ 1 kg q.i./ha and Quizalofop ethyl 5 E.C. PoE @ 50 g a.i./ha at 3-5 leaves stages of weeds followed by mechanical weeding by hand hoe at 30-35 DAT significantly increased the number of branches than other herbicide treatments. In dry matter accumulation, weed-free conditions produce high amounts among the weeds. Combined treatment with both Pendimethalin and Quizalofop ethyl and Pendimethalin 30 E.C. PE @ 1 kg q.i./ha and Quizalofop ethyl 5 E.C. PoE @ 50 g a.i./ha showed similar dry matter accumulation. The statistical result suggested that the production of increased higher plant height, leaf area index, plant dry weight/m^2, and dry herbage yield per hectare of *A. paniculata* was obtained by plot 1 with 30 × 20 cm along with treatment with Pendimethalin 30 E.C. PE @ 1 kg q.i./ha + Quizalofop ethyl 5 E.C. PoE @ 50 g a.i./ha with mechanical weeding by hand hoe at 30-35 DAT.

Patidar *et al.* [26] studied the influence of row spacing and nitrogen levels on the biochemical constituents of *A. paniculata*. The work was carried out in a split-plot design with replication thrice. The study included five nitrogen levels (0, 40, 60, 80, and 100 kg/ha) and three-row spacings (15, 30, and 45 cm) (Figs. **3** & **4**). The result revealed maximum magnitudes of biochemical constituents such as protein, nitrogen, fiber, fat, ash, potassium, phosphorus, and andrographolide content at 80 kg N/ha and 30 cm row spacing.

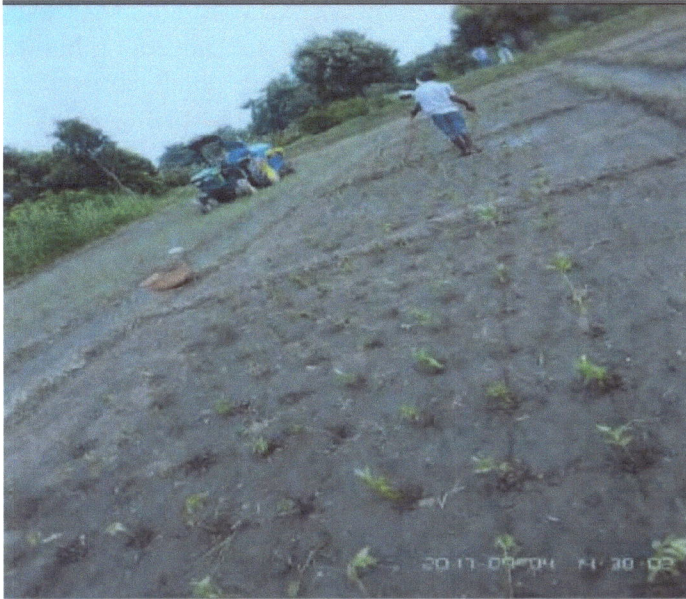

Fig. (3). **Plant geometry of *A. paniculata*** (Source: Verma *et al.* [7]).

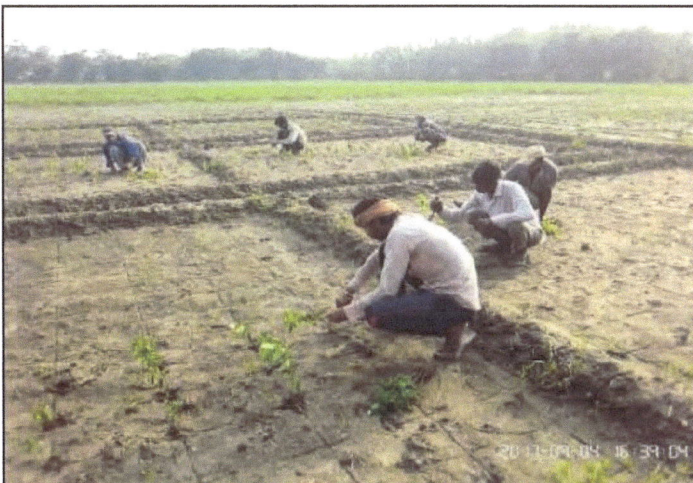

Fig. (4). **Transplanting of *A. paniculata* seedlings** (Source: Verma *et al.* [7]).

Effect of Planting and Harvesting Time

An experiment was designed to study the effect of time of planting and harvesting on growth, herbage yield, and andrographolide content in Kalmegh. The work was conducted at the Vegetable Research Station, Rajendranagar, Hyderabad. It was performed on four different planting dates (1st July, 16th July, 1st August, and 16th August) during the Kharif season. It included 3 stages of harvesting time, *i.e.*, pod setting, flowering, and pre-flowering. Factorial RBD with thrice replications was used for the experiment. CIM-Megha was used for sowing. HPLC procedure was employed to measure the andrographolide content, and further statistical analysis was performed. The result showed increased plant height (54.16), maximum number of branches per plant (16.5), and leaves per plant (262.84), which were recorded in the planting time of 1st August. The maximum herb weight, dry herb weight, and dry herbage yield were recorded in the planting time of 1st August with the respective values of 72.54, 24.32, and 3804.7. The flowering stage of harvest showed a maximum number of leaves per plant (249.15), and the pod-setting stage was recorded with a minimum number of leaves per plant (194.62). Maximum fresh herb weight, dry herb weight, and dry herbage yield were obtained at the pod setting stage with respective values of 83.21, 30.29, and 4644.4. The flowering stage of harvest was noted to have the maximum andrographolide content (2.55) [16].

Detpiratmongkol and Liphan [15] studied the effects of harvesting times on the growth, yield, and quality of *A. paniculata*. Prachinburi, Nakhon Prathom, and Pistanulok 5-4 seed cultivars were used for sowing. The experiment was laid out in a split-plot design, and for the subplot, four harvesting times *viz* , 120, 135, 150, and 170 days after planting (DAP) were used. The height of the plant, branches per plant, number of capsules per plant, leaf and stem dry weight, and andrographolide content were enumerated at the time of harvesting. Plant height was significantly affected by different cultivars. Prachinburi cultivar was recorded with maximum plant height (47.57 cm). NakhonPrathom and Pitsanulok 5-4 were noted with 29.95 and 24.86 cm, respectively. Plants harvested at 170 DAP noted great plant height (39.39 cm), whereas plants harvested at 120 DAP recorded lesser plant height (30.92 cm) respective to harvesting times. In stem dry weight, plants harvested at 170 DAP recorded maximum stem dry weight (3.77 g plant^{-1}), while plants harvested at 120 DAP showed minimum stem dry weight. Pranchiburi cultivar was recorded with a maximum number of branches per plant (48.38), and a minimum number of branches per plant was obtained at Pitsanulok 5-4 cultivar (30.00). Plants harvested at 170 DAP displayed the highest number of branches per plant (40.33), whereas plants harvested at 120 DAP showed the lowest number of branches per plant. The leaf dry weight of Pranchiburi, Nakhon Prathom, and Pitsanulok 5-4 was 2.34 g plant^{-1}, 1.31 g plant^{-1}, and 1.14 g plant^{-1}, respectively. Crop harvested at 135 DAP obtained the highest leaf dry weight (2.15 g plant^{-1}). The lowest leaf dry weight was 1.15 g plant^{-1} recorded at 170 DAP harvesting time. Regarding capsules per plant, the number of capsules per plant for Pranchiburi, Nakhon Prathom, and Pitsanulok 5-4 was 382 and 302. The crop harvested at 170 DAP displayed the highest number of capsules per plant (377), whereas the minimum was recorded in the crops harvested at 120 DAP (269). Pranchiburi cultivar showed a maximum seed dry weight yield (3.61 gm-2), and Pitsanulok displayed a minimum yield (2.08 gm^{-2}). The highest seed dry weight yield was 3.44 gm^{-2}, obtained at 170 DAP. Regarding leaf dry weight, three cultivars showed significant effects. The Prachinburi cultivar displayed maximum andrographolide content (2.93%), while the minimum was recorded at 1.86% in Pitsanulok 5-4 cultivar. Regarding harvesting time, crop age of 135 DAP displayed the highest andrographolide content (2.54%). The lowest andrographolide content was noted at a crop age of 170 DAP (2.07%). The researcher suggested that the Pranchiburi cultivar and the plants harvested at 135 DAP were the best variety and harvesting times for the cultivation of *A. paniculata*.

Work was conducted to study the role of traits for higher production of andrographolide and neo-andrographolide in *A. paniculata* at the pre-flowering harvesting stage. The experiment was carried out in randomized block design with twenty-five treatments and thrice replications at 30 × 30 cm spacing. The plants were harvested at the pre-flowering stage, and further, it was estimated for diterpenoid lactone, andrographolide, and neo-andrographolide content. The obtained result exhibited andrographolide content at 0.634% and neo-andrographolide content at 0.539%. Andrographolide and diterpenoid lactones yield was recorded at 0.634% and 0.523%, respectively. The percentage of andrographolide in plants exhibited a significantly positive correlation with the rate of neo-andrographolide content, diterpenoid lactones yield, andrographolide yield. The multiple regression analysis of biochemical parameters revealed that diterpenoid lactone yield was significantly increased by andrographolide and neo-andrographolide yield in *A. paniculata* at the pre-flowering stage. Neo-andrographolide yield's highest direct positive effect (0.572) on diterpenoid lactone yield was recorded in path value analysis of biochemical parameters. The maximum genetic advance was obtained in neo-andrographolide at 111.34%, andrographolide at 79.81%, and diterpenoid lactones at 90.66% in the analysis of the principal component of biochemical characters at the pre-flowering stage [27].

Kumar and Kumar [28] experimented with spatial and harvesting influences on the growth, quality, yield, and andrographolide content of *A. paniculata*. The experiment was carried out in a split-plot design, with a subplot as planting design and the main plot as harvesting time with three replications. Four harvesting times were recorded at 120, 135, 150, and 170 DAP, and four planting densities were as follows: 30 × 15 cm, 30 × 10 cm, 20 × 15 cm, and 20 × 10 cm. The highest net returns (760.00 EUR ha^{-1}), dry herbage yield (5.14 t ha^{-1}), andrographolide content (2.63%), B: C ratio (2.59), and total yield were obtained with an optimum planting distance of 30 × 15 cm at 135 days DAP. Besides, the maximum dry herbage yield (4.58 t ha^{-1}) and the highest seed yield (19.7 kg ha^{-1}) were registered at plant spacing 20 × 10 cm. The highest iron content was estimated at 120 DAP.

Parashar *et al.* [29] evaluated the morphological and physiological parameters of *A. paniculata* at different growth stages. The work was carried out in a randomized complete block design with four replications. The plants were collected 30, 45, 60, 75, 90, 105 and 120 days after sowing. The researcher evaluated the number of leaves, number of branches, herbage yield, fresh and dry weight of the plant, leaf area index, leaf area duration, specific leaf area, and Biomass duration. The result revealed that all the parameters increased relatively with crop growth stages, but the particular leaf area gradually decreased with the crop's maturity.

Effect of Soil Health on Germination and Crop Productivity

The effect of bioinoculants on promoting soil health, germination, and crop productivity was investigated by Premalatha *et al.* [18]. *Paenibacillus glycanilyticus, Cohnella* sps., *Chryseobacterium taklimakanense,* and *Lysobacter soli* were isolated from *Hemidesmus indicus*. Vermicompost was used as a carrier material for bioinoculants. Vermicompost was finely powdered, and pH was neutralized using $CaCO_3$. It was autoclaved for 20 minutes at 121^0 C. For the single culture, 100 ml of bacterial culture was used per kg of the carrier material. About 50-100 ml of bacterial culture was used for mixed biofertilizer inoculum. CIM- Megha was sown on the sterilized soils on the pot. Plant height, number of branches, fresh weight, and dry weight of the plants' stages, including vegetative (60 days after sowing – DAS), flowering (90 DAS), and maturation phases (120 and 150 DAS). Bacterial colonization at the rhizosphere was also enumerated. For seed germination, seedling growth and vigor were analyzed by separating seeds from all treatments after harvesting (120 DAS). The quantification of andrographolide and neo-andrographolide content was also estimated for seeds treated with single and bacterium consortiums. The result revealed increased plant height, dry weight, fresh weight, and number of branches compared to control plants. Maximum plant height was obtained in single inoculum application (*Cohnella* sp.) with 95.8 cm on the 150th day after sowing. *P. glycanilyticus* with *Cohnella* sp. and *C. taklimakanense + P. glycanilyticus + L. soli* with *Cohnella* sp. were recorded with 90.2 and 91.5 cm, respectively. After the 150th day of sowing, the maximum number of branches was recorded. 39.5% fresh and dry plant weight was recorded with *Cohnella* sp., *C. taklimakanense*, *P. glycanilyticus*, and *L. soli*. Seed germination results showed significant variations in the germination percentage of all seeds treated with single and bacterial consortiums over non-inoculated control. The analyzed dried herbage samples for phytochemical compounds noted the highest andrographolide content at 3.50% in plants inoculated with *Cohnella* sps. Whereas multiple inoculations of *Cohnella* sps. with *P. glycanilyticus*, *C. taklimakanense*, and *L. soli* were noted with 3.06% over control at 60 DAS. Seeds treated with *Cohnella* sps were recorded with 1.01% neo-andrographolide content after 60 days of sowing. The result concluded that seeds treated with *Cohnella* sps. Alone or with other compatible strains, better plant height, number of branches, dry and fresh weight, seed germination, andrographolide, and neo-andrographolide content than the non-inoculated control were observed.

Influence of Fertigations

A study was conducted to develop a standard procedure for cultivating *A. paniculata* using a fertigation technique. Two growth media and six treatments were studied in total. T1, T3, and T5 were treated with coconut-RHA (70:30), and T2, T4, and T6 were treated with 100% coco peat. T1 and T2 were treated with 10 ppm, T3 and T4 with 50 ppm, and T5 and T6 with 70 ppm magnesium compositions. Maximum plant height was recorded at T1 (32.51 cm), T3 (32.51 cm), and T5 (31.75 cm) treatments. The andrographolide content corresponded to the control 1 and 2 (0.67 – 0.70 µg/mL). The dry herb yields of T5 and T6 decreased from 2.4 g to 1.6 g and 2.4 g to 1.2 g because of the higher magnesium compositions of the nutrient solution. T3 and T5 treatments showed a higher yield than T4 and T6 comparatively. The quantity of andrographolide content is equivalent to that of conventional techniques in the incorporated fertigation technique, and the value ranges from 0.67 – 0.70 µ/mL. Eventually, maximum plant height (31.75 cm), maximum number of leaves (141 number), dry herb yield (2.2 g), and andrographolide content (0.7 µg/mL) were obtained for the T3 standard procedure. Hence, the researcher concluded that combining coco peat-RHA medium and 50 ppm magnesium composition in the nutrient solution was the best method for cultivating *A. paniculata* [13].

Mishra and Jain [12] studied the impact of integrated nutrient management on the fruiting, flowering, and vegetative growth of *A. paniculata*. The experiment was laid out in a randomized block design with eight treatments that include vermicompost, biofertilizers, chemical fertilizers, combined therapy of biofertilizers and vermicompost, combined treatment of biofertilizers and chemical fertilizers, combined treatment of chemical fertilizers and vermicompost, combined treatment of biofertilizers, chemical fertilizers, and vermicompost and control. Combined therapy of biofertilizers, chemical fertilizers and vermicompost recorded maximum plant height (51.64 cm), number of leaves (91.6), number of branches (66), land area occupied by per plant (20.3 cm), leaf area (24.46 cm^2), leaf length and breadth (9.8 cm LL, 2.7 cm LB), leaf area index (1.30) and number of fruits (27.8) and flowers (75.2) of *A. paniculata* at 135 DAS. The result concluded that the integrated use of chemical fertilizers, biofertilizers, and vermicompost treatments raised the growth parameters of *A. paniculata* significantly.

Nishchitha *et al.* [30] determined the effect of integrated nutrient management on the quality and yield of *A. paniculata*. The experiment was carried out in randomized block design with three replications. Vermicompost, poultry manure, and Azatobacter enriched in farm yard manure and NPK mixture were applied to different compositions. The result revealed the highest fresh herb yield per hectare, andrographolide content, plant spread, and plant height were recorded with the application of 100:75:50 kg NPK/ha + *Azatobacter* (1 q) enriched in FYM (5 t ha^{-1}) + vermicompost 1 t per ha at harvest. No significant variation was observed in andrographolide content in plants.

Kumar and Topal [31] experimented with the potential of organic fertilizers on the shoot growth of *A. paniculata*. The work enclosed different treatments, such as biocompost, farmyard manure, and vermicompost, which were added to the soil with 1-2 ratios. The experiment was conducted at the three nurseries of the Forest Department located at different elevations in Tehri Garhwal, India. The result revealed maximum shoot height in vermicompost (13.73 cm) than farmyard manure (12.44 cm), biocompost (10.78 cm), and control (9.07 cm). The researcher concluded that vermicompost was the most suitable medium for the significant growth of *A. paniculata*.

Kalariya *et al.* [32] studied the effect of foliar exogenous methyl jasmonate and salicylic acid on andrographolide yield in *A. paniculata* under a semi-arid climate. The plant was subjected to deficit soil moisture stress imposed during 90-140 DAT. The result exhibited declined chlorophyll and carotenoid content and dry herbage yield to 14% in 6% soil moisture content and showed upregulated antioxidant enzyme activity. The concentration of andrographolide varied from 1.40% to 1.54%. Because of soil moisture stress, the andrographolide yield decreased to 8.21%, but the concentration increased to 6%. Increased methyl jasmonate and salicylic acid doses declined chlorophyll and carotenoid content and raised antioxidant enzyme activity moderately. However, it could have been more effective in losing dry herbage yield or total andrographolide yield in any morphotype.

Impact of Shading Level

Liphan and Detpiratmongkol [17] performed experiments on the impact of shading levels on the growth, yield, andrographolide content of *A. paniculata*. Three varieties of Kalmegh *viz* ., Prachinburi, NakhonPrathom, and Saraburi were applied, and their responses to varying shade levels (0%, 25%, 50%, and 75%) were studied under greenhouse conditions. The test was conducted in a split-plot design with three replications from March to July 2018 in Thailand. The number of leaves per plant, stem height, dry weight of stem, leaf, root, andrographolide content, and leaf and seed dry weight yield were documented. The Prachinburi variety yields better results, followed by NakhonPrathom and Saraburi. The highest growth, root, stem, leaf, andrographolide content, seed dry weight yield, and total dry weight yield were obtained at 25% shading levels, followed by 0%, 50%, and 75%. The author recommended that the Prachinburi variety and 25% shading levels would be helpful in the better yield of cultivation of *A. paniculata*.

Liphan and Detpiratmongkol studied the response of *A. paniculata* to shading at different growth stages [33]. A field experiment was conducted from January to April 2018. Prachinburi, Phisanulok 5-4, and Phitchit 4-4 were used for the experiment. Split plot randomized complete block designs with three replications were carried out. The main plot was divided into four subplots, where each received 20% shading at different growth stages of *A. paniculata*. The subplot treatments encompassed shading treatment (control), shading for 30 DAP till harvest, shading for 60 DAP till harvest, and shading for 90 DAP till harvest. Plant height, dry weight of leaf and root, stem, leaf dry weight yield, and total dry weight were recorded. Maximum plant height, dry weight of leaf and root, stem, leaf dry weight yield, and total dry weight were obtained for the Prachinbuti cultivar, followed by Phisanulok 5-4 and Phichit 4-4. Shading at different growth stages revealed the least growth and yield at no shading, some growth and yield at 90 DAP, and good growth at 30 and 60 DAP. The highest growth and yield were recorded at 30 DAP under 20% shading.

Role of Endophytes for the Production of Plant Growth Promoters, Enzymes, and Antimicrobial Compounds

An experiment was performed to study the effect of endophytes of *A. paniculata* on the production of plant growth promoters, antimicrobial compounds, and enzymes. One g of root, stem, and leaf were surface sterilized with tween 20 and sodium hypochlorite solution, followed by washing with sterile distilled water and Milli-Q water. Using 0.85% sterile saline water, the sterilized samples were made to slurry and various dilutions. 0.1 ml was taken from the prepared dilutions, introduced into Czapex Dox agar plates and Nutrient agar, and incubated at 37^0 C for 24 h. After the incubation period, bacterial and fungal strains were isolated. Further, it was screened for IAA production, phosphate solubilization, nitrogen fixation, cellulose activity, and amylase activity for the production of antimicrobial compounds against *E. coli, Staphylococcus* sps., and *Vibrio* sp. Six fungal and nine bacterial endophytes were isolated from *A. paniculata*. Most of the endophytes produced IAA ranging from 2-45 µg/ml. APS2-B (stem isolate) enabled phosphate solubilization, and APL3-B (leaf isolate) was capable of nitrogen fixation. All six fungal endophytes exhibited amylase and cellulase activity. The antimicrobial activity result showed that 4 bacterial isolates showed potential activity against *E. coli, Staphylococcus* sp., and *Vibrio* sp. The stem isolates APS3-B exhibited a broad spectrum of antimicrobial activity among the four bacterial isolates. APL1-F, APR3-F, APS3-F, and APS2-B fungal isolates were active against test pathogens. APR3-F, APS3-F, and APS2-B fungal isolates inhibited *Staphylococcus* sp. and *Vibrio* sp. significantly. The quality of *A. paniculata* for largescale cultivation could be improved using endophytes [34].

Role of Growth Regulators

Shekhada *et al*. [35] studied the function of different plant growth regulators on the quality and yield of *A. paniculata*. Different concentrations (50, 100, and 200 mg) of phytohormones (GA$_3$, NAA, and Paclobutrazol) were prepared as spray solutions. Phytohormones were sprayed 30 days after the transplantation of a crop and observations were made during that time period. Dry herbage yield and andrographolide content after the harvesting period were recorded. The highest dry herbage yield (4913.84 kg ha^{-1}) was obtained significantly at GA$_3$ 100 mgl^{-1} followed by paclobutrazol 100 mgl^{-1}(4901.68 kgha^{-1}) and paclobutrazol 200 mgl^{-1}(4884.48 kg ha^{-1}). The highest andrographolide content (1.453%) was obtained at GA$_3$ 200 mgl^{-1} followed by GA$_3$ 100 mgl^{-1}(1.403%) and paclobutrazol 100 mgl^{-1}(1.395%) as compared to the control. Andrographolide percentage at harvest was positively correlated with growth parameters *viz* . total dry weight (0.654) and leaf dry weight (0.688). Physiological parameters were positively correlated with the quality of the andrographolide *viz* . SLW (0.699), CGR (0.692), RGR (0.677), BMD (0.651), and NAR (0.655).

Work was conducted to determine the effect of Kunapa Jala (KJ) and Panchagavya (PG) application on crop growth rate (CGR), net assimilation rate (NAR), relative growth rate (RGR), leaf area index (LAI), total leaf area, leaf area duration (LAD), and production of 14-deoxy-11,12-didehydroandrographolide, neoandrographolide, and andrographolide. The experiment was laid out in a randomized block design with control, PG, KG, inorganic fertilizer, farmyard manure, and humic acid. RP-UFLC was used to estimate and detect the content. The parameters were carried out 30, 60, 90, and 120 days after sowing. The highest leaf area and leaf area index were obtained for KJ at 90 DAS. Leaf area duration was obtained between 90 -120 DAS. Higher CGR, RGR, and NAR were obtained between 60 and 90 DAS for PG-treated plants. RP-UFLC showed a high amount of 14-deoxy-11,12-didehydroandrographolide, neoandrographolide, and andrographolide in PG-treated plants at 120 DAS and also recorded the maximum amount of ingredients at 120 DAS in both treatments. Hence, the researcher suggested that Kunapa Jala (KJ) and Panchagavya (PG) applications yielded better results in physiological parameters and production of andrographolide content [36].

Impact of Weed Control Technique in Yield and Economics For *A. paniculata*

Meena *et al*. [37] assessed yield and economics for *A. paniculata* using different weed control techniques. The experiment was conducted during the Kharif season of 2015 and was laid out in a randomized block design with three replications and ten treatments. The highest fresh and dry herbage yield was 25.070 t/ha, which was noted in weed-free treatment. All the treatments showed increased fresh and dry herbage yield compared to the weedy check treatment. The maximum and minimum net return, gross return, and B: C ratio were recorded in weed-free treatment and weedy check.

Dhanush *et al*. [38] estimated the growth, yield, and economics of *A. paniculata* under ratooning as influenced by nutrient levels. The experiment was carried out in a factorial complete block design with nine treatments and three replications. The treatments include recommended dosage of farmyard manure along with nitrogen at three levels (N_1- 75%, N_2- 50%, N_3- 25%) and muriate potash at three levels (K_0- no potassium, K_1-50%, K_2-100%). The recommended dose of nutrients (75:75:50 Kg N: P2O5: K2O ha-1) was applied for the main crop. The andrographolide content was analyzed using HPLC grade ethanol and andrographolide standard. The result recorded maximum plant height, plant spread, number of primary branches, fresh and dry weight of leaves, stems, herb yield, and andrographolide content at the application of FYM at 25 t ha^{-1} with 75% nitrogen and 100% potassium. Andrographolide content was equivalent to 50% nitrogen and potassium, and the highest net returns and maximum B: C ratio were also obtained at the application of FYM at 25 t ha^{-1} with 75% nitrogen and 100% potassium.

Impact of Plant Density on Yield and Medicinal Substance Accumulation

An experiment was designed to study the effect of plant density and harvest date on yield, physiological responses, and andrographolide accumulation under controlled environmental conditions. Different planting densities *viz* . 15, 20, 25,

30, 35, and 40 plants m^{-2} were applied, and physiological responses were estimated at 30 (vegetative stage), 60 (initial stage of flowering), and 90 (flowering stage) DAT. The result revealed no significant differences in *Andrographis*, harvested at 30 days of transplanting (Vegetative stage) and 60 DAT (initial flowering stage). The highest photosynthetic rates were recorded at flowering stage harvest time (90 DAT) at a plant density of 15 plants m^{-2}. At a more moderating planting density (30 plants m$^{-2)}$, the highest number of leaves, andrographolide content, and yield were obtained. Eventually, a high correlation (r = 0.8 to 1.0 and r = -0.8 to -0.1, P<0.01) was acquired in five out of seventeen indices of leaf reflectance. Hence, the author concluded that 30 plants m-2 planting density and harvest time at 90 DAT provided good andrographolide content, yield, and plant growth in PFAL technology [14].

Influence of Different Accessions of Seed Raised *A. paniculata* in Growth and Yield.

Prathanturarug *et al.* [39] determined variations in andrographolide, 14-deox--11,12-didehydroandragropholide content, and morphological characteristics of seed-raised *A. paniculata* in 28 accessions. The experiment was laid out in a randomized complete block design, and plant height, number of nodes, leaf width, leaf length, and number of nodes were recorded. The average amount of dried leaves ranged from 2.13 to 8.23 g. The average andrographolide and 14-deox--11,12-didehydroandrographolide content was between 12.44 and 33.52 mg/g and 0.23 and 2.08 mg/g, respectively. Variations in andrographolide, 14-deoxy-11,-2-didehydroandrographolide content, and morphological characteristics of seed-raised *A. paniculata* were statistically significant. Further, the researcher isolated the plants that produced high amounts of andrographolide (up to 52.57mg/g dried leaves) and 14-deoxy-11,12-didehydroandrographolide (up to 3.46 mg/g dried leaves). The author concluded that these were potentially essential sources for breeding and improving cultivars.

Co-cultivation

Kirthi *et al.* [11] experimented with the co-cultivation of *A. paniculata* with food crops, such as *Zea mays* (Maize), *Pennisetum glaucum* (Pearl millet), *Cajanus cajan* (Pigeon pea), and *Abelmoschus esculentus* (Okra) for enhancing field productivity and resource use efficiency. The experiment was laid out in randomized block design with thrice replication. All food crops were intercropped with *A. paniculata* at 50% (27,777 plants ha^{-1}), 75% (37,037 plants ha^{-1}), and 100% (55,555 plants ha^{-1}) with a total population of *A. paniculata* (55,555 plants ha^{-1}). Intercropping with *Cajanus cajan* (Pigeon pea) exhibited the highest dry herb yield of *A. paniculata* at 4412 kg, followed by *Abelmoschus esculentus*

(Okra) at 50% plant population yield of 4412 kg ha^{-1} and 75% plant population in the intercropping of *A. paniculata* and *Cajanus cajan* (Pigeon pea), yielding at 4011kg ha^{-1}. The highest net returns were obtained at *Cajanus cajan* (2016-2208 USD ha^{-1}), followed by *Abelmoschus esculentus* (1465-2001 USD ha^{-1}), *Pennisetum glaucum* (1.64-1265 USD ha^{-1}) and *Zea mays* (1123-1241 USD ha^{-1}). The researcher concluded that *A. paniculata*, with a 50% plant population, was suitable for the highest productivity, andrographolide content, and monetary returns.

Effect of Aging on Yield of Andrographolide Content

Work was conducted to determine the impact of aging on andrographolide content in *A. paniculata* and determine the best harvesting time. Plant height, number of leaves per plant, number of branches per plant, fresh weight of the plant, dry weight of the plant, leaf-to-stem ratio, and andrographolide content were recorded at 30,60, 90, 120, and 150 days after sowing. Further, it was statistically analyzed by ANOVA. The best harvesting time was recorded at 150 days after sowing with plant height (45.6 ± 1.33 cm), number of leaves per plant (110.90 ± 2.41), number of branches per plant (47.80 ± 2.04), fresh weight of plant (115.37 ± 0.77), dry weight of plant (56.49 ± 1.23), and leaf to stem ratio (1:3.35). The maximum andrographolide content was noted 90 days after sowing and was a minimum of 150 days. This might be due to the loss of leaves. Although the maximum andrographolide content was at 90 days, other parameters, such as the dry matter content of plants, were high in 120 DAS. So, the author concluded that harvesting the crop at 120 DAS could be beneficial [40].

The present review summarized works of different researchers involving different factors that influence the physiological, morphological parameters and andrographolide content of *A. paniculata*, which include plant geometry, planting density and harvesting time, soil health, fertigation, shading level, endophytes, plant growth regulators, weeding control techniques, different accessions of seeds, plant density, co-cultivation, and aging (Fig. **5**). Plant geometry with a plot measuring 30 × 20 cm, coco peat-RHA medium, 50 ppm magnesium composition, integrated use of chemical fertilizers, and biofertilizer and vermicompost treatments were optimum conditions for better yield. Among different seed cultivars, Pranchiburi cultivars showed a good percentage of germination and growth, and the highest andrographolide content was recorded at 135 DAP in the flowering stage. In different concentrations, GA$_3$ treated plants recorded the highest dry herbage yield andrographolide content. 25% shading level was suitable for plant growth compared to all other shading percentages. Co-cultivation with *Cajanus cajan* exhibited better yield and quality of *A.*

paniculata. In the case of dry storage, 1 to 3 months and 25^0 C temperature were recommended.

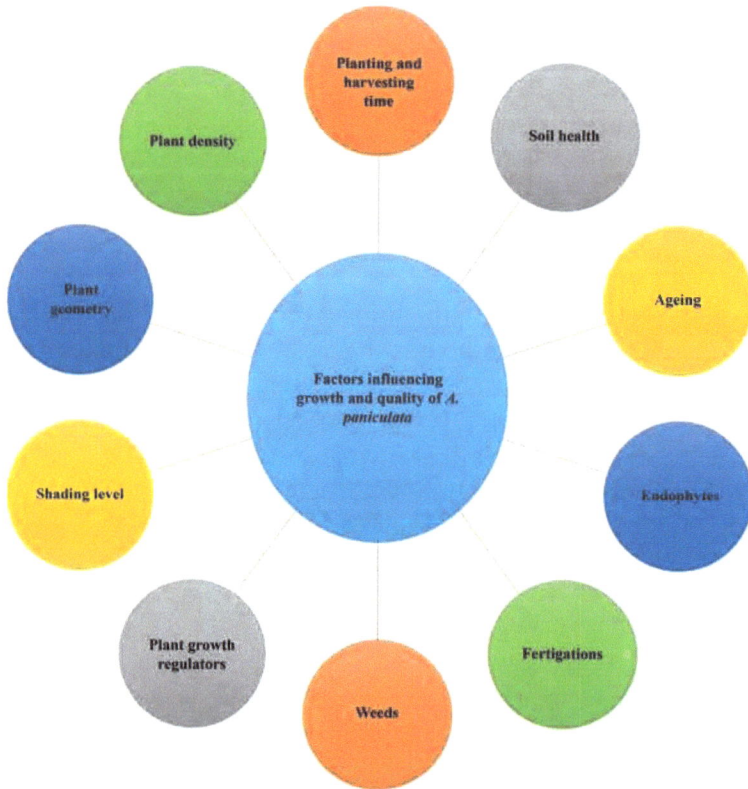

Fig. (5). Factors influencing the growth and quality content of *Andrographis paniculata*.

CONCLUSION

Plenty of work has been carried out to explore *A. paniculata* for medicinal purposes. Subsequent large-scale cultivation of *A. paniculata* has yet to be standardized, and in deprived areas, very few works have been carried out. The seed of *A. paniculata* possessed dormancy and a low germination rate. Even though vegetative propagations yield the highest survival percentage in a short period compared to seed propagation, most workers used different seed cultivars. Thus, further work on vegetative propagation is needed, and a substantial amount of importance ought to be given to optimize the propagation of *A. paniculata* on a large scale.

LIST OF ABBREVIATIONS

DAT   Days after transplanting

DAS   Days after sowing

PEG   Polyethylene glycol

GA$_3$ Gibberellic acid

HPLC   High Performance Liquid Chromatography

IAA   Indole Acetic Acid

NAA   Naphthalene Acetic Acid

PFAL   Plant Factory with Artificial Lighting

REFERENCES

[1]   Milkuri CR, Indu K, Bhargavi C, Rajendra MP, Babu HB. A review on vegetative propagation and applications in forestry. J Plant Dev Sci 2022; 14(3): 265-72.

[2]   Lakhiar IA, Gao J, Syed TN, Chandio FA, Buttar NA. Modern plant cultivation technologies in agriculture under controlled environment: a review on aeroponics. J Plant Interact 2018; 13(1): 338-52.
[http://dx.doi.org/10.1080/17429145.2018.1472308]

[3]   Ved DK, Goraya GS. Demand and supply of medicinal plants in India. FRLHT, 2008; Bangalore and National Medicinal Plants Board, New Delhi.

[4]   Integration of Medicinal and Aromatic Crop Cultivation and value chain management for small farmers. National academy of agricultural sciences, New Delhi. 2016; Policy Paper 79.

[5]   Intharuksa A, Arunotayanun W, Yooin W, Sirisa-ard P. A comprehensive review of *Andrographis paniculata* (Burm. f.) Nees and its constituents as potential lead compounds for COVID-19 drug discovery. Molecules 2022; 27(14): 4479.
[http://dx.doi.org/10.3390/molecules27144479] [PMID: 35889352]

[6]   WHO Monographs on Selected Medicinal Plants. Geneva, Switzerland: World Health Organization 2002; Vol. 2.

[7]   Verma H, Negi MS, Mahapatra BS, Shukla A, Paul J. Evaluation of an emerging medicinal crop Kalmegh [*Andrographis paniculata* (Burm. f.) Wall. ex Nees] for commercial cultivation and pharmaceutical & industrial uses: A review. J Pharmacogn Phytochem 2019; 8(4): 835-48.

[8]   Jayawardhane J, Damunupola JW, Jayasuriya KMGG. Propagation of three important medicinal plants in Aacanthaceae; *Andrographis paniculata, Barleria prionitis* and *Rhinacanthus polonnaruwensis*. Ceylon Journal of Science 2021; 50(2): 129-37.
[http://dx.doi.org/10.4038/cjs.v50i2.7874]

[9]   Hossain MS, Urbi Z. Z. Effect of Naphthalene acetic acid on the adventitious rooting in shoot cuttings of *Andrographis paniculata* (Burm.f.) Wall. ex Nees: An important therapeutical herb. Intern J Agronomy, 2016; 2016: 1617543, 6.
[http://dx.doi.org/10.1155/2016/1617543]

[10]   Saffie N, Ariff FFM, Bahari SNS, Abdullah MZ, Taini MM. Germination, propagation and selection of *Andrographis paniculata* for future breeding programme. Intern J Agric Forestry and Plantation 2019; 8: 168-74.

[11]   Kirthi V, Kushal PS, Anjali S, Nikil BL. Nilofer, Devendra K, Anil KS, Rakesh K, Puja K, Saudan S. Co-cultivation of a medicinal plant kalmegh [*Andrographis paniculata* (Burm. f.) Wall ex Nees] with

food crops for enhancing field productivity and resource use efficiency. Industrial Crops & Products 2021; 159(2021): 113076.

[12]   Mishra S, Jain A. Effect of INM on vegetative growth, flowering and fruiting of *Andrographis paniculata*. Univers J Agric Res 2014; 2(3): 93-6.
[http://dx.doi.org/10.13189/ujar.2014.020302]

[13]   Suhaini MA, Hawaji MH, Che Man SH, Baharulrazi N, Yunus NA. Characterization of Andrographolide in *Andrographis paniculata* under different cultivation conditions. Chem Eng Trans 2020; 78: 127-32.
[http://dx.doi.org/10.3303/CET2078022]

[14]   Chutimanukul P, Mosaleeyanon K, Janta S, Toojinda T, Darwell CT, Wanichananan P. Physiological responses, yield and medicinal substance (andrographolide, AP1) accumulation of *Andrographis paniculata* (Burm. f) in response to plant density under controlled environmental conditions. PLoS One 2022; 17(8): e0272520.
[http://dx.doi.org/10.1371/journal.pone.0272520] [PMID: 35925998]

[15]   Detpiratmongkol S, Liphan S. Effects of different harvesting times on growth, yield and quality of Kalmegh (*Andrographis paniculata* Wall ex Nees). Intern J Agric Technol 2018; 14(7): 1161-70.

[16]   Himbindu T, Hariprasad Rao N, Satyanarayana Reddy G, Sastry KP. Effect of time of planting and harvesting on growth, herbage yield and andrographolide content in Kalmegh (*Andrographis paniculata* Nees.). Bull Env Pharmacol Life Sci 2017; 6(10): 46-9.

[17]   Liphan S, Detpiratmongkol S. Influence of shading levels on growth, yield and andrographolide content of Kalmegh. Plant Arch 2020; 20(1): 1349-54.

[18]   K Premalatha, Botlagunta N, D Santhosh, *et al.* Enhancement of soil health, germination and crop productivity in *Andrographis paniculata* (Burm.f.) Nees, an important medicinal crop by using a composite bio inoculant. J Plant Nutr 2021; 1-16.
[http://dx.doi.org/10.1080/01904167.2021.1899207]

[19]   Sareer O, Ahmad S, Umar S. *Andrographis paniculata*: a critical appraisal of extraction, isolation and quantification of andrographolide and other active constituents. Nat Prod Res 2014; 28(23): 2081-101.
[http://dx.doi.org/10.1080/14786419.2014.924004] [PMID: 24912126]

[20]   Semwal MP, Sunita TP, Pratap SV, *et al.* Influence of planting geometries and weed control practices on growth and herbage yield of Kalmegh (*Andrographis paniculata* Nees.). J Med Plant Studies 2016; 4(6): 162-6.

[21]   Singh V, Singh RK. Effect of season, time of planting and plant density on the growth, yield and andrographolide content of Kalmegh (*Andrographis paniculata* Nees) under north Indian condition. Int J Plant Sci 2006; 1(1): 6-9.

[22]   Sujata B, Sunil P, Arti J, Shikha S. Studies on seed germination and seedling growth in Kalmegh (*Andrographis paniculata* Wall. ex Nees) under abiotic stress conditions. Int J Sci Environ Technol 2012; 1(3): 197-204.

[23]   Kumar B, Verma SK, Singh HP. Effect of temperature on seed germination parameters in Kalmegh (*Andrographis paniculata* Wall. ex Nees.). Ind Crops Prod 2011; 34(1): 1241-4.
[http://dx.doi.org/10.1016/j.indcrop.2011.04.008]

[24]   Shruthi K, Balakrishna P, Naveena K. Studies on seed quality parameters of Kalmegh (*Andrographis paniculata* Wall. ex Nees) in relation to seed deterioration under accelerated ageing conditions. Res J Agric Sci 2018; 9(2): 372-4.

[25]   Talei D, Valdiani A, Abdulla MP, Hassan SA. A rapid and effective method for dormancy breakage and seed germination of King of Bitters (*Andrographis paniculata* Wall. ex Nees) seeds. Maydica electronic publication, 2012; 57: 98-105.

[26]   Patidar S, Gontia AS, Upadhyay A, Nayak PS. Biochemical constituents in Kalmegh (*Andrographis paniculata* Nees.). World Appl Sci J 2011; 15(8): 1095-9.

[27]   Kumar J, Sinha A, Sah RB, Nayak H, Nirala DP. Screening of traits for higher biochemical constituents' production in Kalmegh (*Andrographis paniculata*) plants harvested at pre-flowering stage. J Pharmacogn Phytochem 2018; SP1: 568-73.

[28]   Kumar S, Kumar A. Spatial and harvesting influence on growth, yield, quality and economic potential of Kalmegh (*Andrographis paniculata* Wall ex Nees). J Agric Rural Dev Trop Subtrop 2013; 114(1): 69-76.

[29]   Parashar R, Upadhyay A, Singh J, Diwedi SK, Noor AK. Morpho-physiological evaluation of *Andrographis paniculata* at different growth stages. World J Agric Sci 2011; 7(2): 124-7.

[30]   Nishchitha M, Hiremath JS, Gireesh A, Mahantesh PS, Pooja MR, Lokesh CH. Effect of integrated nutrient management on yield and quality of Kalmegh (*Andrographis paniculata* Nees.). J Pharmacogn Phytochem 2018; SP3: 122-5.

[31]   Kumar B, Topal D. Effect of organic fertilizers on the growth of shoot of Kalmegh (*Andrographis paniculata*). Intern J Novel Res in Life Sciences 2015; 2(2): 9-11.

[32]   Kalariya KA, Shahi D, Saran PL, *et al.* Effect of genotypes and foliar spray of methyl jasmonate and salicylic acid on andrographolide yield in *Andrographis paniculata* (Burm. f.) Wall. ex Nees. under semi-arid climate. Bull Natl Res Cent 2023; 47(1): 34.
[http://dx.doi.org/10.1186/s42269-023-01009-w]

[33]   Liphan S, Detpiratmongkol S. Response of Kalmegh (*Andrographis paniculata* (Burm. f.) Nees) to shading at different growth stages. Plant Arch 2019; 19(2): 2093-8.

[34]   Adhikari M, Mukhopadhyay M. Potentials of endophytes of *Andrographis paniculata* for the production of plant growth promoters, enzymes and antimicrobial compounds. SAARC J Agric 2022; 19(2): 157-70.
[http://dx.doi.org/10.3329/sja.v19i2.57678]

[35]   Shekhada RR, Macwan SJ, Patel NJ, Gajbhiye NA. Growth regulators on quality and yield of Kalmegh (*Andrographis paniculata* Nees). International Journal of Economic Plants 2022; 9(Nov, 4): 294-8.
[http://dx.doi.org/10.23910/2/2022.IJEP0482c]

[36]   Ankad GM, Hiremath J, Pai SR, Hegde HV. Evaluation of *Vrikshayurveda* treatments on physiological attributes and production of diterpenoids in *Andrographis paniculata* (Burm.f.) Nees. Ayu 2021; 42(1): 45-51.
[http://dx.doi.org/10.4103/ayu.ayu_311_21] [PMID: 36743276]

[37]   Meena BR, Meena SS, Kala DC. Assesment of yield and economic for Kalmegh (*Andrographis paniculata* Nees) by using different weed control techniques. Int J Curr Microbiol Appl Sci 2017; 6(5): 2303-8.
[http://dx.doi.org/10.20546/ijcmas.2017.605.257]

[38]   Dhanush SL, Mallikarjuna Gowda AP, Kademani AJ, Praneeth C, Chandramohan Reddy G. Growth, yield, quality and economics of Kalmegh (*Andrographis paniculata* Nees.) under ratooning as influenced by nutrient levels. Int J Pure App Biosci 2018; 6(1): 753-7.
[http://dx.doi.org/10.18782/2320-7051.6245]

[39]   Prathanturarug S, Soonthornchareonnon N, Chuakul W, Saralamp P. Variation in growth and diterpene lactones among field-cultivated *Andrographis paniculata*. J Nat Med 2007; 61(2): 159-63.
[http://dx.doi.org/10.1007/s11418-006-0115-6]

[40]   Ashok K, Amit A, Sujatha M, Murali B, Anand MS. Effect of ageing on andrographolide content in *Andrographis paniculata*. J Nat Rem 2002; 2(2): 179-81. Available from: https://globinmed.com/conservation/hempedu-bumi-79366/

CHAPTER 15

Micropropagation of *Andrographis* Species - A Review

Varimadugu Aruna[1,*], **M. Johnson**[2,*], **Medagam Tejaswini Reddy**[1], **Vadakavila Geethikalal**[1], **S. Preethi**[2], **B. Shivananthini**[2], **I. Silvia Juliet**[2] and **Vidyarani George**[2]

[1] *Department of Biotechnology, Chaitanya Bharathi Institute of Technology, Hyderabad, Telangana, India*

[2] *Centre for Plant Biotechnology, Department of Botany, St. Xavier's College (Autonomous), Palayamkottai – 627002, Tamil Nadu, India*

Abstract: The *Andrographis* of the Acanthaceae family is one of the potential sources for many pharmacological drugs with a wide array of essential phytochemicals. The present review summarizes the micropropagation of several *Andrographis* species viz., *A. affinis* Nees, *A. alata* (Vahl) Nees, *A. echioides* (L.) Nees, *A. lineata* Nees, *A. lobelioides* Wight, *A. macrobotrys* Nees, *A. neesiana* Wight, *A. paniculata* (Burm. f.) Wall. ex Nees, and *A. producta* Gamble. Nodal and shoot tip explants were suitable for *in vitro* shoot regeneration, whereas, for callus induction and indirect regeneration studies, cotyledonary leaf and hypocotyl segments were better choices as explants. The major surface sterilants used were alcohol (70%) and mercuric chloride (0.1-0.2%). Murashige and Skoog (MS) medium was the prime choice for *in vitro* regeneration studies of *Andrographis*.

Keywords: *Andrographis*, Acanthaceae family, *In vitro* regeneration, Micropropagation, Phytochemicals, Surface sterilants.

INTRODUCTION

Andrographis – A Medicinal Genus

Andrographis is a crucial medicinal genus of Acanthaceae with 26 species native to India [1]. *Andrographis* spp. possesses some chief phytochemical compounds like andrographolide, neoandrographolide, 14-deoxy-andrographolide, 14-deox--11, 12 -didehydroandrographolide, andrographolide, and serpyllin accountable for several biological and pharmacological activities [1]. *Andrographis* spp. are well known for their pharmacological activities. Their major activities include antidiabetic, anti-inflammatory, antimicrobial, anticancer, anti-venom, antioxi-

* **Corresponding authors Varimadugu Aruna and M. Johnson:** Department of Biotechnology, Chaitanya Bharathi Institute of Technology, Hyderabad, Telangana, India;
Centre for Plant Biotechnology, Department of Botany, St. Xavier's College (Autonomous), Palayamkottai – 627002, Tamil Nadu, India; E-mails: varuna_biotech@cbit.ac.in, aruna429@gmail.com; cpbsxc@gmail.com; ptcjohnson@gmail.com

S. Karuppusamy, Vinod K. Nelson & T. Pullaiah (Eds.)

dant, antipyretic, antifertility, anthelminthic, immunomo-dulatory, antiviral, and hepatoprotective [1]. This work aimed to compile several micropropagation works accomplished by various researchers on different *Andrographis* species. The *Andrographis* species to be reviewed are *Andrographis affinis* Nees, *Andrographis alata* (Vahl) Nees, *Andrographis echioides* (L.) Nees, *Andrographis lineata* Nees, *Andrographis lobelioides* Wight, *Andrographis macrobotrys* Nees, *Andrographis neesiana* Wight, *A. paniculata* (Burm. f.) Wall. ex Nees, and *Andrographis producta* (C.B.Clarke) Gamble.

Need for Micropropagation

Plant conservation is an excellent strategy for preventing plants from extinction and maintaining their status in the ecosystems. Increasing commercial and pharmacological demands for these natural resources have degraded their habitats and created a threatened status in this environment. Further, the reproductive status of many plants undergoes various natural and anthropogenic barriers that lead the way toward sterility. Seed and vegetative propagation were influenced by many internal and external factors like predation, desiccation, pathogenic activities, extended dormancy, unfavorable seasons, *etc* [2]. The distribution of *A. lineata* by natural propagation through rootstocks and seeds was restricted due to biotic pressure such as cattle grazing, forest fires, *etc* [3]. Most of the species reported are endemic, but their need in pharmacological aspects is inevitable, so conservation becomes a significant challenge. Overcoming such adversity in conservation and large-scale propagation with minimum period and small area *in vitro* micropropagation can be a better alternative.

Need for Updation in Micropropagation.

Micropropagation is a revolutionary technique for the prompt multiplication of plants [4]. Micropropagation is the large-scale propagation of true-to-type propagules throughout the year in varying climates and with minimized time and space [5]. Micropropagation is an efficient, proven method for commercially exploiting aromatic and medicinal plants [6]. High-quality plant-based medicines can be tremendously achieved through plant tissue cultures *via* micropropagation. The documentation of various advantages of micropropagation over other conventional methods was executed [7]. Some significant benefits are the extensive propagation of plants from a single explant in a short time and space; species can be micropropagated throughout the year. Pathogen-free plant production, increased multiplication rate, and meristem culture yield genetically identical plants, secondary metabolites production, *etc* [7]. Micropropagation is an alternate method to propagate and conserve medicinal plants by selecting high-yield lines and their efficient cloning. The above-stated works have strongly endorsed that micropropagation can be an alternative to conventional vegetative propagation [7].

MICROPROPAGATION- *ANDROGRAPHIS* SPP.

Explants and Surface Sterilization

Micropropagation works on different *Andrographis* species were studied, and the explants used in these works were given as a compilation. On an MS basal medium, 94 percent of *A. paniculata* seeds germinated within five days of inoculation. Within fifteen days, the seeds had grown into plantlets [8]. Following that, explants from these plantlets were utilized. Pods, leaves, and nodal segments were surface sterilized by first washing them under running tap water for 20 minutes to remove adhering particles such as dust and soil, then rinsing them with a 0.1 percent (v/v) aqueous solution of Tween 20 for 30 minutes. To completely eradicate microbiological contamination over the surface, the samples were rinsed with 70 percent ethanol solution for 2-3 minutes, followed by treatment with 1.2 percent sodium hypochlorite solution (chlorine bleach) for 5-7 minutes. To reduce the effect of chlorine bleach on living plant tissues, all samples were immediately rinsed four times with sterile autoclaved distilled water. After the pods had been sterilized, they were dried on sterilized blotting paper and gently dissected with tweezers to expose seeds for micropropagation. The damaged ends of the leaflets were cut off with a knife. Using a knife, the outer covering of nodal buds and the ends of nodal segments were also removed [9]. Elongated shoots (20-40 mm long) were obtained from Kalmegh plants growing in the field, brought to the lab with the cut ends immersed in distilled water, and then washed in a 2% (w/v) Teepol solution. Surface sterilization was also performed for 5 minutes in a 0.1% (w/v) mercuric chloride solution. The stem (1 to 1.2 cm in length) and leaf segment (2.5 mm 2) were utilized as explants after cleaning the trice with sterile distilled water [10].

For multiple shoot regeneration of *A. paniculata*, shoot tips and nodal segment explants were cultured on MS medium supplemented with varying concentrations of BAP, Kn, and NAA alone or in various combinations [11]. Purkayastha *et al.* [8] devised a speedy and efficient approach for large-scale propagation of *A. paniculata*, using *in vitro* culture of nodal explants obtained from 15-day-old aseptic seedlings. In nodal explants cultivated on MS media supplemented with BAP, high-frequency direct shoot growth was observed. BAP was one of the most efficacious cytokinins (BAP, Kn, TDZ, and 2-iP) examined. The shoot-generating capacity of the nodal explants was impacted by the BAP concentration (1–12.5 M), with 10 M BAP producing an average of 34 shoots in 94% of the cultures within four weeks. There were significant differences in the average number of shoots per explant (8.6–34.1) amongst the three BAP concentrations studied. Concentrations of all cytokinins examined reached a level that can be deemed above optimal, as evidenced by a decrease in the frequency of shoot proliferation. Even after being transferred to hormone-free MS media, the numerous shoots obtained on varying concentrations of BAP failed to elongate. The induced shoots were elongated within two weeks on MS basal medium supplemented with 1.0 M GA$_3$. After each harvest of freshly developed shoots, the original nodal explants were subcultured on a shoot multiplication medium to generate a proliferating shoot culture. Even after three harvests, the explants kept their morphogenic capacity. As a result, a single nodal explant produced approximately 60–70 shoots in 90 days, while nodal explants from primary shoots regenerated an identical number of shoots, demonstrating their high-frequency regeneration capability in *A. paniculata*. Roy *et al.* [12] devised an efficient approach for the *in vitro* regeneration of plantlets from *A. paniculata* shoot tip and nodal segment explants. When nodal segment explants were cultivated on MS supplemented with 11.10 M/l BAP, they produced the most shoots (181.24). The number of shoots (30) per culture increased by adding 10% coconut water and 2.0 g/L activated charcoal to the medium mentioned above. In the same medium, the shoot tip explant also performed well. The medium was supplemented with 100 mg/L urea and 2.0 g/l activated charcoal, which resulted in appropriate shoot elongation; on half-strength MS medium supplemented with 9.80 M IBA, the isolated shoots rooted successfully (90%).

An *in vitro* study on *A. alata* was carried out with different explants. Mature seeds raised in a soil bed were used as a source for explants such as cotyledon, epicotyls, hypocotyls, root segments, tender leaves, nodal and internodal segments, and mature and immature seeds. Surface sterilization was initiated with 10 minutes of tap water washing, liquid detergent Teepol, and 0.1% mercuric chloride, and the sterilization time varied with explants. For seeds, it was 8-10 minutes; for cotyledon, hypocotyls, epicotyls, and radicle explants, it was 5-6 minutes; and for tender leaf and stem segments, it was 6-7 minutes. Then, the explants were rinsed with double distilled sterilized water 7-8 times. Shoot bud organogenesis and callogenic potency were high with hypocotyl explants. Shoot differentiation from the callus of leaf explants was high. The regenerants from the callus of cotyledon, hypocotyls, root, and leaf of *A. alata* showed morphological variation compared with *in vivo* plants. The regenerates from cotyledon showed reddish brown pigmentation on leaves; from hypocotyl showed larger, ovate, glabrous, and obtuse leaves; stem glabrous, narrow inter node and stout node; from root callus showed short internodes and large, ovate leaves [13]. Efficient regeneration of *A. alata* through leaf callus culture was documented. Leaf explants produced luxuriant callus mass [14]. Juvenile explants were used to induce *in vitro* flowering in *A. lineata*. The mature plants underwent *de novo* flowering morphogenesis. Mature nodal explants showed a high percentage of flowering—cotyledonary node-produced multiple flower bud induction [15].

In vitro, the response of *A. alata* and *A. lineata* was recorded using mature plants' nodes, shoot tips, leaves, and petioles. The surface sterilization was started with tap water washing for 15 minutes, 5% Teepol detergent for 15 minutes, and repeated tap water and distilled water washing, followed by sterilization with 70% alcohol for 15 seconds and 0.1% mercuric chloride ($HgCl_2$) for 2 minutes and then rinsed with distilled water for 5-6 times. Nodal and tender leaf explants showed good shoot multiplication [16]. A well-organized protocol for *in vitro* regeneration of *A. affinis* was carried out, and the experiment resulted in the highest shoot regeneration (100%) with nodal explants [17]. Mass propagation of *A. lineata* through *in vitro* culture of nodal explants was studied, where multiple shoot proliferation was obtained at the highest percentage of 94.2% [18].

In *A. paniculata*, Tween 20 was used to treat the seeds, which were washed for 15-20 minutes under tap water. Seeds were surface sterilized for 4-5 minutes with a 0.1% (w/v) mercuric chloride solution and then washed 8 to 10 times with sterile distilled water. Surface-sterilized seeds were inoculated aseptically into MS media for germination and developing aseptic cultures. All cultures were kept in a controlled environment at 25 ± 2°C with a 16-hour photoperiod and a 50 μmol/m²/s¹ irradiance. All the studies were carried out thrice with 20 explants per treatment [12]. The explants were treated with mercuric chloride (0.1) for 1-2 minutes and washed with sterilized distilled water and then with ethanol (50%) for 2-3 minutes, followed by sterilized distilled water. After adding the MS medium, sucrose (3%), and myoinositol (0.1%), the pH was adjusted to 5.6-5.8 using HCl (0.1N) or NaOH (0.1N) and then adjusted agar (8 gm/l) was added. After autoclaving at 121°C for 20 minutes at 1.06 kg/cm² pressure, the cultures were incubated at 25±2°C with a relative humidity of 70-80% and a photoperiod of 16/8 hours (Light/Dark) beneath photon flux thickness [19]. The *in vitro* propagation procedure is depicted in Fig. (**1**).

An evaluation of aseptic seed germination studies on *A. echioides* was carried out. Mature seeds were used as explants. Seeds were surface sterilized with ethyl alcohol (70%) for 25 seconds and 0.1% mercuric chloride for 3 minutes. The evaluation achieved the maximum seed germination percentage (67.10%) and 79.93% survival percentage. For micropropagation studies, shoot tips, nodal segments, stem bits, and root bits were used as explants. Of these, shoot tips showed a high response (85.72%), followed by nodal segments (70.63%) [19]. *In vitro* plant regeneration of *A. neesiana* was reported, where mature capsules were used for aseptic plantlet generation. The capsules were surface sterilized with running tap water for 30 minutes, then with 0.1% aqueous solution of Tween 20 for 30 minutes, 70% ethanol for 2 minutes, and finally with 0.2% HgCl$_2$ solution for 5 minutes. The seed germination obtained was 96%. Nodal segments from the germinated seedlings were used for further study, and shoot proliferation results showed good when supplemented with various plant growth hormones [6].

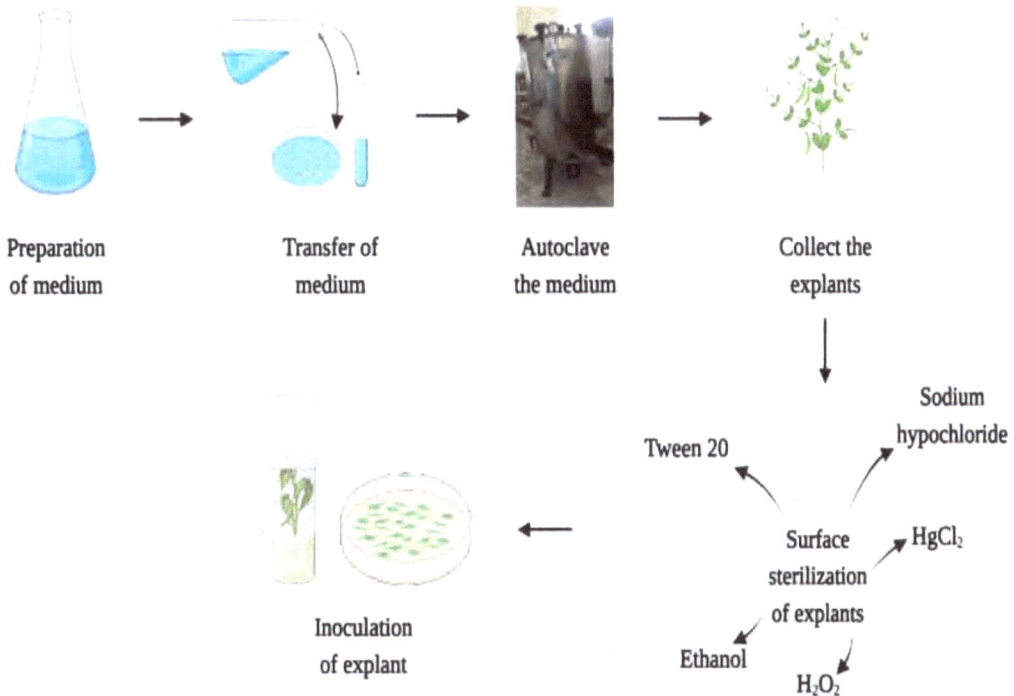

Fig. (1). Surface sterilization and inoculation of *Andrographis* species.

The standardization of micropropagation of *A. echioides* using different explants and media was documented. Of the studied explants, shoot tips showed a positive response for shoot induction [20]. Micropropagation of *A. lineata* was carried out. The eight-month-old plant was used for shoot tips and nodal segment explant selection and then surface sterilized with distilled water for 30 minutes, 70% alcohol for 1 minute, commercial bleach (5.25% sodium hypochlorite) for 15 minutes. It is then washed thrice with distilled water, then with 0.1% mercuric chloride for 8 minutes, and finally with sterile distilled water for 5 minutes. High-frequency shoot proliferation was obtained from shoot tip explants, and the final survival rate was about 70% [21]. *In vitro* production of Echioidinin, 7-O-Methylwogonin from callus cultures of *A. lineata* was investigated. Mature leaves were used for this study. Surface sterilization was done with 70% ethanol for 30 seconds, sterile distilled water rinsing, 0.1% mercuric chloride for 2 minutes, and sterile distilled water washing. Callus proliferation was achieved with the selected explants [22].

In *in vitro* shoot multiplication studies on *A. lineata* where mature seeds were washed with tap water for 5 minutes, 1% Tween 20 for 30 minutes, rinsed with sterile distilled water, and then sterilized with 70% alcohol for 60 seconds, 30% hydrogen peroxide for 5 minutes was used to sterilize the explants. The plants collected from 30 days of seedlings were shoot tips, cotyledonary nodes, nodal explants, leaves, internodes, and root segments. Nodal explants showed maximum response [23]. *In vitro* plant regeneration, flowering, and fruiting were reported in *A. lineata*. Nodal explants from mature plants were initially washed with running tap water and 4-5 times with distilled water, sterilized with 70% alcohol for 15 seconds and 0.1% mercuric chloride ($HgCl_2$) for 2 minutes, and rinsed with sterile distilled water for 5-6 times. Higher regeneration frequency (91.4%) was achieved with nodal explants [24]. Indirect organogenesis protocol was recorded for *A. echioides*. Mature seeds were used for initial aseptic seedlings, a source for explants selection. Seeds were washed with tap water for 15-20 minutes, then sterilized with 70% alcohol for a few seconds and rinsed thrice with distilled water. Final sterilization took place with 0.1% mercuric chloride for 3-5 minutes and then with sterile distilled water 3-7 times. Seed germination was achieved at 90% after one week of inoculation. Leaf and nodal explants were sourced from 35-day-old seedlings for micropropagation. The response of leaf and nodal explants to various supplements for callus induction was about 90% and 95%, respectively. Shoot formation recorded with leaf callus explants was 84%, and shoot callus explants was 89%. The final survival rate was around 70% [25].

The influence of plant growth regulators on *in vitro* propagation of *A. echioides* was carried out. Explants chosen from healthy mother plants were shoot tips (1.5-2 cm), nodal segments (2-2.5 cm), leaf bits (0.5-1.0 cm^2), root bits (1.0-2.0 cm), and stem bits (1-1.5 cm). The explants were rinsed with liquid detergent for 5 minutes, then with distilled water for 3-4 times and sterilized with 70% ethyl alcohol for 25 seconds, and then with 0.1% mercuric chloride for 2-6 minutes, depending on the explant type. Shoot tip explants showed a more positive response (85.72%) and a survival percentage (68%) with a low contamination percentage. Explants with organized structures like shoot tips and nodal segments were highly responsive [26]. Direct regeneration and genetic fidelity studies of *A. echioides* were documented. Mature seeds from 2-year-old plants were used as initial explants for raising aseptic seedlings. Initial washing was done with tap water, then with 0.1% mercuric chloride for 2 minutes, followed by sterilized double distilled water rinsing 2-3 times. *In vitro* seedlings germinated after three weeks of culture. Aseptic leaf explants were cultured from 25-day-old seedlings for direct regeneration studies [27].

In vitro propagation of *A. macrobotrys* was recorded. A mature one-year-old plant was used as a source of nodal explants. Explants were washed with 10% Tween 20 for 5 minutes, then 0.1% aqueous mercuric chloride for 5 minutes, and 95% alcohol wash for 30 seconds, followed by sterile distilled water rinsing and culturing. In the initial stage, the axillary buds of explants started bulging, and additional shoot primordia were induced after two weeks of culture [28]. *In vitro* propagation of *A. alata* was carried out with nodal explants. Nodal explants were collected and sterilized with 0.1% mercuric chloride for 5 minutes. Multiple shoots were formed from the cultured nodal explants [29]. A work on the practical and rapid *in vitro* regeneration of *A. echioides* was recorded. Nodal explants were selected and washed in running tap water and then with 10% Tween 20, surface sterilized with 0.1% mercuric chloride for 1-2 minutes, and then rinsed with sterile double distilled water 4-6 times. Nodal explants showed a good percentage of shoot multiplication [30] for micropropagation of *A. producta* seeds, which were used as initial explants for *in vitro* seedling production. Shoot tips (1-3 m) and nodal explants (5 mm) were excised from 6-week-old seedlings and employed as explants for *in vitro* propagation. Nodal explants and shoot tip explants undergo direct regeneration of shoots. Shoot tip explants produce multiple shoots and are ideal for the micropropagation of *A. producta* [31]. Micropropagation of *A. lineata* var. *lawii* was carried out with various explants, shoot tip, nodal, and cotyledonary segments. Shoot tips and nodal explants were used for multiple shoot direct regeneration. Cotyledonary leaf explants produced callus-mediated multiple-shoot buds [32].

Medium and Plant Growth Regulators

The influence of several plant growth regulators and different strengths of MS medium on various *Andrographis* species was studied and collated. A remarkable work on the *in vitro* propagation of *A. alata* was reported. The preliminary effects of MS medium, Linsmaier and Skoog's medium, Gamborg's medium, White medium, and Nitsch medium were determined in both mature and immature seeds. MS medium showed a maximum positive response. The effect of various growth regulators 2,4-D, NAA, IAA, BAP, and Kn was studied for their callogenic potential on different explants, such as immature seed, cotyledon, hypocotyls, root, leaves, and stem—the BAP and NAA combination induced maximum callogenic response. For shoot bud organogenesis, the BAP and NAA combination was more conducive. The callogenic potency was high with hypocotyls-derived calli. The highest number of shoot buds per callus was differentiated at a combination of BAP (2.5μM) and NAA (0.5μM) in *A. alata*. In

A. alata, root explants and seedling explants showed caulogenic competence. For rhizogenesis, the shoot buds were cultured in ½ strength MS medium with 0.25μM- 1μM NAA [13].

An efficient protocol for plantlet regeneration of *A. alata* through leaf calli was developed. MS medium supplemented with NAA produced abundant calli. The BAP and NAA (2 μM and 0.5 μM NAA) at optimal concentration induced callogenesis. The effect of the BAP and NAA combination caused shoot buds from calli. The micro shoots rooted well on MS medium with 1μM BAP and 0.75 to 1.25 μM NAA. The plantlets were then acclimatized in the soil [14]. *In vitro* flowering and differential accumulation of andrographolide from young explants of *A. lineata* were investigated. The explants from both mature and seedlings showed flowering morphogenesis on MS medium supplemented with BA and IAA. MS medium with two mg/l BA + 2mg/l IAA + 0.01% polyvinylpyrrolidone (PVP) showed a higher percentage of flowering, and cotyledonary nodes also showed multiple bud induction. Andrographolide content from different *in vitro* plantlet tissues was estimated using HPLC methods [15].

In vitro response of *A. alata* and *A. lineata* studies was executed with suitable explants, viz., nodal and tender leaves. The effect of various cytokinins (BA, TDZ, and Kn) alone and combined with auxins (NAA, IAA, and IBA) in MS medium on shoot induction and multiplication was studied. Additionally, growth adjuvants like tender coconut milk, casein hydrolysate, and antioxidants like ascorbic acid, PVP, and activated charcoal were used to improve shoot initiation and multiplication. Mature seeds were selected, sterilized, and cultured in half-strength MS liquid and semisolid nutrient media. Various explants were studied, and nodes and stumps of *A. alata* and *A. lineata* were used for further study. From the cytokinins tested, BA and TDZ showed increased shoot number and shoot length. Nodal explants cultured at 2.5 mg/l BA and 0.2 mg/l IBA combination in *A. alata* and at 3.0 mg/l BA and 0.2 mg/l IAA combination in *A. lineata* produced a higher number of shoots. *In vitro* flowering was achieved with MS medium fortified with BA + IAA/NAA along with 0.01% of PVP. In *A. alata*, 1.0 mg/l BA, along with 0.5 mg/l NAA and 1.0 mg/l IAA in *A. lineata*, produced better morphogenic callus. *In vitro* rooting of microshoots was observed on ½ and full MS basal medium without auxins [16].

The development of an efficient protocol for *in vitro* regeneration of *A. affinis* from nodal explants was reported. MS medium with BA and Kn at various concentrations was tested for the proliferation of shoots. 100% of shoot regeneration was obtained with MS medium containing 2 mg/l BA and 1 mg/l Kn. The regenerated plantlets were transferred to soil and maintained in a greenhouse [17].

In vitro propagation of *A. lineata* was attempted, where nodal segments were chosen as explants, and the surface was sterilized. The effect of different media, amino acids, and carbohydrates at various concentrations with plant growth regulators was tested on the nodal explants. Maximum percentage of shoot proliferation was 94.2% with 7.8 shoots per explants from the cultures on MS medium fortified with B5 vitamins + 1.5 mg/l of 2-iP + Kn (0.6 mg/l) + 20 mg/l Glutamine. The shootlets were then transferred to an MS medium fortified with different concentrations (0.5 to 3 mg/l) of IBA, IAA, and NAA. Root length was best attained with MS containing 2.0 mg/l IBA, and the percentage was about 95.6%. The plantlets were then subjected to hardening [18]. An efficient *in vitro* method for mass propagation of an endemic medicinal plant, *A. neesiana*, from nodal explants was developed. The authors proliferated high-frequency direct shoots on MS medium supplemented with TDZ from nodal explants. They also recorded that TDZ at 10μM concentration developed an average of 34 shoots in 94% of cultures in 4 weeks. Induced shoots were transferred to MS medium supplemented with 1.0μM Gibberellic acid (GA$_3$) for shoot elongation and were repeatedly subcultured. An average of about 60-70 shoots were obtained from a single explant, and rooting was induced in about 94% of shoots cultured in MS medium with 2.5 μM IAA. Rooted plantlets underwent hardening and were transferred to soil [6].

The evaluation of the *in vitro* seed germination and micropropagation of *A. echioides* was carried out successfully. The earliest seed germination (8.67 days) was recorded in the seed cultures on MS medium with 1mg/l of BAP. For direct regeneration, the shoot tip showed greater positive induction. Greater shoot induction takes place in MS medium enriched with 2.5mg/l of BAP. For shoot elongation, an MS medium with BAP (3.0 mg/l) showed a more positive response. Root induction (94.85%) was achieved with ½ MS medium supplemented with IAA (0.5 mg/l) + IBA (1.0mg/l). Hardening was carried out for the resultant plantlets [28]. The standardization of the micropropagation technique of *A. echioides* was achieved using different explants and media, of which shoot tips responded positively for shoot induction. MS medium with 2.5 mg/l BAP was found to be more effective for shoot induction. Multiple shoots were achieved with MS medium + BAP (3.0 mg/l); for shoot elongation, BAP (2.0 mg/l) + GA$_3$ (1.0 mg/l) showed a better response. For better rooting, ½ MS + IAA (0.5 mg/l) + IBA (1.0 mg/l) was used. The plantlets were subjected to optimum substrate hardening [20].

A report on the *in vitro* propagation of the endemic medicinal plant *A. lineata* was documented using shoot tips and nodal explants. The explants were surface sterilized and cultured aseptically on sterilized MS medium enriched with 30g/l sucrose and 0.8% agar. The inoculated cultures were incubated at 25±2°C with a light intensity of 16/8 hr (light/dark) cycle and 60-65% humidity. Different cytokinins (BAP, Kn, TDZ, and 2-iP) at various concentrations (5.0 to 50.0 mg/l) were tested for their effect on shoot proliferation from nodal cultures. The culture medium was additionally supplemented with AdS for adventitious shoot formation. Maximum shoots (25 ± 0.11) per explant were attained from the cultures with 1.5 mg/l BAP. The induced shoots were transferred to MS medium with GA_3 (0.5 -2.5 mg/l). A higher percentage of shoot elongation (87.0%) was induced with GA_3 at 0.3 mg/l. The effect of different concentrations (0.5, 1.0, and 2.0 mg/l) of various auxins like IAA, IBA, and NAA on root proliferation of elongated shoot cultures was analyzed. The developed plantlets were relocated in paper cups with suitable substrate for hardening [22].

Work on *in vitro* shoot multiplication of *A. lineata* was accomplished using cotyledonary nodes, shoot tips, leaves, nodal explants, internodes, and root segments from the 30 days old *in vitro* raised *A. lineata* from seeds cultured on ½ strength of MS medium with 0.6% agar. Explants were inoculated on MS medium fortified with BA 8.87µm. Nodal explants showed better results and were used for further *in vitro* studies. MS medium with various concentrations of cytokinins, BA, 2-iP, and Kn separately and in combination with NAA and IBA was used for *in vitro* cultures of nodal explants. The cultures were incubated at 25±2°C with 16 hrs of photoperiod. MS medium with BA 8.87µm + IBA 6.54 µm showed maximum results of 32.04 shoots per nodal explant in 30 days. They were sub-cultured to fresh MS medium with BA 8.87 µm for further proliferation. The developed shootlets with 5-6 nodes were cultured in full, 1/2, and 1/4 strength MS basal medium, Gamborg's B_5 medium, and woody plant medium with 0.6% agar for root proliferation. Of these, 1/2 strength MS medium showed greater rooting efficiency. The plantlets were shifted to pots for acclimatization [24].

In vitro plant regeneration, flowering, and fruiting of *A. lineata* with nodes as explants were studied. The explants were surface sterilized and inoculated in MS medium fortified with BA at varying concentrations (0.5-3.5 mg/l). Regeneration frequency (80.2%) was achieved maximum on MS medium with 2.5 mg/l of BA. Then, the developed cultures were tested with various media (Woody plant medium, B5 medium, and MS medium) in combination with BA for shoot induction and multiplication, and MS medium showed the best results. Then, an MS medium with different cytokinins (BA, TDZ, and Kn) with and without auxins (NAA, IAA, and IBA) was used to study shoot induction and multiplication. MS medium with 2.0 mg/L BA + 0.1 mg/L IAA showed good results with the explants. To improve the shoot initiation and multiplication, the medium was supplemented with growth adjuvants such as tender coconut milk, casein hydrolysate, and antioxidants like ascorbic acid, polyvinyl pyrrolidone, and activated charcoal. For root proliferation, the microshoots were cultured in full, ½, and 1/4 strength MS medium with and without auxins. Maximum frequency (74.2%) root formation was observed in 1/2 strength MS medium. *In vitro* flowering was studied with a single nodal explant on MS medium with growth regulators (BA, IAA, NAA, and IBA). Maximum flowering [5.5 flowers /explants (70%)] was seen in cultures supplemented with 2.0 mg/l BA and 1.5 mg/l NAA, along with 3% sucrose and 0.01% PVP. *In vitro* flower morphology was similar to *in vivo* flowers. Pollen morphology was studied for pollens from *in vitro* flowers through SEM, and they were similar to *in vivo* pollen grains. The plantlets were subjected to hardening with optimal autoclaved substrates [24].

Roy *et al.* [12] worked on improving the methods for high-frequency plantlet regeneration in *A. paniculata* by direct organogenesis. Plant regeneration *via* organogenesis from stem base explants of *A. paniculata* was standardized using an effective methodology. MS basal media was used to germinate the seeds. On MS media supplied with various quantities of cytokinin such as BAP, Kn, TDZ, and Zn, shoot multiplication occurred. On MS media supplemented with 2.0 mg/L Zn, however, high-frequency direct organogenesis produced the most adventitious shoots (62.0 ± 4.2/ explant). The organogenic path of regeneration was discovered through histological investigations. On MS media supplemented with BA (2.0 mg/L), shoot elongation from proliferated shoots was seen. After being dipped in IBA (1000 mg/L) and then transferred to MS basal media, the shoots were rooted.

Dandin and Murthy [33] tested the efficiency of shoot regeneration in *A. paniculata* on MS medium supplemented with a BAP, TDZ, Kn, and 2-iP at concentrations of 0.5, 1.0, 2.0, and 5.0, respectively. On MS medium supplemented with BAP (1.0 M) and Kn (5.0 M), the greatest number of 39 shoots per explant was reported. An anatomical study confirmed shoot regeneration *via* direct organogenesis.

Bansi and Rout [10] suggested a protocol for *A. paniculata* plant regeneration. Leaf and stem explants on MS basal media supplemented with 1.5 to 3.0 mg/l BA, 50 mg/l adenine sulfate (Ads), and 3% (m/v) sucrose resulted in rapid direct plant regeneration of *A. paniculata*. When 1.0 mg/l NAA was added to the culture media together with BA + Ads, the rate of shoot bud regeneration increased. MS medium supplemented with 3.0 mg/l BA, 50 mg/l Ads, and 1.0 mg/L NAA generated the highest mean number of shoot buds per explant after six weeks of development (28.6). Depending on the culture media, the percentage of regeneration varied. On half-strength MS medium supplemented with 0.5 mg/LIBA or NAA acid and 2% percent sucrose, the elongated shoots were rooted in 9 to 11 days.

Al-Mamun *et al.* [34] designed an *in vitro* micropropagation of *A. paniculata* to explore and establish a cost-effective methodology for quick *in vitro* regeneration. The study used MS media supplemented with BAP, Kn NAA, and IBA, either alone or in combination, for *in vitro* shoot development, shoot multiplication, root induction, and establishment of complete plantlets from Kalmegh shoot tips and nodal segments. At a dosage of 0.5 mg/L, BAP alone showed maximum (100%) shoot regeneration from the nodal segment. Axillary shoot proliferation was shown to be greatest in a medium containing 0.5 mg/L BAP and 0.1 mg/L NAA (90%).

Multiple shoot cultures of *A. paniculata* were studied by Zaheer and Giri [35]. Cotyledonary node (seedling devoid of root portion) explants were used to induce *A. paniculata* on full-strength MS media supplemented with 30 g/L sucrose and 1.0, 2.0, 3.0, and 4.0 mg/L BAP; 1.0, 2.0, 3.0, and 4.0 mg/L Kn; and 1.0, 2.0, 3.0, and 4.0 mg/L zeatin (Zt). After 8 weeks of culture, they discovered that *A. paniculata* cotyledonary node explants on MS media supplemented with 2.0 mg/L BAP and Zeatin produced multiple shoots at an average of 15.25 ± 2.128 and 16.16 ± 3.851 shoots/explant. After three subcultures (84 days) *in vitro* passages, single cotyledonary node explants proliferated further in MS+BAP media, yielding a maximum of 150 ± 18.40 multiple shoots.

Jindal *et al.* [36] investigated the proliferation and multiplication of *A. paniculata* nodes. By employing nodal explants, regeneration was performed on MS media supplemented with BAP, Kn, and 2iP at concentrations of 0.5-2.5 mg/L and BAP (2.0 mg/L) in conjunction with cytokinins like Kn (0.5-2.0 mg/L) and auxins such NAA and IAA at values of 0.1-0.5 mg/L. MS supplemented with BAP (2.0 mg/L) and NAA (0.5 mg/L) produced the most shoots per explant of all the combinations tested.

Kataky *et al.* [37] conducted micropropagation and antioxidant potential screening of *A. paniculata*. In full and half-strength MS media with varied concentrations of growth regulators, high-frequency shoot proliferation *via* nodal explants of *A.paniculata* was attained. After 45 days of culture, half MS medium supplemented with BAP 1mg/L + AdS 0.5mg/L produced a maximum average of 18.36 shoots, whereas Kn 0.5mg/L + AdS 0.5mg/L produced a maximum average of 16.66 shoots.

Arpita *et al.* [9] studied *A. paniculata* micropropagation from various sections. They used set concentrations of IAA and Kn in MS media to examine varied patterns of callus stimulation and nodal segment growth during micropropagation. The Kn and IAA concentrations utilized were 0.3 mg/L and 3 mg/L, respectively. The results showed that 18 of the 25 nodal segments produced a callus of 4-6 mm with a 72%t efficiency. With an efficiency of 84%, 21 of 25 seedlings developed a callus of 2-3 mm. A few seedlings showed some shoot growth during callus development. With a 44%t efficiency, 11 of 25 explants prepared from leaves developed a callus of 3-5 mm.

Deshmukh *et al*. [38] researched *in vitro* multiple shoot induction in *A. paniculata*. For additional research, *in vitro*-grown 30-day-old seedlings were used. Internodal and nodal sections of the plant were transferred into shoot induction media (BAP (1-3 mg/L). Among all growth hormone treatments, BAP 1.5mg/L demonstrated the greatest shoot induction (4-5 shoots per plant) (4-5 shoots per plant).

Mohammed [39] used mature zygotic embryonic explants to regenerate *A. paniculata in vitro*. Within 30 days of embryonic explant induction, a high frequency of adventitious shoot formation was observed, and shoot induction was followed by either direct regeneration on MS medium supplemented with BAP or indirect adventitious shoot regeneration in TDZ. BAP was more effective than other cytokinins for direct adventitious shoot induction or direct organogenesis from both embryonic explants of *A. paniculata*, with BAP 1.5 mg/L producing 73% shoot induction and 12.3 shoots per explant, while BAP 3.0 mg/L produced 52% shoot induction and 9.3 shoots per explant in the cotyledons study. Among the numerous concentrations studied, TDZ 1.0 mg was successful in indirect shoot regeneration or indirect organogenesis, with 26% shoot regeneration from the embryonic axis with 3.3 shoots and 76% from cotyledons with 6 shoots per explant.

Callus Induction and Indirect Organogenesis

A suitable protocol for indirect organogenesis in *A. echioides* was optimized. For this study, seeds from healthy disease-free plants were used to develop *in vitro* seedlings. Leaves and nodes from the raised *in vitro* seedlings were the sources of explants for callus induction. The culture was raised on MS medium supplemented with (3.0mg/l 2, 4-D) + (2.0 mg/l NAA) and showed higher callus induction of about 90% for leaf explants and 95% for nodal explants. Shoot regeneration from leaf callus explants was 93%, and it was 87% from shoot callus explants. Then, the regenerated shoots were sub-cultured on MS medium with BAP (3.0 mg/l). The growth rate from leaf callus and shoot callus was 84% and 89%, respectively. The shoots were rooted well in MS medium supplemented with IAA (2.0 mg/l) and IBA (1.5mg/l). The plantlets were successfully acclimatized and hardened [25].

The impact of growth regulators on the micropropagation of *A. echioides* was studied using different explants. The explants used were shoot tips, nodal segments, stem bits, leaf bits, and root bits, of which shoot bits showed the highest response of 85.72%. The highest direct shoot regeneration (83.22%) was on MS medium supplemented with BAP (2.5 mg/l). On MS medium + BAP (3.0 mg/l), cultured shoots showed multiple shoot induction, and shoot elongation was better observed in MS medium with BAP (2.0 mg/l) + GA_3 (1.0 mg/l). The highest rooting (94.85%) was recorded in ½ MS + IAA 0.5 mg/l + IBA 1.0 mg/l [26]. Savitikadi *et al.* [27] reported the micropropagation and genetic fidelity analysis of regenerated plants of *A. echioides*. *In vitro* seedlings leaf explants were excised and inoculated on MS medium with plant growth regulators. The highest frequency of direct shoot regeneration (24.48 ± 1.54) was observed with cultures in MS medium supplemented with TDZ + IAA at 0.5 and 0.2 mg/l. The highest rooting percent (90.42%) was observed in the MS medium with IAA (1.0 mg/l) and IBA (1.0 mg/l). The plantlets of *A. echioides* were hardened. PCR-based molecular analysis using ISSR and rbcL primers confirmed the genetically cloned nature of regenerated plantlets [27].

In vitro propagation method for *A. macrobotrys* mass multiplication was successfully achieved using nodal segments. The explants were cultured on MS medium augmented with different cytokinins like BAP, Kn, 2-iP, and TDZ at concentrations 2.5, 5, 7.5, and 10 μM L^{-1}. An average of about 32 shoots per explant was regenerated from a culture containing MS medium with 7.5 μM L^{-1} BAP. Root induction was effective with 5 μM L^{-1} IBA. The plantlets were transferred to pots with a 1:1 ratio of soil and coco peat at 25±2°C, 80% humidity, and 16 h photoperiod. The plants were transferred to the field after 8 days [28]. A study on the *in vitro* regeneration, genetic fidelity analysis, and neoandrographolide content of *A. alata* was reported. For the propagation of nodal explants, MS medium fortified with 10μM BAP was used, and multiple shoots were proliferated. Roots were generated in ¼ concentrated MS medium augmented with 1μM IBA. Genetic fidelity was analyzed with RAPD and ISSR markers. Neoandrographolide presence was confirmed with reverse-phase high-performance liquid chromatography, and it was equivalent to that of the mother plant [28].

An effective *in vitro* propagation of *A. echioides* from mature nodal explants was executed. The culture medium used was MS medium supplemented with 3% sucrose. Plant growth regulators used were two different cytokinins, BAP and Kn, combined with NAA. Highest shoot bud induction (90 ± 2.88%) was in MS medium with BAP (2.0 mg/l) + NAA (0.5 mg/l). In this medium, the maximum number of shoots per explant was 5 ± 1.00, with the highest shoot length of 2.0 ± 0.57 cm. MS medium supplemented with BAP (2.0 mg/l) + optimum concentration of NAA (0.5 mg/l) + GA_3 (1.0 mg/l) promoted shoot elongation as well as enhanced shoot regeneration. This combined MS medium produced the highest shoot proliferation percentage (95 ± 5.00), number of shoots per explant (9 ± 1.00), and maximum shoot length (6.8 ± 1.11 cm). MS medium with IAA (1.0 mg/l) + IBA (0.5 mg/l) promoted the highest root percentage (90 ± 5.77), number of roots per explant (12 ± 1.15), and root length (6.5 ± 1.26 cm) The micropropagated plantlets were established in the field through acclimatization [30].

Young leaves, internodes, nodes, and roots of *A. paniculata* seedlings were removed and inoculated in disposable Petri -dishes containing solid MS media supplemented with various combinations of auxins and cytokinin at varying doses. Parameters such as the percent of explants demonstrating callus induction and the color and texture of the callus induced were monitored and documented for each explant type and media composition employed up to 4 weeks of culture. Changes in diameter, height, and fresh weights of cultures (in g) throughout the next 6 weeks of culture were used to measure callus proliferation. Callus cultures were cultured in the dark at 25 °C ± 1 °C and under a 16-hour photoperiod. Cool white fluorescent tube lamps with a light intensity of 100 µmol m^{-2} s^{-1} were employed as the light source [40].

For callus induction, explants were inoculated in an MS medium containing IAA and Kn growth regulators. At a consistent concentration of several hormones, such as Kn and IAA, callus induction was detected in all three parts. In comparison to other portions of *A. paniculata*, callus development was shown to be highest in seeds and over 84% at a specific concentration of growth agents. The effect of this range of growth regulators on callus development was shown to be less effective in nodal segments and leaflets. Due to the presence of active parenchymatous cells, the potential of callus induction in the nodal buds was also above average, at 72%. On the other hand, due to the scarcity of undifferentiated cells in leaflets, the likelihood of callus formation was lower than typical, at roughly 44%. The graphical observation also showed that the totipotency of other portions of the plant to grow callus was lower than that of seeds. Cellular damage is possible during the sterilizing process. The seed, on the other hand, is sealed within the pods, which protects them from severe contamination. Seed viability and internode viability towards callus formation are somehow similar at a given point. Both of these can be considered for a healthy callus formation [9].

The development of a protocol for micropropagation of *A. producta* using nodal and shoot tips as explants was accomplished. Seeds were sterilized and cultured in MS medium supplemented with 3% sucrose. The raised *in vitro* seedlings (6-week-old) were used as a source for shoot tips and nodal explants. They were cultured in MS medium with 3% sucrose and different concentrations (2.5, 5.0, 7.5, and 10.0 µM) of BAP, Kn, 2-iP, and TDZ separately. The optimum temperature was 25± 2°C and with 60% relative humidity under a photoperiod of 6 h light. At 10μM of 2-iP in MS medium, the highest number of axillary shoots (14.60) were regenerated from nodal explants, whereas at 5μM of BAP, the highest number of shoots (17.50) were regenerated from shoot tip explants. Shoot tip explants cultured in MS medium fortified with 10μM 2-iP regenerated an average of 27.66 adventitious shoots. Maximum rooting of shoots was observed in ¼ strength MS medium amended with 10μM IBA. The results showed that shoot tips were the better explants for the micropropagation of *A. producta* [31].

Micropropagation of *A. lineata* var. *lawii* was studied using shoot tip and nodal explants. MS medium supplemented with BAP was used for culture inoculation. Shoot tips and nodal explants produced an average of 24.83 and 21.41 shoots, respectively. TDZ-supplemented medium-induced callus mediated multiple shoots from cotyledonary leaf explants. Proliferation and elongation of callus-mediated shoot buds were achieved on MS medium fortified with 2 μM BAP. Root induction was observed with MS medium containing 10μM IBA [32]. *In vitro* regeneration protocol of *A. lobelioides* was carried out on MS medium through callus and shoot induction studies. For root induction, half-strength MS medium was utilized. Maximum percentage of callus was obtained with BAP (1.0 mg/l) + 0.1 mg/l Kn fortified MS medium. Maximum shoot regeneration was obtained (10.3 ±0.41 shoots per explant) with BA (0.5 mg/l) and IAA (0.05 mg/l). Root induction was high (95.9 ± 0.51 roots per shoot) with IBA (0.6 mg/l) [41].

In vitro Rooting

Purkayastha *et al.*'s [8] investigation of rapid *in vitro* multiplication and plant regeneration from nodal explants of *A. paniculata* revealed that the plant has a high frequency of regeneration potential. In 94% of shoots cultivated on MS media supplemented with 2.5 M IBA, rooting was induced within a week. After hardening, the plantlets were successfully moved to the soil, with a survival rate of 92%. The system is quick; from the commencement of shoot buds to the transplantation of regenerants into the soil, it takes only 8–9 weeks.

In their investigations on *in vitro* propagation of *A. paniculata*, Roy *et al.* [12] reported that isolated shoots rooted successfully (90%) on half-strength MS fortified with 9.80 M/l IBA, with an average number of roots per shoot of 28-30. In poly bags containing a 2:1:1 ratio of soil, sand, and compost, the plantlets were effectively acclimatized. After that, the acclimatized plantlets were moved to the experimental field.

When Dandin and Murthy [33] investigated *A. paniculata* regeneration, they found that regenerated shoots were cultured on MS medium supplemented with NAA, IAA, and IBA at concentrations of 0.5, 1.0, 2.0, and 5.0 M for the induction of roots. After being transferred to half-strength MS medium supplemented with IBA (2.0 M), 100% of the shoots formed roots. The rooted plantlets were acclimatized and established in the soil successfully.

Bansi and Rout 2013 [10] attempted to establish an *A. paniculata* plant regeneration protocol, reporting that the elongated shoots were rooted within 9 to 11 days on half-strength MS medium supplemented with 0.5 mg/L IBA or NAA acid and 2% sucrose. On a medium containing 0.5 mg/L IBA and 2% sucrose, the highest percentage of rooting (76.24%) was achieved. When exposed to higher concentrations of either IBA or NAA, the microshoots basal region became callused. In the greenhouse, the rooted plantlets made it. Under normal soil conditions, the *in vitro*-produced plantlets were grown. The preservation and propagation of this vital medicinal plant will be made easier as a result of this discovery.

In his research on efficient *in vitro* micropropagation of *A. paniculata*, Al-Mamun *et al.* [34] discovered that the medium containing 0.2 mg/L of IBA resulted in a maximum rooting of 100 percent with 12.4 roots per explant.

When Jindal and Choudhary [36] researched shoot proliferation and multiplication from nodes of *A. paniculata*, they found that when cultivated on MS medium supplemented with NAA, IAA, and IBA at concentrations of 0.5- 3.0 mg/L, shoots were regenerated for the induction of roots. When the cultures were transferred to full-strength MS media supplemented with IBA (3.0 mg/L), 100% rooting was observed.

Deshmukh *et al.* [38] observed that well-grown shoots were subcultured on the media IAA (1-3 mg/L) and NAA (1-3 mg/L) for root initiation in their *in vitro* multiple shoot induction research on *A. paniculata*. Maximum roots were found in IAA 1.5 mg/L and 2.0 mg/L.

Acclimatization

Acclimatization and hardening are major steps in transplanting an *in vitro* developed plantlet to an *ex vitro* condition. *In vitro* cultured plantlets are exposed to various special conditions such as large doses of growth regulators, high air humidity, and limited inflow of CO_2 which results in abnormal morphology, physiology, anatomy, *etc.* So, *ex vitro* transplantation can impair the plantlets due to sudden environmental changes, which coerce the acclimatization process ineluctably. Acclimatization is usually carried out with gradual levels of humidity, temperature, irradiance, CO_2 concentration, and airflow rate [30]. The resultant plantlets of micropropagated *A.neesiana* were subjected to acclimatization in greenhouse conditions. The plantlets were reared in pots filled with soil, vermiculite, and vermicompost at a ratio of (1:1:1). In order to prevent moisture loss, the plants were covered with polythene bags for a week. Then, the plants were transferred to greenhouse at optimum conditions, such as 28°C day, 20°C night, 16 hrs day length, and 70% relative humidity. The plastic covering was gradually removed after a week, and the plants were transferred to the nursery. The micropropagated plants showed a 92% survival rate. The *in vitro* plants showed normal growth and morphology [6].

Micropropagated *A.alata* plantlets were transferred to plastic containers with sterile sand and soil at a 1:1 ratio and covered with thin, perforated transparent polythene bags. MS medium at 1/10th strength was supplemented along with watering. The plantlets were incubated at culture room conditions for 1 week and then transferred to field conditions for hardening. The acclimatization percentage of plantlets derived from various explants was studied separately. A 65% survivability rate was observed in regenerants from leaf callus. The regenerants showed slight morphological variation in the shape and texture of leaves [13]. The microshoots of *A. alata* and *A. lineata* propagated in aseptic conditions were acclimatized by planting in plastic trays with vermiculite as substrates. The trays were covered with plastic sheets and maintained in a mist chamber for one week. After a week, during morning hours, the regenerants were allowed to be exposed to direct sunlight. The plantlets were relocated to root trainers with a mixture of vermicompost and sand at a 1:1 ratio and 10 ml of autoclaved ¼ MS salts for 10 days. Then, they were maintained in plastic bags containing soil, organic manure, and sand at a 2:1:1 ratio in open shade. The plantlets were watered twice a day for 1 week and transferred to field conditions. Acclimatized *A. alata* plants showed a 70-85% survivability rate in a natural environment. The *in vitro* plantlets were morphologically similar to *in vivo* plants [16, 22]. In *A. lineata*, 86% of the *in vitro* plants were successfully acclimatized in garden conditions [22].

For acclimatization of *A. lineata*, *in vitro* plantlets pot with garden soil and farmyard manure at a (2:1) ratio was used and kept in an environmental plant growth chamber. The plants showed a 78% survivability rate in an *in vivo* environment [18]. *In vitro* derived plantlets of *A. echioides* were acclimatized in different substrates such as vermiculite, red earth, sand, and a combination of vermiculite+ sand+ red earth at 1:1:1. Of the tested substrate combination, the substrate showed better a survivability of 60.38% [19]. Aseptically cultured plantlets of *A. lineata* were subjected to hardening in paper cups with autoclaved sand, vermiculite, and soil mixture at a (2:1:1 *v/v/v*) ratio. For persistent moisture content, the plants were covered with polythene bags and maintained in the plant growth chamber at 25±2°C and 85% relative humidity. After 3 weeks, the plants were transferred to greenhouse conditions. About 70% survivability rate was recorded with acclimatized plantlets. RAPD analysis revealed consistent genetic stability in the *in vitro* culture of *A. lineata* [16].

A. lineata plantlets developed *in vitro* were transferred to plastic pots with sterile peat moss, farmyard manure, and soil mixture at a (1:1:1) ratio and covered with polythene sheets for acclimatization. For watering, ¼ strength MS basal salt solution without sucrose was used. Watering was done for every 3 days. After 3 weeks, the plants were relocated to shade for 4 weeks. They were then transferred to field conditions. The survivability rate achieved was 75% under field conditions [18]. The plantlets of *A. echioides* were acclimatized by transferring them to paper cups with sand, red soil, and vermicompost in a (1:1:1) ratio. They were watered once in 2 days and maintained under environmental conditions. The survival rate was recorded as 70% [20].

In vitro plantlet of *A. echioides* was hardened in poly cups with compost and garden soil at a (1:2) ratio as substrate. Polythene sheet covering of plants prevents moisture and humidity loss. The plantlets were irrigated with ½ strength MS salt solution for four weeks and maintained at 50-70% humidity. The hardening was carried out in greenhouse conditions and then acclimatized in field conditions. The survivability was recorded as 80%. Genetic fidelity was studied with ISSR and rbcLa DNA barcoding primers, and it was revealed that micropropagated plantlets of *A. echioides* were genetically stable to *in vivo* plants [22]. The plantlets of *A. macrobotrys* propagated in aseptic conditions were acclimatized in pots with a substrate mixture of soil and coco peat at a (1:1) ratio. The transferred plants were kept in a growth chamber at 25±2°C, 80% relative humidity, 100µmol m^{-2} s^{-1} for 16 hrs of photoperiod. For irrigation, the Hoagland solution was used once every 4 days. After 8 weeks, the plants were relocated to soil with farmyard manure and sand in the field [28].

Acclimatized *A. alata* plantlets were transferred to the substrate with equal amounts of soil and coco peat in pots. They were maintained at 25± 2°C temperature, 16 h of light, and 60% of relative humidity. The genetic fidelity of the acclimatized plants was analyzed using RAPD and ISSR primers. The results showed three monomorphic bands in both *in vitro* and *in vivo* plants, which revealed their similarities in morphology [24]. *In vitro* microshoots of *A. echioides* developed were transferred to paper cups containing a mixture of garden soil, vermiculite, and sand in a ratio of 2:1:1 for hardening. The humidity was maintained at 60-70% and covered with polythene covers to prevent moisture loss. The incubated temperature was around 25± 2°C, and the light intensity was about 16/8 h photoperiod. The plants were then transferred to a glass house after 4 weeks. Finally, they were relocated to a garden where plants were gradually exposed to direct sunlight. The plants had better survivability of about 80% [25].

Micropropagated plants of *A. producta* were acclimatized in pots with equal volumes of coco peat and vermiculite. The plants were kept in a growth chamber at a temperature of $25 \pm 2°C$, light 16/8 h photoperiod, and 60% humidity. They were transferred to a pot mixture of soil and coco peat in greenhouse conditions. The survival percentage was recorded as 95% [31].

Plantlets with four to five completely developed leaves and rooted micropropagules of *A. paniculta* were properly rinsed to remove the clinging gel before being planted in earthen pots with a mixture of soil, sand, and dry cow-dung manure (1:1:1, w/v) and placed in the greenhouse to acclimate. Watering was done every two days on the plants. One month after being transferred into pots, the survival rate was measured [11]. About 92% of the micropropagated plants survived and displayed typical morphological and growth features. On MS media supplemented with 10 µM BAP, 94% of the explants proliferated, with an average of 34 shoots per explant. This valuable medicinal plant would benefit from such a high regeneration frequency for widespread propagation and multiplication. Explants created from *in vitro* raised plantlets to eliminate contamination associated with *ex vitro* explants, ensuring the clonal proliferation of selected species. *In vitro* cultures are capable of producing a consistent supply of phytoconstituents. Furthermore, this efficient and dependable plant regeneration system based on direct shoot organogenesis can be used in genetic manipulation research to boost biomass growth and, ultimately, bioactive chemical production, according to Purkayastha *et al.* [8].

CONCLUSION

Andrographis is a key medicinal genus with various therapeutically important species. Most of the research works were focused on the commonly known *Andrographis* species *A. paniculata* and *A. lineata*. Even though other species have high therapeutic values, they still remain untouched for micropropagation studies. Also, there is a need for conservation because most of the species are endemic to India. Future research works on the micropropagation of these *Andrographis* species will be helpful for the commercialization of the active principles, sustainable utilization, and conservation from exploitation.

LIST OF ABBREVIATIONS

2,4-D 2, 4, Dichlorophenoxy acetic acid

BA 6- benzyl adenine

BAP 6-Benzyl Amino Purine

GA Gibberellic acid

HgCl₂ mercuric chloride

IAA	Indole Acetic Acid
IBA	Indole 3 Butyric Acid
ISSR	Inter Simple Sequence Repeats
Kn	Kinetin
MS	Murashige and Skoog
NAA	Naphthalene Acetic Acid
RAPD	Randomly Amplified Polymorphic DNA
TDZ	Thidiazuron
PVP	Polyvinylpyrrolidone
AdS	Adenine Sulphate
2-iP	6-(γ,γ- Dimethylallylamino)purine

REFERENCES

[1] Karmegam N, Nagaraj R, Karuppusamy S, Prakash M. Biological and pharmacological activities of *Andrographis* spp. (Acanthaceae) distributed in southern Eastern Ghats, India. Int J Curr Res Biosci Plant Biol 2015; 2(9): 140-53.

[2] Panda PC, Mohanty SK, Bal P, Kamila PK. Macro-propagation of threatened plants of India and its conservation implications. Frontiers in Plant Sciences 2019.

[3] Balu S, Algesaboopathi C. Propagation of *Andrographis lineata* Nees by stem cuttings. Anc Sci Life 1995; 14(4): 235-9.
[PMID: 22556703]

[4] Frankenberger EA, Hasegawa PM, Tigchelaar EC. Influence of environment and developmental state on the shoot-forming capacity of tomato genotypes. Z Pflanzenphysiol 1981; 102(3): 221-32.
[http://dx.doi.org/10.1016/S0044-328X(81)80224-3]

[5] Abdalla N, El-Ramady H, Seliem MK, *et al.* An academic and technical overview on plant micropropagation challenges. Horticulturae 2022; 8(8): 677.
[http://dx.doi.org/10.3390/horticulturae8080677]

[6] Karuppusamy S, Kalimuthu K. Rapid *in vitro* multiplication and plant regeneration from nodal explants of *Andrographis neesiana*: A valuable endemic medicinal plant. Biol Res 2010; 4(4): 211-6.

[7] Debnath M, Malik C, Bisen P. Micropropagation: a tool for the production of high quality plant-based medicines. Curr Pharm Biotechnol 2006; 7(1): 33-49.
[http://dx.doi.org/10.2174/138920106775789638] [PMID: 16472132]

[8] Purkayastha J, Sugla T, Paul A, Solleti S, Sahoo L. Rapid *in vitro* multiplication and plant regeneration from nodal explants of *Andrographis paniculata*: a valuable medicinal plant. In Vitro Cell Dev Biol Plant 2008; 44(5): 442-7.
[http://dx.doi.org/10.1007/s11627-008-9156-8]

[9] Arpita SAAD, Singh A, Awasthi A. Study of in-vitro micropropagation of medicinally important plant *Andrographis paniculata* from its different parts. Int J Sci Res 2017; 6(5): 1060-3.

[10] Bansi TS, Rout GR. Plant regeneration protocol of *Andrographis paniculata* (Burm. f.) - an important medicinal plant. Afr J Biotechnol 2013; 12(39): 5738-42.

[11] Roy PK. *In vitro* propagation of *Andrographis paniculata* Nees.-A threatened medicinal plant of Bangladesh. Jahangirnagar University Journal of Biological Sciences 2016; 3(1): 67-73.
[http://dx.doi.org/10.3329/jujbs.v3i1.28279]

[12] Roy S, Giri A, Bhubaneswari C, Narasu ML, Giri CC. High frequency plantlet regeneration *via* direct organogenesis in *Andrographis paniculata*. Med Aromat Plant Sci Biotechnol 2009; 3: 94-6.

[13] Nagaraja YP. *In vitro* studies on *Andrographis paniculata* Nees. and *Andrographis alata* Nees. Ph D Thesis, Kuvempu University 2002.

[14] Nagaraja YP, Krishna V, Maruthi KR. Rapid micropropagation of *Andrographis alata* Nees. through leaf callus culture. Plant Cell Biotechnol Mol Biol 2003; 4: 117-24.

[15] Mohammed A, Gopal G. *In vitro* flowering and differential accumulation of andrographolide in cultures of *Andrographis lineata* Nees - an important medicinal plant of India. In Vitro Cell Dev Biol Anim 2005; 41: 54A-A.

[16] Arifullah Md. 2006.

[17] Govindaraj S, Thangaswamy S, Hariprasad S, Alagesaboopathi C. *In vitro* regeneration and mass multiplication of *Andrographis affinis* Nees - An endemic medicinal species from India. Asian J Microbiol Biotechnol Environ Sci 2008; 10: 173-7.

[18] Lakshmiprabha A, Chandrasekar B, Nandagopalan V, Jayabalan N. *In vitro* mass propagation of *Andrographis lineata* Nees. through nodal explant-an important ethnomedicinal plant. J Swamy Bot Club 2008; 25: 1-4.

[19] Sumitha J, Saritha B, Arjun P. *In vitro* biomass accumulation and regeneration of potential medicinal plant green chiretta-*Andrographis paniculata* (Burm. f.) Nees. Intern J Bot Studies 2022; 7(1): 109-13.

[20] Hemalatha P, Vadivel E. Evaluation of *in vitro* seed germination and micropropagation techniques in *Andrographis echioides* (L.) Nees. Int J Agric Sci 2010; 6(1): 209-12.

[21] Deepa V. Micropropagation and antidiabetic effect of *Andrographis lineata* Wall. ex. Nees - an endemic medicinal plant. Ph D Thesis, Anna University 2011.

[22] Mohammed A, Chiruvella KK, Rao YK, Geethangili M, Raghavan SC, Ghanta RG. *In vitro* production of echioidinin, 7-O-methywogonin from callus cultures of *Andrographis lineata* and their cytotoxicity on cancer cells. PLoS One 2015; 10(10): e0141154.
[http://dx.doi.org/10.1371/journal.pone.0141154] [PMID: 26488879]

[23] Aruna V, Pullaiah T. *In vitro* shoot multiplication of medicinally important plant *Andrographis lineata* Nees *via* nodal explants. European J Med Plants 2016; 17(3): 1-7.
[http://dx.doi.org/10.9734/EJMP/2016/30411]

[24] Mohammed A, Chiruvella KK, Ghanta RG. *In vitro* plant regeneration, flowering and fruiting from nodal explants of *Andrographis lineata* Nees (Acanthaceae). J Crop Sci Biotechnol 2016; 19(3): 195-202.
[http://dx.doi.org/10.1007/s12892-016-0003-x]

[25] Xavier TF, Kumar S. Indirect organogenesis of *Andrographis echioides* (L.) Nees. World J Pharm Res 2018; 7(5): 1655-64.

[26] Hemalatha P, Sivakumar V, Rajamani K, Praneetha S. Studies on influence of growth regulators on *in vitro* propagation of *Andrographis echioides* (L.) Nees. J Pharmacogn Phytochem 2020; 9(6): 233-6.
[http://dx.doi.org/10.22271/phyto.2020.v9.i6d.12888]

[27] Savitikadi P, Jogam P, Rohela GK, *et al*. Direct regeneration and genetic fidelity analysis of regenerated plants of *Andrographis echioides* (L.) - An important medicinal plant. Ind Crops Prod 2020; 155: 112766.
[http://dx.doi.org/10.1016/j.indcrop.2020.112766]

[28] Kadapatti SS, Murthy HN. *In vitro* micropropagation of *Andrographis macrobotrys*. J Herbs Spices Med Plants 2022; 28(1): 89-98.
[http://dx.doi.org/10.1080/10496475.2021.1964012]

[29] Kadapatti SS, Murthy HN. Rapid plant regeneration, analysis of genetic fidelity, and

neoandrographolide content of micropropagated plants of *Andrographis alata* (Vahl) Nees. J Genet Eng Biotechnol 2021; 19(1): 20.
[http://dx.doi.org/10.1186/s43141-021-00122-5] [PMID: 33496903]

[30]   Kolar AB, Sheik Mohamed S, Shareef Khan M, Ghouse Basha M. Direct plant regeneration from mature nodal explants of *Andrographis echioides* (L.) Nees–a valuable medicinal plant. Plant Arch 2021; 21(1) (Suppl. 1): 1842-8.
[http://dx.doi.org/10.51470/PLANTARCHIVES.2021.v21.S1.296]

[31]   Kadapatti SS, Murthy HN. Micropropagation of *Andrographis producta* through axillary and adventitious shoot regeneration. J Genet Eng Biotechnol 2022; 20(1): 152.
[http://dx.doi.org/10.1186/s43141-022-00438-w] [PMID: 36318363]

[32]   Kadapatti SS, Murthy HN. Micropropagation of threatened medicinal plant *Andrographis lineata* var. *lawii*. Vegetos 2023; 37(1): 202-10.
[http://dx.doi.org/10.1007/s42535-023-00585-6]

[33]   Dandin VS, Murthy HN. Regeneration of *Andrographis paniculata* Nees: Analysis of genetic fidelity and andrographolide content in micropropagated plants. Afr J Biotechnol 2012; 11(61): 12464-71.

[34]   Al-Mamun M, Akhter R, Rahman A, Ferdousi Z. Efficient *in vitro* micropropagation of *Andrographis paniculata* and evaluation of antibacterial activity from its crude protein extract. European J Med Plants 2015; 6(4): 231-41.
[http://dx.doi.org/10.9734/EJMP/2015/15663]

[35]   Zaheer M, Giri CC. Multiple shoot induction and jasmonic versus salicylic acid driven elicitation for enhanced andrographolide production in *Andrographis paniculata.* Plant Cell Tissue Organ Cult 2015; 122(3): 553-63.
[http://dx.doi.org/10.1007/s11240-015-0787-2]

[36]   Jindal N, Chaudhury A, Kajla S. Shoot proliferation and multiplication from nodes of *Andrographis paniculata.* International Research Journal of Pharmacy 2015; 6(9): 654-7.
[http://dx.doi.org/10.7897/2230-8407.069128]

[37]   Kataky A, Handique PJ. Micropropagation and screening of antioxidant potential of *Andrographis paniculata* (Burm. f) Nees. J Hill Agriculture 2010; 1(1): 13-8.

[38]   Deshmukh AS, Pawar SD, Nirgude MS, Pingle A S. *In vitro* multiple shoot induction in *Andrographis paniculata.* Intern J Current Microbiol Appl Sci 2018; (6): pp. 791-795.

[39]   Mohammed A. *In vitro* plant regeneration of *Andrographis paniculata* Nees using mature zygotic embryonic explants. Agric Res Technol 2017; 5(5)
[http://dx.doi.org/10.19080/ARTOAJ.2017.05.555674]

[40]   Das D, Bandyopadhyay M. Manipulation of DXP pathway for andrographolide production in callus cultures of *Andrographis paniculata.* Planta 2021; 254(2): 23.
[http://dx.doi.org/10.1007/s00425-021-03674-5] [PMID: 34223986]

[41]   Samydurai P, Rajendran A. *In vitro* regeneration of an endemic medicinal plant *Andrographis lobelioides* Wight. Plant Cell Biotechnol Mol Biol 2018; 26: 85-90.

CHAPTER 16

In vitro Production of Medicinally Potential Andrographolides from *Andrographis* Species

S. Karuppusamy[1,*]

[1] *Department of Botany, The Madura College, Madurai-625011, Tamil Nadu, India*

Abstract: *Andrographis* L. (Acanthaceae) is a vital genus that produces the most potential secondary metabolites, such as labdane diterpenoids called andrographolides. Pharmaceutical requirements for andrographolides are sustained through habitat collection and limited cultivation of *Andrographis paniculata*. However, in India, the genus is represented by about 26 species distributed in the southern Peninsula, most of which are endemic to the region. Commercial exploitation for andrographolide extraction is met with *A. paniculata* alone. The low rate of seed production in this plant and enormous variation in andrographolide content were found in the natural population. Tissue culture techniques help us to produce commercially viable andrographolides on a large scale. The present review analyzes the alternative sources of andrographolides from diverse species of *Andrographis*. Also, the review describes *in vitro* culture of callus and suspension cultures, the development of adventitious and hairy root cultures, the addition of biotic and abiotic elicitors for enhancing andrographolide production, and also the production of valuable compounds by utilizing bioreactors, *Agrobacterium*-mediated transformation, and genetic engineering for increasing biosynthesis of andrographolides.

Keywords: Andrographolide, *Andrographis paniculata*, *In vitro* production, Plant tissue culture, Secondary metabolite.

INTRODUCTION

Secondary plant products are low molecular weight compounds with significant pharmaceutical potential. Besides using them as food, humans are constantly exploring and exploiting these natural plant products for use as medicines, cosmetics, dyes, flavors, and food. *Andrographis* (Acanthaceae) comprises 26 species predominantly native to India [1]. This genus displays high diversity, particularly in Peninsular India and the Himalayas, with many species endemic to India. This genus, *Andrographis*, has been highly integrated with the maintenance of the human healthcare system since time immemorial. Several of these species

* **Corresponding author S. Karuppusamy:** Department of Botany, The Madura College, Madurai-625011, Tamil Nadu, India; E-mail: ksamytaxonomy@gmail.com

are extensively used in ethnomedicinal systems in tribal areas of Western Ghats [2]. Many of the species of *Andrographis* found in India are used in various industries and form an integral part of the traditional system of medicine. The critical compound andrographolide varies within different plants and by geographical location. In wild and conventionally propagated plants, the andrographolide content is typically around 2-3% based on fresh weight. The traditional propagation method through vegetative means needs to be improved to meet the pharmaceutical industry's demand, leading to reliance on wild plants. Variations of phytochemical contents in the wild population and delayed rooting response of seedlings may affect the propagation of this plant only through the seeds [3, 4]. The ever-increasing demand for andrographolides in the pharmaceutical market solely depends on extracting drugs from wild-grown plants. This overharvesting poses a risk of extinction. However, commercial exploitation of andrographolide is hampered due to the limited availability of wild-grown plants [5]. The substantial demand for andrographolide in Indian and international markets has been increasing through commercial cultivation by Indian farmers. Several medicinal potentials of *Andrographis* include carminative, febrifugal, anthelmintic, antirheumatic, antidiabetic, antihyperglycemic, antipyretic, anti-inflammatory, antinociceptive, and antioxidant effects [6]. Sustainable production methods are crucial given the high demand and limited availability of wild plant sources. *In vitro*, producing valuable secondary metabolites using biotechnological methods is a viable alternative for maintaining natural diversity and continuously utilizing plant drugs. In recent decades, *in vitro* techniques have been extensively used to produce secondary metabolites [7] commercially. These techniques used bioreactor, biotic and abiotic elicitors, and cell immobilization for scaling up the production of natural compounds [8]. However, bioreactor trials fail to yield the desired quantities of target compounds due to a lack of understanding of biosynthetic pathways and mechanisms. Enhancing productivity involves overcoming the limitation of precursor availability by adding specific additives to cultured cells or organs. Techniques such as elicitation, immobilization, and metabolic engineering can improve phytocompound production.

SOURCES OF ANDROGRAPHOLIDE – *ANDROGRAPHIS* SPECIES

Andrographis comprises 43 species globally, with 26 species in India [9]. In the southern parts of Eastern Ghats, more than ten species of *Andrographis*, including *A. affinis*, *A. alata*, *A. beddomei*, *A. elongata*, *A. echioides*, *A. glandulosa*, *A. lineata*, *A. ovata*, *A. paniculata*, and *A. serpyllifolia*, are distributed. Among these, *Andrographis paniculata* holds significant potential traditional medicinal value due to its broad spectrum of biological activities. The pharmacological efficacy of *Andrographis* is attributed to their content of flavonoids, terpenoids, and flavonoid glycosides such as andrographolide, echiodinin, and echiodinin 5-o-β-D-glucopyranoside. Notably, andrographolide, neoandrographolide, and deoxyandrographolide are identified as the most bitter compounds among these. While other *Andrographis* species also contain andrographolides, the rarity of several species has limited their exploration as phytopharmaceutical sources. The primary phytochemical responsible for the medicinal properties of these plants is andrographolide [1].

ANDROGRAPHOLIDE AND ITS ANALOGS

Andrographolide, a labdane diterpenoid, is produced by *A. paniculata*. It is a significant component in over 26 Ayurvedic formulations and is primarily used for treating liver diseases. Among secondary plant products, andrographolides are the most pharmacologically active compounds. However, they are only sourced from conventionally propagated or wild-grown plants, which represent a mere 2-3% of the total, and are insufficient to meet the growing pharmaceutical demand, which is increasing annually by 3.1% [4]. *A. paniculata* also synthesize various other compounds including 5,7-tetramethoxyflavanone, 5-hydroxy-7 trimethoxy-flavone, numerous flavonoids, and polyphenols [10 - 12]. The andrographolide content varies across different plant parts: approximately 4% in the dried whole plant, 0.8-1.2% in the stem, and 0.5-6% in leaf extracts. Other significant diterpenoids in *A. paniculata* include deoxyandrographolide, neoandrographolide, 14-deoxy-11,12-didehydroandrographide, and isoandrogra-pholide [13]. From the EtOAC-soluble fraction of ethanol or methanol extracts, several main flavonoids have been identified, such as 5-hydroxy-7,8-dimethoxyflavone, 5-hydrox-7,8,2',5'-tetramethoxyflavone, 5-hydroxy -7,8,2',3'-tetramethoxyflavone, 5-hydroxy-7,8,2'-trimethoxyflavone, 7-O-methyl wogonin, and 2'-methyl ether [14]. As illustrated in Fig. (1), these compounds underscore the chemical diversity and potential therapeutic significance of *A, paniculata*.

A. paniculata is a plant known for its medicinal properties and contains various bioactive compounds. The principal constituent include andrographolide and its derivatives such as andrographiside , neoandrographolide, 6-acetylneo andrographiside , 2,3,14-deoxy-11,12-didehydroandrographolide,14-deoxy-11 ,12-didehydro andrographiside , 14-deoxy andrographolide,14-deox--andrographiside, 4-andrographaninandropanoside, isoandrographolide, andrographato-side, andropanolide, and bis-andrographolides A, B, C and D. Additionally, several 2-oxygenated flavonoids have been identified in *A. paniculata*: 5-hydroxy-7,8,2-trimethoxy-flavone, 5,2-dihydroxy-7-8-dimethoxyflavone, 5-hydroxy-7, 8-dimethoxy-flavone,13 5-hydroxy-7-8-dimethoxyflavanone, and andrographidine A. To date, detailed biological investigations have primarily focused on andrographolide, 14-deoxy-11,-

2-didehydroandrographolide, and neoandrographolide. Other andrographolide derivatives' biological activities remain unexplored [15 - 17]. The structures of some of the andrographolides are shown in Fig. (**1**).

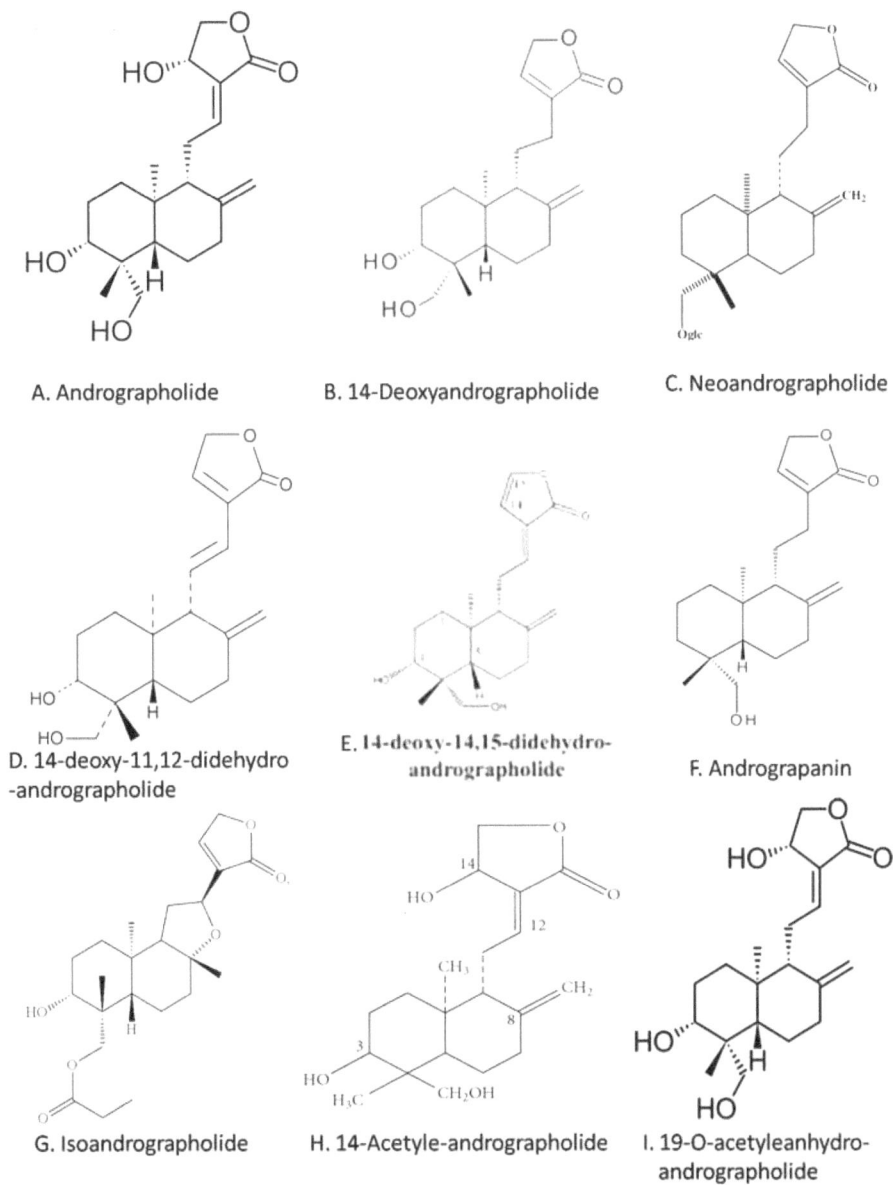

Fig. (1). Andgrographolide and it analogs isolated from *Andrgraphis paniculata*.

ANDROGRAPHOLIDE ACCUMULATION IN THE INTACT PLANTS

The sustained production of andrographolide from *A, paniculata* is challenged by several factors. 1. Limited harvesting: The flowering season of *A. paniculata* occurs from late September to December, sometimes extending to mid-February. During this peak flowering season, the plant reaches its maximum biomass yield and highest andrographolide accumulation. Post flowering, the plants shed their leaves and die off, completing their annual cycle. Thus, andrographolide extraction is confined to about three months annually, necessitating the harvest and drying of the entire plant during the flowering stage, which hampers ongoing propagation effort [18].

2. Problematic seed setting: The seeds of *A. paniculata* are very small and have a dormancy period of 5-6 months post-dispersal, resulting in low germination rates [19]. This characteristic makes large-scale commercial propagation challenging. Reliable seed propagation is complex, limiting the cultivation and production of andrographolide.

3. Variability in andrographolide content: The andrographolide content in field-grown *A. paniculata* varies significantly. Factors contributing to this variability include seasonal changes, geographical differences, time of harvest, and environmental factors such as climate, soil type, and fertilizer dosage [20 - 22]. Due to these factors, achieving a consistent and high yield of andrographolide from *A. paniculata* is challenging. These limitations necessitate careful planning and management of cultivation practices to optimize andrographolide production, including exploring alternative propagation methods, optimizing harvest timing, and possibly developing more reliable cultivation techniques or selecting high-yielding varieties through breeding programs [23 - 26].

IN VITRO RESPONSES OF *ANDROGRAPHIS* SPECIES

In a study focused on the propagation and organogenesis of *A. paniculata*, various explants, including leaf, shoot tip, embryonic tissues, and transverse thin cell layers (TTCL), were used. The goal was to establish a rapid and reliable method for *in vitro* callus production using these different explants. The explants were assessed for their callus production capabilities on different media supplemented with plant growth regulators [27]. Among the explants tested, leaf and nodal explants demonstrated superior responses for callus induction on MS medium, which was enhanced with various combinations of plant growth regulators [28]. Specifically, leaf explants exhibited optimal callus production on MS medium supplemented with one mg/L 2,4-dichlorophenoxyacetic acid (2,4-D) and 0.5 mg/L kinetin (Kn). Increasing the concentration of 2,4-D to 1.5 mg/L and Kn to 1 mg/L further improved the callus production from the leaf explants. Similarly, nodal explants showed the best results for callus initiation on MS medium fortified with 1..5 mg/L 2,4-D and one mg/L Kn [29].

The study investigated the regeneration of multiple shoots from various explants cultured on MS media supplemented with plant growth regulators, specifically cytokinin alone or combined with auxins. The findings are as follows: Explants and shoot regeneration – Nodal TTCL explants: Produced the highest number of multiple shoots, averaging 16 shoots per explant. Embryo explants – produced 12 shoots from decapitated embryonic axes and nine from cotyledons. Shoot tips and leaves generated an average of 6 shoots per explant. The following criteria are the effectiveness of cytokinin: Thidiazuron (TDZ) is identified as the most effective cytokinin-like substance for inducing multiple shoot formation. 6-Benzylaminopurine (BAP) and Kinetin (Kn) are also effective but less so than TDZ. 2-Isopentyladenine (2iP) was the least effective in including organogenic response. Shoot elongation and rooting – shoots were elongated successfully on the medium containing one mg/L Kn and 0.5 mg/L Indole-3-butyric acid (IBA). Rooting was achieved *in vitro* on half-strength MS medium with 0.5 mg/L IBA, resulting in an average of 7.4 roots per shoot and an average root length of 4 cm. Somatic embryogenesis – zygotic embryo explants were used to induce somatic embryogenesis. The highest embryogenic response (75%) and average number of embryos (23 embryos per explant) were observed on media fortified with 1.5 mg/L Naphthalene acetic acid (NAA) and 1.5 mg/L Kn [30].

In the studies on the *in vitro* proliferation of shoots from *A. affinis* and *A. echioides*, various concentrations and combinations of plant growth regulators were tested to optimize shoot regeneration. For *A, affinis,* the optimal medium for achieving the highest shoot regeneration frequency (100%) involved using MS medium fortified with two mg/L benzyl adenine (BA) and one mg/L Kinetin (Kn) from nodal segments. The regenerated shoots were healthy when transferred to an MS medium containing two mg/L indole-3-butyric acid (IBA) [31].

In the case of *A. echioides*, shoot tips were used as explants for direct regeneration. The MS medium fortified with 2.5 mg/L BAP showed a high response for shoot induction. For multiple shoot induction, MS medium containing three mg/L BAP was effective. Furthermore, for shoot elongation, the combination of 2 mg/L BAP and one mg/L gibberellic acid (GA$_3$) was more efficacious [32].

Nodal and internodal explants *A. paniculata* were cultured onto MS medium fortified with BAP (1-3 mg/L) for shoot multiplication. The higher rate of multiplication frequency was observed at 1.5 and 2mg/l BAP with the result of four shoots per explant within 30 days of culture [33]. Researchers have developed an efficient protocol for the micropropagation of *A. paniculata* from nodal explants [34]. They observed the highest number of multiple shoots (4-6) on MS medium fortified with four mg/l BAP and 0.5 mg/l NAA. The rooting efficiency of *in vitro* shoots was rooted on MS medium fortified with IBA (2 mg/L). It is a proven method for the regeneration of *A. paniculata*. *In vitro* plant regeneration *via* micropropagation [35 - 37] and somatic embryogenesis have been reported in *A. paniculata* [3].

High-frequency shoot multiplication was observed on an MS medium fortified with various concentrations of cytokinins, including benzyl adenine (BA), kinetin (Kn), thidiazuron (TDZ), and zeatin (Zn). Notably, high-frequency direct organogenesis was achieved on an MS medium containing two mg/L Zn, resulting in 62 ± 4.2 shoots per explant. Additionally, shoot elongation was successfully induced on MS medium supplemented with two mg/L BA. For *A. neesiana*, nodal explants cultured on MS medium with BA, Kn, and TDZ exhibited rapid proliferation of axillary shoots with over 60 shootlets per explant within 35 days of culture. This protocol holds the potential for the mass multiplication of shootlets and the extraction of andrographolides.

IN VITRO PRODUCTION OF ANDROGRAPHOLIDES

The passage outlines findings on producing two specific compounds, paniculides and andrographolides, in various tissue cultures compared to intact seedlings. In tissue culture, methods interpreted the accumulation of paniculides from leaves, stems, hypocotyls, roots, and embryo explants but did not produce andrographolides [38]. Extracts from the intact plant parts, such as leaves, stems, roots, and seedlings, contained andrographolides but not paniculides. Modifying the culture medium, such as using synthetic auxins and replacing coconut milk with Kn and casein hydrolysate, did not affect paniculide production from hypocotyl cultures. Root cultured for nine months on a simple artificial medium devoid of auxin, meso-inositol, or coconut milk synthesized significant paniculides. There is a clear differentiation in the production of paniculides and andrographolides between tissue cultures and intact seedlings. This suggests that intact plant physiology, possibly involving complex interactions between different tissues and their biochemical pathways, is required for andrographolide production. Conversely, tissue cultures might favor or exclusively produce paniculides due to altered or simplified metabolic states. The unchanged production of paniculides despite various alterations in the medium composition implies that the synthesis of paniculides in hypocotyl cultures is robust and not significantly influenced by these changes. This might indicate a constitutive pathway for paniculide biosynthesis in these cultures. The ability of root cultures to produce significant quantities of paniculides on a simple medium for an extended period suggests that minimal nutritional requirements are sufficient for their production, potentially simplifying the cultivation process for industrial purposes. Investigating the specific metabolic pathways and regulatory mechanisms leading to the exclusive production of paniculides in tissue cultures and andrographolides in intact seedlings can provide deeper insights into plant secondary metabolism. Further research must aim to optimize the culture conditions specifically tailored to enhance the production of desired compounds, whether paniculides or andrographolides, by manipulating environmental factors, nutrient availability, or genetic modifications [38]. Understanding these processes may have significant implications for the biotechnological production of these compounds, potentially leading to more efficient and cost-effective methods for producing valuable phytochemicals used in pharmaceuticals and other industries.

Biomass Production and Andrographolide Extraction

In the study on the seedling culture of *A. paniculata*, introducing aspartic acid and casein hydrolysate into the growth medium increased biomass. However, this increase in biomass was inversely related to the accumulation of andrographolides, a secondary metabolite [39]. This suggests a correlation where biomass accumulation is associated with primary metabolism while andrographolide production is linked to secondary metabolic processes. Further examination of untreated seedling cultures revealed that although biomass consistently increased over four months, the accumulation of andrographolide was most significant during the first two months. The highest concentration of andrographolides was observed after two months of culture, and although high levels persisted into the third month, a notable decline was recorded in the fourth month. Throughout the four-month culture period, the andrographolide content ranged from 2.06 mg/g dry weight (DW) to 2.99 mg/g DW [39]. The influence of different auxins on callus formation was also studied, showing that the combination of 1.5 mg/L NAA and 0.75 mg/L BAP produced the highest amount of callus from leaf explants. Further analysis indicated that andrographolide content in rhizogenic callus grown on MS medium containing three mg/L NAA was 2.4 mg/g DW [30]. These findings suggest that organogenic cultures could be optimal for the *in vitro* production of andrographolides.

The accumulation of andrographolides in *A. paniculata* varies significantly between *in vivo* and *in vitro* grown plants. In stems of *in vivo* grown plants, the andrographolides content was 16.76 mg/g DW; in the leaves, it was 30.51 mg/g DW. Interestingly, the stems of *in vitro* regenerated plants showed a marked increase to 50.62 mg/g DW, and the leaves had 34.51 mg/g DW. This indicates that *in vitro* cultivation can lead to higher andrographolide concentrations than *in vivo* cultivation [40]. Efforts to enhance further andrographolide production involve various plant growth regulators. Notably, the synthetic cytokinin 1-(--chloro-4-pyridyl)-3-pheylurea (CPPU) was tested at concentrations of 0, 5, and 10 mg/L for seven days. CPPU significantly boosted leaf biomass and andrographolide production in *A. paniculata*. It promoted axillary bud formation and increased branching by 4.6 to 5.6 times, which resulted in higher fresh and dry weights. Although a ten mg/L concentration of CPPU caused some leaf stress and reduced chlorophyll content, the five mg/L concentration effectively enhanced andrographolide content without detrimental effects [41].

Leaf Explant and Adventitious Root Cultures

The study focuses on the induction, multiplication, and enhancement of andrographolide content in adventitious root cultures of *A. paniculata* using MS media with various concentrations of auxin and naphthaleneacetic acid (NAA). Researchers found that leaf explants of *A. paniculata* were cultured on MS media fortified with auxins at concentrations ranging from 0.5 to 5 mg/L [26]. The highest number of adventitious roots (26.66 ± 1.52) was induced on a modified MS medium containing one mg/L NAA, followed by full-strength MS with one mg/L NAA (24 ± 2.64). Mass multiplication of adventitious roots achieved on one-month-old adventitious roots was excised and subcultured on MS liquid medium fortified with one mg/L NAA. After five weeks, the dry weight (DW) recovery was 11.27 ± 0.15 g/L in full-strength MS and 10.94 ± 0.60 g/L in modified MS medium [42]. The highest andrographolide content was recorded at 133.28 ± 1.52 mg/g DW from a modified MS medium with one mg/L NAA after 42 days of culture. This andrographolide content was 3.5 to 5.5 times higher than natural sources [43]. Modified MS medium was most effective for root growth and andrographolide accumulation, showing the highest root growth (26.7 ± 1.52 g/L) and andrographolide content (133.3 ± 1.5 mg/g DW). Half-strength and full-strength MS media were less effective than the modified MS medium. Among different auxin treatments, only NAA could induce adventitious roots effectively [43]. Andrographolide content in suspension cultures was 3.5 times higher than in natural sources. Overall, the study demonstrates that using a modified MS medium with one mg/L NAA is optimal for inducing and cultivating adventitious roots of *A. paniculata*, leading to significantly higher andrographolide production than natural sources.

Initiation of Callus Cultures

Leaf discs were cultured on MS medium for callus induction with various concentrations of 2,4-D alone and with combinations of 2,4-D + Kn, 2,4-D + NAA, and BAP + NAA [44]. Callus production was observed at lower concentrations of 2,4-D (0.5 and 1 mg/l) and with a combination of 2,4-D + NAA

(1+1mg/l), 2,4-D + Kn (1 + 0.5mg/l) and BAP + NAA (1+ 1mg/l). Callus cultures were also initiated from 3-week-old plantlets of *A. paniculata*. Leaf, stem, and root sections from *in vitro*-grown plantlets were excised and used for callus induction [45]. One mg/l NAA and one mg/l 2,4-D greatly enhanced the frequency of callus formation. The age of the explants positively influences the callus induction. Optimum callus induction was observed in the presence of 1 mg/l IAA and used to isolate bioactive compounds [46]. Callus induction was achieved on MS + 1 mg/l 2,4-D + 1 mg/l NAA from *A. paniculata*. Calli were obtained from *A. paniculata* leaf explants on MS medium fortified with 2mg/l NAA, 1mg/l Kn, and 50mg/l phenylalanine. With the incorporation of 0.01g/l sodium azide in the medium for 5 hours, callus induction frequency was 83.3%±5.7%, and fresh and dry weights of callus recorded were 1.67± 0.18g and 0.13±0.01 g/culture, respectively.

Accumulation of Andrographolide in Callus Cultures

The callus cultured on MS medium fortified with one mg/L 2,4-D and 1.5 mg/l NAA noticed the highest amount of andrographolide content (7.64 mg/g FW), followed by the response from media containing 1 mg/l 2,4-D with 1.5 mg/L Kn, 2.5 mg/l BAP, and 0.5 mg/L NAA. It indicates that specific plant growth regulator combinations enhanced the accumulation of andrographolide *in vitro* [47]. In another investigation, the amount of andrographolide detected was high in the case of 1 mg/L each of 2,4-D and NAA, followed by one mg/L 2,4-D with 0.5 mg/L Kn. The lowest accumulation (4.21 ± 0.03 mg/g FW) was recorded in 1 mg/L BAP and one mg/l NAA, indicating that this combination suppresses the accumulation [44]. Andrographolide content in 2,4-D with NAA (1 mg/L) was 13.50 ± 2.31 mg/g on FW basis followed by 12.66 ± 1.13 mg/g on 1 mg/L 2,4-D and one mg/L Kn containing medium [48]. Callus was also initiated from mature leaf explants of *A. lineata* on MS medium containing one mg/L IAA. The dried callus was subjected to solvent extraction with acetone. This analysis revealed the occurrence of two known flavones, namely 7-methylwogonin (MW) and echioidinin (ED) [46]. Treatment of sodium azide at 0.01g/L concentration for 3 hours resulted in a 7-fold increase in andrographolide production compared to control in callus cultures. This study also proved that sodium azide's concentration and treatment time influenced the FW and DW of callus, callus induction frequency, and andrographolide production. Most effective and significant results were obtained when callus was treated with 0.01g/L concentration of sodium azide [49]. Photoperiod influenced the callus proliferation and andrographolide accumulation in leaf-derived calli of *A. paniculata*. Callus induction was initiated within 12 h of incubation, which showed 6.2 mg/g of andrographolide, whereas under normal photoperiodic conditions, 4.2 mg/L was observed [50]. The influence of γ-irradiation and L-phenylalanine significantly impacted callus proliferation and andrographolide production; andrographolide accumulation enhanced up to 0.0072% w/w. Maximum callus growth and proliferation recorded was 19.24 mg on an FW basis. An increase in the dose of γ-irradiation also appeared to increase andrographolide accumulation [50]. The effect of various concentrations of 2,4-D (6 and 9 mg/L), NAA (0-2 mg/L), IAA (6 mg/L), and benzyladenine (BA) (6 mg/L) were studied on hypocotyl callus for the production of paniculides. Different auxins influenced the degree of coloration of the tissues, which markedly affected the accumulation of paniculides. Considerable variation in yield was noticed for each treatment depending on the type of auxin used [38].

The Effect of Mutations on Callus and Suspension Cultures

Mutation techniques can be applied to *in vitro* generated seeds, plants, and callus to broaden the genetic variations and then utilize them as material for chemotypic investigations. An induced mutagenesis resulted in *A. paniculata* by T-DNA insertion-mediated *Agrobacterium tumefaciens* [51]. Colchicine treatment and γ-irradiation methods for transforming callus cultures initiated from *A. paniculata* and rapid screening and selection of transformants using cell suspension cultures to enhance andrographolide production [52]. Arsenic-resistant callus line proliferated on MS medium fortified with various concentrations of As_2O_3 (0.0-9.0 μM) along with BA (2.5 mg/L) and NAA (3 mg/L) induced the development of shoots. Shoot organogenesis was slightly inhibited by arsenic metal stress. The rate of adventitious rooting of plantlets gradually decreased with higher concentrations of arsenic (7 μM As_2O_3) in the medium (11.1 ± 1.4 rootlets per plantlet). Further, accumulation of andrographolide was found to be relatively high (4.41 mg/g) in intolerant plants grown at 7μM As_2O_3 compared with untreated control [53].

Ethyl Methane Sulfonate (EMS)

Calli were derived from *A. paniculata* leaf explants inoculated onto MS medium fortified with two mg/L NAA, one mg/L Kn, and 50 mg/L phenylalanine. Treatment with 0.01% EMS for 5 hours resulted in good growth of fresh (1.55 ± 0.06 g) and dry weights (0.12± 0.01g) of callus and also the callus initiation frequency (73.33%) [54]. Treatment with 0.01% EMS resulted in a 6-fold increase in andrographolide production compared to control cultures. The output of andrographolides was analyzed after 70 days of culture. While the control calli produced 0.1mg/g andrographolide, the same was 0.6 mg/g in the calli originating from the explants treated with 0.01% EMS for one h. Explants treated with the same concentration for five h produced calli, which accumulated 0.6 mg/g andrographolide. Treatment cultures with 0.01% EMS for one hour and five hours positively influenced the production of andrographolides. Culturing callus in this concentration produced 0.6mg/g andrographolide compared to the control calli (0.1mg/g). Treatment with 0.01% EMS profoundly affected andrographolide accumulation in callus cultures [54].

Initiation of Suspension Cultures

The initiation of cell suspension cultures of *A. paniculata* was established by inoculating fresh, friable callus on MS medium fortified with one mg/l each of 2,4-D + NAA. Cells were successfully subcultured every 20-21 days on liquid MS medium fortified with the same plant growth regulators. The increase in biomass was analyzed by harvesting the suspensions at 3-day intervals that continued until the culture reached a decline phase by 24 days. The stationary phase for *A. paniculata* suspensions was observed between 12-18 days. Maximum biomass was observed on the 15th day (5.11 mg/g DCW) [55]. Suspension culture was initiated by the inoculation of 0.5g of callus, which was proliferated on 25 ml of MS liquid medium containing 2,4-D (0.5 mg/l), 2,4-D, and BAP (1 + 1 mg/l), 2,4-D and NAA (1 + 1 mg/l).

Accumulation of Andrographolide in Suspensions

The amount of andrographolide recorded was 32.40 ± 2.22 mg/g FW in MS liquid medium containing one mg/l each of 2,4-D + NAA followed by 2,4-D+Kn (1+0.5 mg/l) (31.95 ± 2.21mg/g FW) [44]. Auxin (2,4-D), in combination with cytokinin (BAP), induced the accumulation of andrographolide. It was 27.21 mg/g in cell suspension medium containing 0.5 mg/l 2,4-D, followed by 2,4-D and BAP (1 + 1 mg/l) and 2,4-D and NAA (1 + 1 mg/l) [49]. Different concentrations (0.01, 0.1, and 1 mM) of pyruvic acid were used in cell suspension cultures to produce andrographolides. The amount of andrographolide accumulated was 9.65 mg/g dry weight in 1 mM of pyruvic acid. However, this content was four times higher than that of the cultures of *A. paniculata* grown devoid of pyruvic acid [56].

Accumulation of Andrographolide by Immobilization

Immobilization is a novel approach through which it is possible to achieve higher secondary metabolite production. Calcium alginate and carrageenan entrapped *A. paniculata* cells were cultivated in MS medium fortified with one ppm 2,4-D and 0.5 ppm Kn for 5-10 days, which improved the production of andrographolides by 3-5-fold [57].

Induction of Hairy Root Cultures from *A. paniculata*

The hairy root cultures of *A. paniculata* were developed, which displayed a higher content of andrographolides than intact plants. Various strains of *Agrobacterium rhizogenes* (R-1000, A4, ATCC 15834), multiple types of explants (cotyledons, hypocotyls, and leaves), and various durations of infection by *A. rhizogenes* (1, 2, 3-days) were tested to induce hairy roots. The results indicated that the strain ATCC 15834 was the best for hairy root induction in *A. paniculata*. Similarly, cotyledonary explants and a 2-day co-culture period were ideal for hairy root induction. For growing hairy roots, a half-strength liquid MS medium fortified with 5μM IBA is suitable compared to other concentrations. The adventitious root culture of *A. paniculata* leaf explants was established using various strengths of MS medium fortified with different concentrations of auxins and a combination of NAA + kinetin for growth and andrographolide production. Whereas, only NAA was able to induce adventitious roots and modified strength MS medium obtained the highest root growth (26.7±1.52), as well as the highest amount of andrographolide (133.3±1.5 mg/g DW) accumulation as compared with full-strength MS medium. The produced andrographolide content was 3.5- 5.5 folds higher than the natural plant's, depending on the medium strength [42].

Andrographolide Accumulation in Hairy Roots

Accumulation of andrographolide was high in the second week of culture on an MS medium containing five μM IBA [51]. The effect of media on the transformation frequency of hairy root cultures of *A. paniculata* was evaluated for the production of andrographolide [58]. Adventitious roots were cultured in an MS liquid medium fortified with 2.7 μM NAA and 30 g/l sucrose. It showed significantly higher biomass and andrographolide accumulation [43]. To increase the andrographolides, hairy root cultures derived from *A. paniculata* were treated with chemical elicitors [59]. The percentage of hairy root induction was 62.83 + 1.69, while the induction time was 10.2 days when apical meristems were co-cultured with *Agrobacterium rhizogenes* (MTCC 532) in half-strength MS fortified with 400μM acetosyringone. MS basal medium was found suitable for mass multiplication of hairy roots with a 40.8-fold increase in total biomass yield (fresh weight) after six weeks of culture. Upon exposure of cultures to 50°C temperature for one hour, andrographolide content reached 4695.9 μg/g DW (a 3-fold increase compared to control). The biomass recorded on this medium was 6.81 g/l (dry weight), which produced 3.2 μg of andrographolide per 6.81 g DW of tissue [58]. Neoandrographolide (161.89%) was observed on a half-strength MS medium fortified with two μM/l IBA from the hairy root cultures of *A. lobelioides* [60].

ELICITOR-INDUCED ANDROGRAPHOLIDE PRODUCTION

The study aimed to enhance andrographolide content in suspension cultures of *A. paniculata* and investigate its stimulation in response to pathogen attacks.

Andrographolide, a critical bioactive compound in *A. paniculata*, reached an accumulation of 1.53 mg/g dry cell weight (DCW) at the end of the stationary phase of the growth curve. Various elicitors were tested to stimulate andrographolide production, including biotic elicitors (Yeast, *Escherichia coli*, *Bacillus subtilis*, *Agrobacterium rhizogenes* 532 and *Agrobacterium tumefaciens* C 58) and abiotic elicitors ($CdCl_2$, Silver nitrate, $CuCl_2$ and $HgCl_2$). Among these, biotic elicitors were more effective. Specifically, yeast elicited the highest andrographolide accumulation of 13.5 mg/g DCW, an 8.82-fold increase compared to untreated cultures. Using microbial culture filtrates from yeast, *E. coli*, *B. subtilis*, *A. rhizogenes,* and *A. tumefaciens* also acted as effective biotic elicitors [55]. Both biotic and abiotic elicitors can activate secondary metabolic pathways and enhance the accumulation of target biomolecules [61], although the precise mechanisms behind these responses remain not fully understood.

Effect of Abiotic Elicitors (Copper sulphate)

The study investigated callus induction and andrographolide production in *A. paniculata*. Callus was successfully induced from cotyledon and hypocotyl explants on Skoog and Hilderbrandt's (SH) medium supplemented with 2μg/ml 2,4-D and 0.1 μg/ml 6-BAP. The callus was then transferred to a half-strength MS medium containing 20 g/L sucrose and maintained under a 20-hour photoperiod, producing a biomass production of 17.96 ± 0.06 g per 50 ml culture medium. The andrographolide yield in these cultures was 4.61 ± 0.688 mg/g dry cell weight (DCW). Dawande and Sahay [62] reported that adding copper sulfate to the medium significantly increased the andrographolide content. Specifically, adding 100, 200, 300, 400, and 500 μM concentrations of copper sulfate led to a respective increase in andrographolide content by approximately 1.3, 2.18, 2.81, 3.18, and 4.21 folds. The corresponding actual concentrations of andrographolide were 6.06 ± 0.08, 10.10 ± 0.12, 12.98 ± 0.14, 14.58 ± 0.36, and 29.42 ± 0.31 md/g DCW.

Effect of Methyl Jasmonate (MJ)

Methyl jasmonate (MJ) has been shown to significantly enhance andrographolide accumulation in various cultures of *A. paniculata*. For instance, adding MJ at a concentration of 100 mM to the medium containing hairy root cultures resulted in andrographolide levels reaching 18.2 mg/g fresh weight (FW). When MJ was used in varying concentrations and added to 10-day-old hairy root cultures, it led to a five-fold increase in andrographolide content over 25 days. In cell cultures of *A. paniculata*, MJ also influenced andrographolide accumulation more effectively at 24 hours compared to 48 and 72 hours of treatment [42]. Furthermore, MJ supplementation in suspension cultures at concentrations of 5, 10, 15, 20, and 25 mg/L showed differential effects on andrographolide production. Low concentrations (5-10 mg/L) positively impacted andrographolide biosynthesis, with 5 and 10 mg/L concentrations significantly ($p=0.05$) increasing andrographolide levels to 4.949 ± 0.06 mg/g (1.07-fold) and 13.13 ± 0.11 mg/g dry cell weight (DCW) (2.84-fold), respectively, compared to control cultures (4.61 ± 0.688 mg/g DCW) [62]. Conversely, higher concentrations (15-25 mg/L) exhibited a negative effect. Additionally, a three-fold increase in andrographolide production was observed in tissue culture treated with MJ, and a 5.25-fold increase was noted at a lower MJ concentration (5 µM) in suspension cultures [63, 64]. The underlying mechanism is hypothesized to involve stimulating genes responsible for andrographolide biosynthesis by MJ in *A. paniculata*, although direct evidence is still lacking [65].

Effect of Salicylic Acid (SA) on Andrographolide Accumulation

The study examines the effects of salicylic acid (SA) and chitosan on the production of andrographolide in the cell suspension of *A. paniculata*. SA and chitosan concentrations significantly influenced the production of andrographolide in that SA was used at concentrations of 0.05 mM, 0.5 mM, and 1.5 mM. Chitosan was applied at concentrations of 5 mg, 10 mg, and 20 mg per 50 ml of cell suspension. SA and chitosan treatments were used for 24, 48, and 72 hours. Additionally, chitosan was tested for 96 hours as well. At 0.05 mM for 24 hours, SA treatment resulted in an 18.5-fold increase in andrographolide content, reaching 37 µg/g. At 100 mM, SA significantly stimulated andrographolide production by 8-fold in cell suspensions compared to hairy root culture, whereas treatment with 20 mg of chitosan for 48 hours led to a significant increase in andrographolide content to 119 µg/g, a 59.5-fold enhancement compared to the control [66]. These findings indicate that both SA and chitosan effectively stimulate andrographolide production in *A. paniculata* cell suspension, with chitosan showing a particularly pronounced effect at higher concentrations and longer durations [59].

Effect of Silver Nitrate, Sodium Azide, and Sodium Chloride (NaCl) on Andrographolide Accumulation

Biomass accumulation was slightly stimulated with one mM silver nitrate over 21 days compared to 0.5 mM. The biomass was 0.68 ± 0.01 g, 1.7 times higher than the untreated control. Previous studies on cell suspension culture reported that silver nitrate positively affects both andrographolide accumulation and biomass [55, 67]. Undifferentiated cultures with limited andrographolide accumulation were noted compared to other plants [39]. Specifically, after 14 days of treatment with 0.5 mM silver nitrate, andrographolide accumulation was 25.88 ± 2.72 mg/g dry weight, a 7.09-fold increase over the control [39]. For callus cultures treated with one mM silver nitrate, andrographolide production reached 5.8 mg/g fresh weight [50].

Treatment with 0.01 mg/L sodium azide for three hours resulted in the callus culture in a 7-fold increase in andrographolide accumulation (0.07% w/w) compared to the control (0.01% w/w). Lower concentrations of sodium azide were more effective than higher ones. On callus culture, different concentrations of sodium chloride (25, 50, 75, and 100 mM) were tested in a medium containing 0.5 mg/L 2,4-D [49]. Callus initiation and andrographolide accumulation were observed at 25 mM and 50 mM NaCl, with accumulation levels of 8.30 mg/g and 6.40 mg/g, respectively. Higher concentrations of NaCl (100 mM) inhibited callus growth and andrographolide accumulation [50]. These findings highlight the nuanced effects of various chemical treatments on the growth and secondary metabolite production in *A. paniculata*, suggesting optimal concentrations for maximizing andrographolide production.

Effect of Biotic Elicitors on Andrographolide accumulation

The study on eliciting andrographolides in *A. paniculata* suspension cultures using fungal extracts from *Aspergillus niger* and *Penicillium expansum* provides exciting insights into optimizing andrographolide production. The effect of *A. niger* extract on 4th-day treatment with one ml/L of the extract resulted in an andrographolide content of 52 µg/g, a 2.47-fold increase over the control. It shows that in 7-day treatment with one ml/L of the extract significantly increased andrographolide content to 331 µg/g, a 3.76-fold increase over the control. Increasing the concentrations to 1.5 ml/L resulted in a negative response, and two ml/L significantly suppressed andrographolide accumulation to 8 µg/g, much lower than the control's 88 µg/g [67]. Similarly, in *Penicillium expansum* extract, 2nd-day treatment with 0.6% extract yielded 22 µg/g, 5th-day treatment with 0.6% extract yielded 35 µg/g, and 8-day treatment with 0.6% extract substantially increased andrographolide content to 81 µg/g, a 6.23-fold increase over the control [67]. The results indicate that longer treatment durations with the fungal extracts generally lead to higher andrographolide content in the suspension cultures of *A. paniculata*. However, there is a threshold for the concentration of *A. niger* extract beyond which the elicitation effect becomes detrimental to andrographolide accumulation. In contrast, *P. expansum* extract shows a more consistent positive impact on andrographolide production with increasing duration, up to 8 days.

BIOREACTORS FOR ANDROGRAPHOLIDE PRODUCTION

Optimizing several parameters is crucial to achieving consistent production of andrographolides in a bioreactor, particularly the rate of aeration, which significantly affects cell growth and secondary metabolite production. Varied inoculum sizes such as 0.55%, 1%, 2%, 3%, 4%, and 5% were used to determine the optimal inoculum size for maximum biomass production. Different agitation rates were tested in 0.66, 0.416, 0.833, 1.25, and 1.66 liters per minute (LPM) to establish the optimal agitation rate for effective aeration and enhanced cell growth. Bubble column reactor used for achieving high cell density suspensions of *A. paniculata*. The inoculum size of 4% was found to be optimal, yielding the highest biomass of 12.10 g/L. This suggests that 4% inoculum provides a balance between nutrient availability and space for growth, leading to maximum biomass production. The precise optimal agitation rate was not specified, but various rates were tested to identify the best condition for aeration. Optimal aeration is critical as it influences oxygen transfer rates, which are vital for cell metabolism and growth. The bubble column bioreactor proved more suitable for large-scale production compared to shake flasks. It also provides better control over aeration and mixing, which is crucial for consistent high-density cell cultures. The study indicates that using a 2L bubble column bioreactor under optimized conditions can significantly enhance the production of *A. paniculata* biomass. The bioreactor's ability to maintain high cell density and consistent aeration makes it a superior choice for large-scale production to traditional shake flasks [68]. For future experiments, focusing on refining the aeration rate and further optimizing other culture conditions with the bubble column bioreactor can lead to even more efficient processes.

GENETIC ENGINEERING AND *IN VITRO* ENHANCEMENT OF ANDROGRAPHOLIDE

The overexpression of genes encoding key enzymes in biosynthetic pathways significantly influences the accumulation of corresponding secondary metabolites. This process can be facilitated by engineering cells and cultivating them in a bioreactor, with the addition of signaling molecules like methyl jasmonate (MJ) to the medium [65, 69, 70]. For instance, MJ treatment enhances the expression levels of several key enzymes involved in the biosynthesis of phenolic acids [71]. These enzymes include phenylalanine ammonia lyase (PAL), hydroxyconnamate coenzyme-A ligase (4CL), cinnamic acid 4-hydroxylase (C4H), tyrosine aminotransferase (TAT), 4- hydroxyphenylpyruvate reductase (HPPR), and rosmarinic acid synthase (RAS) (Fig. **2**). Notably, after six days of MJ treatment, these genes exhibit increased expression, resulting in a substantial increase in phenolic compounds withing hairy root cultures. Moreover, MJ treatment also upregulates genes involved in the methylerythritol phosphate (MEP) pathway, such as DXS (1-deoxy-D-xylulose 5-phosphate synthase), DXR (1-deoxy-D-xylulose 5-phosphate reductoisomerase), HDS (4- hydroxy-3-methylbut2-e-yl-diphosphate synthase), and ISPH (1-hydroxy-2-methyl-2-(E)-butenyl 4-diphosphate reductase). Similarly, MJ enhances the expression of genes in the mevalonic acid (MVA) pathway, particularly HMGS (3-hydroxy-3-methylglutaryl-CoA synthase) and HMGR (3-hydroxy-3-methylglutaryl-CoA reductase). The biosynthesis of andrographolide in *A. paniculata* involves both the MVA and MEP pathways. Studies have shown that although the MVA pathway contributes to andrographolide biosynthesis, the MEP pathway plays a more significant role, as indicated by the higher enrichment of specific carbon positions from 1,6-(13C) glucose [72]. Overall, MJ treatment effectively influences both the MEP and MVA pathways, thereby enhancing secondary metabolite biosynthesis [73].

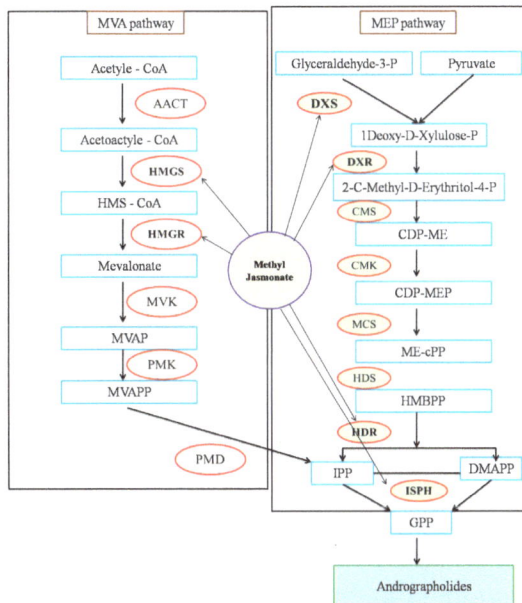

Fig. (2). Andrographolide biosynthetic pathway activation by methyl jasmonate in *Andrographis paniculata*. Light arrows show the relationship between methyl jasmonate signaling and andrographolide biosynthetic pathway enzymes. HMG-CoA, 3-Hydroxy-3-methylglutaryl CoA;MVA, mevalonic acid; MVAP, mevalonic acid 5-phosphate; MVAPP, mevalonic acid 5-diphosphate; IPP, isopentenyl diphosphate; DMAPP, dimethylallyl diphosphate; MEP, 2-C-methyl-D-erythritol 4-phosphate; CDP-ME, 4-diphosphocytidyl--C-methyl-d-erythritol; CDP-MEP, 4-diphosphocytidyl-2-C-methyl-D-erythritol 2-phosphate; ME-cPP, 2--methyl-D-erythritol 2,4-cyclodiphosphate; HMBPP, 1-hydroxy-2-methyl-2-(E)-butenyl 4-diphosphate; Enzymes of the MVA pathway: HMGS, HMG-CoA synthase; HMGR, HMG-CoA reductase; MVK, MVA kinase; PMK, MVAP kinase; PMD, MVAPP decarboxylase; Enzymes of the MEP pathway: DXS, DOXP synthase; DXR, DOXP reductoisomerase; CMS, CDP-ME synthase; CMK, CDP-ME kinase; MCS, ME-2,4cPP synthase; HDS, HMBPP synthase; HDR, HMBPP reductase; ISPH, 1-Hydroxy-2-methyl---(E)-butenyl 4-diphosphate reductase (Modified from Sinha *et al.* 2008 and Thanh-Tom *et al.* 2020).

ENDOPHYTE CULTURE AND ANDROGRAPHOLIDE PRODUCTION

A. paniculata is known for its rich consortia of endophytic microbial diversity, which produce a variety of secondary metabolites [74]. Within its inner tissues, endophytic fungi such as *Aspergillus niger*, *A. flavus*, *Fusarium* species, *Alternaria* species, and yeast-like fungi have been identified. Among these, *A. niger*, *A. flavus,* and *Alternaria* species exhibit protease, lipase, and amylase activities. *Fusarium* species also produce amylase and lipase, while yeast-like fungi are notable for their elevated amylase activity [75]. In addition to fungi, 23 endophytic bacteria have been isolated from *A. paniculata*. One significant isolate, *Aspergillus* species (SbDS), was obtained from the leaves of *A. paniculata*. This fungus was cultured in potato dextrose broth (PDB) medium under static conditions for seven weeks. The culture was then extracted with ethyl acetate, leading to the characterization of three pure compounds: a benzochromen derivative, 1-(3,8-dihydroxy-4,6,6-trimethyl-6H-benzochromen-2-yloxy) propan-2-one, and two known compounds, 5-hydroxy-4-(hydroxymethyl)-2H-pyran 2-one (2) and (5-hyeroxy-2-oxo-2H-pyran-4-yl)methyl acetate [76].

CONCLUSION AND WAY FORWARD

In vitro plant cell cultures are a highly effective means of producing large quantities of secondary metabolites. These cultures provide a renewable, affordable source of valuable compounds and can achieve high production rates irrespective of geographical and seasonal limitations. Notably, the metabolite accumulation in cell cultures often surpasses that of wild plants. For instance, both biotic and abiotic elicitors have been employed to stimulate secondary metabolite production in suspension cultures of *Andrographis* species. Specifically, the biotic elicitor yeast has been shown to increase the accumulation of andrographolides by up to eightfold compared to control cultures. The potential for molecular analysis of these responses is significant as it can inform metabolic engineering strategies aimed at further enhancing andrographolide production. Tissue culture methodologies thus hold substantial promise for meeting the demand for natural products while minimizing environmental impact and preserving biodiversity. Strategies to enhance the yield of pharmaceutically important compounds include overexpressing genes involved in secondary product biosynthesis and suppressing competitive metabolic pathways. Additionally, global regulation approaches that manipulate transcription factors, endogenous phytohormones, and primary metabolism can also significantly boost yields. These methods collectively offer great potential for increasing the supply of rare and valuable secondary metabolites [61]. This chapter highlighted the viability of using tissue culture methods to establish a continuous and enhanced production of andrographolides, potentially meeting global demands more effectively.

REFERENCES

[1]   Karmegam N, Nagaraj R, Karuppusamy S, Prakash M. Biological and pharmacological activities of *Andrographis* spp. (Acanthaceae) distributed in Eastern Ghats, India. Int J Curr Res Biosci Plant Biol 2015; 2: 140-53.

[2]   Samydurai P, Rajendran A, Sarvalingam A, Rajasekar C. Ethnobotanical knowledge of threatened plant species *Andrographis* in Nilgiris Biosphere Reserve, Tamil Nadu, India. Int J Herb Med 2017; 5: 103-7.

[3]   Martin KP. Plant regeneration protocol of medicinally important *Andrographis paniculata* (Burm. f.) Wallich ex Nees *via* somatic embryogenesis. In Vitro Cell Dev Biol Plant 2004; 40(2): 204-9.
[http://dx.doi.org/10.1079/IVP2003520]

[4]   Pandey G, Rao CH. Andrographolide: its pharmacology, natural bioavailability and current approaches to increase its content in *Andrographis paniculata*. Int J Complement Altern Med 2018; 11(4): 355-60.
[http://dx.doi.org/10.15406/ijcam.2018.11.00425]

[5]   Akbar S. *Andrographis paniculata*: a review of pharmacological activities and clinical effects. Altern Med Rev 2011; 16(1): 66-77.
[PMID: 21438648]

[6]   Alagesaboopathi C. Evaluation of antibacterial properties of leaf and stem extracts of *Andrographis elongata* T. Anders. – An endemic medicinal plant of India. Int J Pharm Bio Sci 2013; 4: 503-10.

[7]   Okhuarobo A, Ehizogie Falodun J, Erharuyi O, Imieje V, Falodun A, Langer P. Harnessing the medicinal properties of *Andrographis paniculata* for diseases and beyond: a review of its phytochemistry and pharmacology. Asian Pac J Trop Dis 2014; 4(3): 213-22.
[http://dx.doi.org/10.1016/S2222-1808(14)60509-0]

[8]   Karuppusamy S. A review on trends in production of secondary metabolites from higher plants by *in vitro* tissue, organs, and cell cultures. J Med Plants Res 2009; 3: 1222-39.

[9]   Mabberley DJ. Mabberley's Plant-Book A portable dictionary of plants, their classification and uses. 3rd ed., Cambridge: Cambridge University Press 2008.

[10] Sareer O, Ahmad S, Umar S. *Andrographis paniculata* : a critical appraisal of extraction, isolation and quantification of andrographolide and other active constituents. Nat Prod Res 2014; 28(23): 2081-101.
[http://dx.doi.org/10.1080/14786419.2014.924004] [PMID: 24912126]

[11] Khan A, Sharma P, Khan F, Vijayakumar PV, Shanker K, Samad A. *In silico* and *In vitro* studies on Begomovirus induced andrographolide synthesis pathway in *Andrographis paniculata* for combating inflammation and cancer. Mol. Inf. 2015>
[http://dx.doi.org/10.1002/minf.201501010]

[12] Rashid PT, Ahmed M. Md. Rahman M, Md. Abdul M. 14-Dexoyandrographolide isolated from *Andrographis paniculata* (Burm.f.) Nees growing in Bangladesh and its antimicrobial properties. Dhaka Univ J Pharm Sci1 2018; 7: 265-267.

[13] Yoopan N, Thisoda P, Rangkadilok N, *et al.* Cardiovascular effects of 14-deoxy-11,-2-didehydroandrographolide and *Andrographis paniculata* extracts. Planta Med 2007; 73(6): 503-11.
[http://dx.doi.org/10.1055/s-2007-967181] [PMID: 17650544]

[14] Chao WW, Lin BF. Isolation and identification of bioactive compounds in *Andrographis paniculata* (Chuanxinlian). Chin Med 2010; 5(1): 17.
[http://dx.doi.org/10.1186/1749-8546-5-17] [PMID: 20465823]

[15]   Kulyal P, Tiwari UK, Shukla A, Gaur AK. Chemical constituents isolated from *Andrographis paniculata*. Indian J Chem 2010; 49B: 356-9.

[16]   Lim JCW, Chan TK, Ng DSW, Sagineedu SR, Stanslas J, Wong WSF. Andrographolide and its analogs: versatile bioactive molecules for combating inflammation and cancer. Clin Exp Pharmacol Physiol 2012; 39(3): 300-10.
[http://dx.doi.org/10.1111/j.1440-1681.2011.05633.x] [PMID: 22017767]

[17]   Tan MCS, Oyong GC, Shen CC, Ragasa CY. Chemical constituents of *Andrographis panicualta* (Burm.f.) Nees. Intern J Pharmacogn & Phytochem Res 2016; 8: 1398-402.

[18]   Arunkumar P, Ashok B, Maiti S. An Assessment of andrographolide production in *Andrographis paniculata* grown in different agroclimatic locations. Afr J Agric Res 2013; 8: 6101-9.

[19]   Pholphana N, Rangkadilok N, Saehun J, Ritruechai S, Satayavivad J. Changes in the contents of four active diterpenoids at different growth stages in *Andrographis paniculata* (Burm.f.) Nees (Chuanxinlian). Chin Med 2013; 8(1): 2.
[http://dx.doi.org/10.1186/1749-8546-8-2] [PMID: 23320627]

[20]   Prathanturarug S, Soonthornchareonnon N, Chuakul W, Saralamp P. Variation in growth and diterpene lactones among field-cultivated *Andrographis paniculata*. J Nat Med 2007; 61(2): 159-63.
[http://dx.doi.org/10.1007/s11418-006-0115-6]

[21]   Patarapanich C, Laungcholatan S, Mahaverawat N, Chaichantipayuth C, Pummangura S. HPLC determination of active diterpene lactones from *Andrographis paniculata* Nees planted in various seasons and regions in Thailand. Thai J Pharm 2007; Sci 31: 91-99.

[22]   Sharma M, Sharma A, Tyagi S. Quantitative HPLC analysis of Andrographolide in *Andrographis paniculata* at two different stages of life cycle of plant. Acta Chim Pharm Indica 2012; 2: 1-7.

[23]   Bhan MK, Dhar AK, Khan S, Lattoo SK, Gupta KK, Choudhary DK. Screening and optimization of *Andrographis paniculata* (Burm.f.) Nees for total andrographolide content, yield and its components. Sci Hortic (Amsterdam) 2006; 107(4): 386-91.
[http://dx.doi.org/10.1016/j.scienta.2005.09.001]

[24]   Mishra S, Tiwari SK, Kakkar A, Pandey AK. Chemoprofiling of *Andrographis paniculata* (Kalmegh) for its andrographolide content in Madhya Pradesh, India. Int J Pharma Bio Sci 2010; 2: 1-5.

[25]   Pandey AK, Mandal AK. Variation in morphological characteristics and andrographolide content in *Andrographis paniculata* (Burm. f.) Nees. of central India. Iran J Energy Environ 2010; 1: 165-9.

[26]   Sharma SN, Sahu S, Jha Z, Sharma DK. Evaluation of seasonal variation in relation to secondary metabolite and biomass production of *Andrographis paniculata*. J Nat Rem 2012; 12: 39-46.

[27]   Butcher DN, Bowes BC. The growth and fine-structure of callus cultures derived from *Andrographis paniculata* Nees. Z PflPhysiol 1969; 58: 80-9.

[28]   Murashige T, Skoog F. A revised medium for rapid growth and bioassays with tobacco tissue cultures. Physiol Plant 1962; 15(3): 473-97.
[http://dx.doi.org/10.1111/j.1399-3054.1962.tb08052.x]

[29]   Bidari S, Anitha S, Rajshekaran PE, Shashidhara S, Tatti PN. *In vitro* regeneration of *Andrographis paniculata* Nees, an important medicinal plant. Pharma sciences. Monitor (Charlottet) 2012; 3: 2321-30.

[30]   Vikram P. *In vitro* propagation and andrographolide analysis of Hempedu Bumi (*Andrographis paniculata* Nees). M.Sc. Dissertation submitted to University of Malaysia Kelantan, Malaysia. 2016.

[31]   Govindaraj S, Thangaswamy S, Hariprasad S, Alagesaboopathi C. *In vitro* regeneration and mass multiplication of *Andrographis affinis* Nees – An endemic medicinal species from India. Scientific Res J 2008; 10: 173-7.

[32]   Hemalatha P, Vadivel E. Evaluation of *in vitro* seed germination and microproapgation techniques in

Andrographis echioides (L.) Nees. Int J Agrisci 2010; 6: 209-12.

[33]   Deshmukh AS, Pawar SD, Nirgude MS, Pingle AS. *In vitro* multiple shoot induction in *Andrographis paniculata.* Int J Curr Microbiol Appl Sci 2018; 6: 791-5.

[34]   Basu J, Yogananth N. *In- vitro* anti-inflammatory activity and tissue culture studies on *Andrographis paniculata* (Burm. f.) Wallich ex Nees.: A medicinal plant. J Pharm Res 2011; 4: 1368-9.

[35]   Purkayastha J, Sugla T, Paul A, Solleti S, Sahoo L. Rapid *in vitro* multiplication and plant regeneration from nodal explants of *Andrographis paniculata*: a valuable medicinal plant. In Vitro Cell Dev Biol Plant 2008; 44(5): 442-7.
        [http://dx.doi.org/10.1007/s11627-008-9156-8]

[36]   Karuppusamy S, Kalimuthu K. Rapid *in vitro* multiplication and plant regeneration from nodal explants of *Andrographis neesiana*: A valuable endemic medicinal plant. Adv Biol Res (Faisalabad) 2010; 4: 211-6.
        [http://dx.doi.org/10.1007/s11627-008-9156-8]

[37]   Jindal N, Chaudhury A, Kajla S. Shoot proliferation and multiplication from nodes of *Andrographis paniculata.* Int J Pharm 2015; 6: 614-9.

[38]   Butcher DN, Connolly JD. An Investigation of factors which influence the production of abnormal terpenoids by callus cultures of *Andrographis paniculata* Nees. J Exp Bot 1971; 22(2): 314-22.
        [http://dx.doi.org/10.1093/jxb/22.2.314]

[39]   Das D, Bandyopadhyay M. Novel approaches towards over-production of andrographolide in *in vitro* seedling cultures of *Andrographis paniculata.* S Afr J Bot 2020; 128: 77-86.
        [http://dx.doi.org/10.1016/j.sajb.2019.10.015]

[40]   Dandin VS, Murthy HN. Regeneration of *Andrographis paniculata* Nees: Analysis of genetic fidelity and andrographolide content in micropropagated plants. Afr J Biotechnol 2012; 11: 12464-71.

[41]   Worakan P, Karaket N, Maneejantra N, Supaibulwatana K. A phenylurea cytokinin, CPPU, elevated reducing sugar and correlated to andrographolide contents in leaves of *Andrographis paniculata* (Burm. f.) Wall. ex Nees. Appl Biochem Biotechnol 2017; 181(2): 638-49.
        [http://dx.doi.org/10.1007/s12010-016-2238-x] [PMID: 27613615]

[42]   Sharma SN, Jha Z, Sinha RK. Establishment of *in vitro* adventitious root cultures and analysis of andrographolide in *Andrographis paniculata.* Nat Prod Commun 2013; 8(8): 1934578X1300800803.
        [http://dx.doi.org/10.1177/1934578X1300800803] [PMID: 24079163]

[43]   Praveen N, Manohar SH, Naik PM, Aayeem A, Jeong JH, Murthy HN. Production of andrographolide from adventitious root cultures of *Andrographis paniculata.* Curr Sci 2009; 96: 694-7.

[44]   Sharma SN, Jha Z. Production of andrographolide from callus and cell suspension culture of *Andrographis paniculata.* J Cell Tissue Res 2012; 12: 3423-9.

[45]   Deshmukh AS, Kadam SR, Belge SA, Nirgude MS, Kharade SS. Initiation of callus culture and estimation of andrographolide from *Andrographis paniculata.* J Cell Tiss Res 2017; 17: 5987-90.

[46]   Mohammed A, Chiruvella KK, Koteswara Rao Y, Geethanjili M, Raghavan SC, Ghanta RG. *In vitro* production of 7-O-Methywogoninfrom callus culture of *Andrographis lineata* and their cytotoxicity on cancer cells. PLoS One 2015; •••
        [http://dx.doi.org/10.1371/journal.pone.0141154] [PMID: 26488879]

[47]   Jindal N, Kajla S, Chaudhury A. Establishment of callus culture of *Andrographis paniculata* for the assessment of andrographolide content. Int J Res Ayurveda Pharm 2016; 7(2): 197-201.
        [http://dx.doi.org/10.7897/2277-4343.07286]

[48]   Sharma SN. Andrographolide production and functional characterization of biosynthetic pathways in *Andrographis paniculata.* Ph.D. thesis, Indira Gandhi Krishi Vishwavidyalaya, Raipur. 2012.

[49]   Chandran NA, Kuruvilla S, Pillai PRK. *In vitro* studies on callus culture and enhanced andrographolide production using sodium azide in *Andrographis paniculata.* Int J Appl Pure Sci Agric

2016; 2: 254-8.

[50] Sharmila R. *In vitro* production of an anticancer drug andrographolide from *Andrographis paniculata.* Ph.D. thesis submitted to Bharathidasan University, Tiruchirappalli, Tamil Nadu, India. 2014.

[51] Marwani E, Tangapo A, Dwivany FM. *Agrobacterium*-mediated stable transformation of medicinal plant *Andrographis paniculata* callus expressing GUS gene. Indones J Biotechnol 2013; 18: 92-100.
[http://dx.doi.org/10.22146/ijbiotech.7873]

[52] Cabang AP, Sapaibulwatana K. Enhancing variations in *Andrographis paniculata* (Bum.f.) Wall. ex Nees by induced mutagenesis. UNESCO Post graduate inter University course in Biotechnology. A research report for the Japanese National Commission for UNESCO: 2007; 942-955.

[53] Vijayakumar J, Ponmanickam P, Samuel P, *et al.* Metabolite profiles of Arsenic tolerant plans regenerated from stem calli of *Andrographis paniculata* (Burm.f.) Nees using HPLC and 1D ^{1}H NMR. Am J Biochem Biotechnol 2017; 13(4): 195-207.
[http://dx.doi.org/10.3844/ajbbsp.2017.195.207]

[54] Chandran NA, Pillai PRK. A comparative study on the *in vitro* effect of treatment time of EMS on secondary metabolite production in *Andrographis paniculata* (Burm.f.) Nees. J Pharmacogn Phytochem 2018; 7: 131-7.

[55] Gandi S, Rao K, Chodisetti B, Giri A. Elicitation of andrographolide in the suspension cultures of *Andrographis paniculata.* Appl Biochem Biotechnol 2012; 168(7): 1729-38.
[http://dx.doi.org/10.1007/s12010-012-9892-4] [PMID: 23001530]

[56] Zahedi MG, Rezaei A, Talei D. Effect of pyruvic acid as a precursor on the production of andrographolide in *Andrographis paniculata* cell suspension culture. 8th National congress on Medicinal Plants. 24Tehran, Iran. 2019; p. : 394.

[57] Chauhan P, Panigrahi MK, Swami H, Rana V. Immobilization of *Andrographis paniculata* leaf cells for enhanced production of andrographolide. Pharm Lett 2010; 2: 198-201.

[58] Mahobia A, Jha Z. Efficiency of method and media composition on transformation of *Andrographis paniculata* for hairy root production. J Cell TissRes 2015; 15: 4897-902.

[59] Sharmila R, Subburathinam KM. Effect of signal compounds on andrographolide in the hairy root culture of *Andrographis paniculata.* Int J Pharm Sci Res 2013; 4: 1773-6.

[60] Samydurai P, Rajendran A. Hairy root culture for mass production of medicinal important compound neoandrographolide from *Andrographis lobelioides* Nees. Research & Reviews: J Biotechnol 2018; 8: 14-9.

[61] Lu X, Tang K, Li P. Plant Metabolic engineering strategies for the production of pharmaceutical terpenoids. Front Plant Sci 2016; 7: 1647.
[http://dx.doi.org/10.3389/fpls.2016.01647] [PMID: 27877181]

[62] A Dawande A, Sahay S. Copper sulphate elicitation of optimized suspension culture of *Andrographis paniculata* Nees yields unprecedented level of andrographolides. J Microbiol Biotechnol Food Sci 2020; 9(4): 688-94.
[http://dx.doi.org/10.15414/jmbfs.2020.9.4.688-694]

[63] Zaheer M, Giri CC. Multiple shoot induction and jasmonic *versus* salicylic acid driven elicitation for enhanced andrographolide production in *Andrographis paniculata.* Plant Cell Tissue Organ Cult 2015; 122(3): 553-63.
[http://dx.doi.org/10.1007/s11240-015-0787-2]

[64] Sharmila R, Subburathinam KM, Sugumar P. Effect of growth regulators on andrographolide production in callus cultures of *Andrographis paniculata.* Adv Bio Tech 2013; 12: 17-20.

[65] Sinha RK, Sharma SN, Verma SS, Zha J. Effects of lovastin, fosmidomycin and methyl jasmonate on andrographolide biosynthesis in the *Andrographis paniculata.* Acta Physiol Plant 2018; 40(9): 165-9.
[http://dx.doi.org/10.1007/s11738-018-2746-0]

[66]   Moinuddin MA, Mendhulkar VD. Salicylic acid and chitosan mediated abiotic stress in cell suspension culture of *Andrographis paniculata* (Burm.f.) Nees for andrographolide synthesis. Int J Pharm Sci Res 2013; 4: 3453-9.

[67]   Vakil MMA, Mendhulkar VD, Mendhulkar VD. Enhanced synthesis of andrographolide by *Aspergillus niger* and *Penicillium expansum* elicitors in cell suspension culture of *Andrographis paniculata* (Burm. f.) Nees. Bot Stud (Taipei, Taiwan) 2013; 54(1): 49.
[http://dx.doi.org/10.1186/1999-3110-54-49] [PMID: 28510886]

[68]   Kumar MA, Navaneetha Krishnan V, Selvamani P. High cell density cultivation of *Andrographis paniculata* in shake flask and bubble column reactor for the production of cell biomass and andrographolide. Asian J Microbiol Biotechnol Environ Sci 2015; 17: 97-102.

[69]   Jha Z, Sharam SN, Sharma DK. Differential expression of 3- hydroxy-3-methylglutaryl-coenzyme a reductase of *Andrographis paniculata* in andrographolide accumulation. J Chem Pharm Res 2011; 3: 499-504.

[70]   Sharma SN, Jha Z, Sinha RK, Geda AK. Jasmonate☐induced biosynthesis of andrographolide in *Andrographis paniculata*. Physiol Plant 2015; 153(2): 221-9.
[http://dx.doi.org/10.1111/ppl.12252] [PMID: 25104168]

[71]   Xing B, Yang D, Liu L, Han R, Sun Y, Liang Z. Phenolic acid production is more effectively enhanced than tanshinone production by methyl jasmonate in *Salvia miltiorrhiza* hairy roots. Plant Cell Tissue Organ Cult 2018; 134(1): 119-29.
[http://dx.doi.org/10.1007/s11240-018-1405-x]

[72]   Srivastava N, Akhila A. Biosynthesis of andrographolide in *Andrographis paniculata*. Phytochemistry 2010; 71(11-12): 1298-304.
[http://dx.doi.org/10.1016/j.phytochem.2010.05.022] [PMID: 20557910]

[73]   Ho TT, Murthy HN, Park SY. Methyl jasmonate induced oxidative stress and accumulation of secondary metabolites in plant cell and organ cultures. Int J Mol Sci 2020; 21(3): 716.
[http://dx.doi.org/10.3390/ijms21030716] [PMID: 31979071]

[74]   Arunachalam C, Gayathri P. Studies on bioprospecting of endophytic bacteria from the medicinal plant of *Andrographis paniculata* for their antimicrobial activity and antibiotic susceptibility pattern. Int J Curr Pharm Res 2010; 2: 63-8.

[75]   Gajalakshmi S, Iswarya V, Ashwini R, Bhuvaneshwari M, Mythili S, Sathiavelu A. Secondary metabolite production by endophytic fungi isolated from *Andrographis panicualta*. Intern J BioSci Tech 2012; 5: 12-7.

[76]   Munawar M, Muharni M, Ivantri I. Chemical constituents of an endophytic fungus *Aspergillus* sp. (Sbd5) isolated from Sambiloto (*Andrographis paniculata* Nees). Microbiol Indones 2015; 9(2): 82-8.
[http://dx.doi.org/10.5454/mi.9.2.5]

SUBJECT INDEX

A

Acid 107, 151, 188, 189, 286, 288, 310, 319
  ascorbic 286, 288
  Gallic 188
  lactic 151
  mevalonic 319
  naphthaleneacetic 310
Action, neuroprotective 132, 203
Activity 5, 6, 59, 85, 108, 130, 158, 160, 182, 189, 191, 239, 241, 242, 243, 244, 245, 246, 247, 249, 270
  anti-breast cancer 243
  anti-inflammatory 59, 108, 239
  anti-neuroinflammatory 130
  anti-prostate cancer 158
  anticorona virus 85
  antiplasmodial 241, 249
  cellulase 270
Acute respiratory syndrome 84
Alanine aminotransferase 90
Amylase activities 270, 320
Androgen 145, 150, 153
  deprivation therapy (ADT) 145, 150
  hormones 145, 153
Andrographolide 4, 57, 204, 205, 210, 223, 224, 228, 229, 306, 308, 309, 310, 311, 312, 313, 314, 315, 316, 317, 318, 319, 320
  anticancer effect 204, 210
  biosynthesis 316, 319
  natural 4, 57, 210
  production 306, 308, 309, 310, 311, 312, 313, 314, 315, 316, 317, 318, 320
  treatment 205, 223, 224, 228, 229
Angiogenesis 187, 191
  lung tumor 191
  inhibitors 187
Anti-bacterial activity 238, 239
Anti-fungal activity 238
Anti-hypertensive mechanism 222
Anti-inflammatory 4, 236, 239

activity 236, 239
effects 4
Anti-microbial peptides (AMPs) 173, 183
Anti-neuroinflammatory responses 128
Anti-oxidant activity 236
Anti-tumor activity 240
Antiatherosclerotic effect 87
Antibacterial 68, 82, 83, 146, 241, 242, 243, 244, 245, 246, 247
  activity 82, 241, 242, 243, 244, 245, 246, 247
  agent 68
  effect 83
  properties 146
Antibodies, monoclonal 174
Anticancer 6, 85, 86, 146, 158, 159, 175, 191, 201, 202, 203, 204, 205, 206, 208, 210, 211, 212, 234, 236, 238, 239, 242, 243, 247, 248
  activity 158, 159, 203, 205, 206, 210, 211, 234, 236, 238, 239, 242, 243, 247, 248
  drugs 6, 146, 201, 202, 203, 205, 208
  effects 85, 86, 175, 191, 204, 205, 206, 210, 212
Antidiabetic 89, 90, 240, 242, 246, 248
  activity 89, 242, 246, 248
  assay 240
  effect 89, 90
Antifibrosis activity 56
Antifilarial activity 239, 249
Antihyperglycemic effects 89
Antihypertensive effects 4
Antimicrobial activity 82, 237, 242, 244, 246, 247, 248, 270
  antioxidant activity 242
Antioxidant(s) 10, 11, 98, 101, 103, 104, 119, 129, 130, 219, 221, 234, 236, 237, 286, 288, 290
  artificial 129
  properties 98, 103, 130
  therapy 119
Antioxidative effects 121

www.ingramcontent.com/pod-product-compliance
Lightning Source LLC
Chambersburg PA
CBHW050805220326
41598CB00006B/126